CLINICAL SKILLS IN INFANT MENTAL HEALTH

SARAH MARES   LOUISE NEWMAN   BEULAH WARREN
WITH KAREN CORNISH

ACER Press

First published 2005
by ACER Press
Australian Council *for* Educational Research Ltd
19 Prospect Hill Road, Camberwell, Victoria, 3124

Copyright © NSW Institute of Psychiatry 2005

All rights reserved. Except under the conditions described in the *Copyright Act 1968* of Australia and subsequent amendments, no part of this publication may be reproduced, stored in a retrieval system or transmitted in any form or by any means, electronic, mechanical, photocopying, recording or otherwise, without the written permission of the publishers.

Edited by Wendy Skilbeck
Cover and text design by R.T.J. Klinkhamer
Printed and bound by Shannon Books Australia Pty Ltd

National Library of Australia Cataloguing-in-Publication data:

Clinical skills in infant mental health.

Bibliography.
Includes index.
ISBN 0 86431 444 2.

1. Infants - Mental health. 2. Infants - Development. 3. Infant psychiatry. 4. Child mental health. 5. Child development. I. Mares, Sarah.

618.9289

Visit our website: www.acerpress.com.au

Foreword

Working with families and babies, toddlers and children is fascinating and rewarding. This is so whether the work is specialised and more focused on the atypical or whether it mostly involves helping families through the normal range of experiences that come with having and raising children.

Because health care for families covers such a wide range of disciplines and fragmentation of services, lack of communication between health workers is an ongoing concern. To minimise this as much as possible, it is crucial for health professionals (and students) to have an understanding of the clinical aspects and theories that underpin the clinical practice of other workers in the field.

In addition, regardless of specific backgrounds, all health workers and practitioners have to learn to look beyond the linear and the external. Whether the work is in paediatric occupational therapy, midwifery, nursing, medicine, psychology or child care, professionals who spend their days helping families need to understand how babies, toddlers and children grow emotionally and the significance of their behaviour—especially as the very young have no words to tell their stories or put forward their points of view. There is a growing realisation in all disciplines that relationships that children have with parents, extended families and any other significant people has a direct affect on human development and overall well-being, not only in the early years but potentially throughout life. The good news is that with effective and early detection and intervention many negative issues in early childhood can be resolved or at least minimised. So, it makes sense that all professionals in the field, from child-care workers to family doctors, should have an understanding of the relevance of infant mental health issues.

Until Sarah Mares, Louise Newman and Beulah Warren put together *Clinical Skills in Infant Mental Health* there wasn't a comprehensive, clearly written book available to help clinicians with the theories underpinning infant mental health or dealing with the practicalities of incorporating an infant mental health approach into their clinical practices. *Clinical Skills in Infant Mental Health* is also invaluable for students, as it is not only accessible and well-referenced but an absorbing read.

Sarah, Louise and Beulah are experts in the field of early childhood development, assessment and intervention, and during my career I have been lucky enough to be able to draw on their expertise. I am delighted that after many years of research, teaching, clinical practice and total commitment to the

FOREWORD

field of infant mental health they have found the time to make such a valuable contribution to this vital perspective of child and family health.

This book will be an incredibly useful working manual for all health professionals to have by their sides as a constant reference whether their fields are 'specialised' or 'general', or somewhere in between.

Robin Barker, Child and Family Health Nurse
Author of *Baby Love, The Mighty Toddler, Baby and Toddler Meals*
April 2005

Contents

Foreword *iii*
Acknowledgements *vi*
Note to readers *viii*
Authors *ix*
Quotations *xi*

PART A
Clinical framework 1

CHAPTER 1 Introduction to infant mental health *3*
CHAPTER 2 Attachment: theory, disruptions and disorders *25*
CHAPTER 3 Principles of assessment in infant mental health *40*
CHAPTER 4 Assessing risk in infancy *58*

PART B
The early infant–parent relationship 67

CHAPTER 5 Pregnancy, labour and birth *69*
CHAPTER 6 Biomedical problems in infancy *87*
CHAPTER 7 Sleeping *111*
CHAPTER 8 Feeding *133*

PART C
The toddler period 153

CHAPTER 9 Behavioural and emotional difficulties in toddlers *155*
CHAPTER 10 Consequences of trauma *173*
CHAPTER 11 Gender development and identity *183*

PART D
Parents and society 199

CHAPTER 12 Perinatal mental illness *201*
CHAPTER 13 Parents abused as children *217*
CHAPTER 14 Parents with personality disorder *231*
CHAPTER 15 Parenting and substance abuse *250*
CHAPTER 16 Adolescent parents *261*
CHAPTER 17 Families with multiple adversity *272*

Glossary *287*
References *291*
Index *311*

Acknowledgements

The NSW Institute of Psychiatry (NSWIOP) is a statutory body dedicated to educating health professionals in all aspects of mental health care. The Institute runs one of only two programs in infant mental health education in Australia, and the course is now delivered to students across Australia and in New Zealand.

This book provides an overview of infant mental health issues in clinical settings from our perspective. There are many experts who contribute as course writers and presenters to this and other programs run by the NSWIOP. Some material has been adapted from work initially written and prepared for a range of courses run by the NSWIOP. The contribution of individual course writers to the Masters of Infant Mental Health program must be acknowledged. These individuals have contributed to both the course program, and to our understanding and approach to clinical work with infants and their families. The book has grown out of our experience in developing and delivering the IMH course, and we hope it addresses what we perceive as a current gap in the relevant literature.

In addition to the authors, the following people have written and presented topics in the Masters program: Ms Elke Andrees, Associate Professor Marie-Paule Austin, Professor Bryanne Barnett, Ms Noel Boycott, Ms Julie Campbell, Dr Judy Cashmore, Dr Ralph Chan, Dr Robyn Dolby, Ms Judith Edwards, Dr Frances Gibson, Dr Louise Gyler, Ms Helen Hardy, Ms Margaret Hope, Dr Nick Kowalenko, Dr Kasia Koslowska, Dr Leo Leader, John Lord, Ms Annette McInerney, Dr Catherine McMahon, Dr Lyn Moore, Dr Marija Radojevic, Dr Christine Robinson, Ms Lorraine Rose, Dr Ruth Selig, Dr Jacqueline Small, Dr Caroline Stevenson, Ms Norma Tracey, Dr Bev Turner, Associate Professor Garry Walter, Ms Jane West, Ms Nicki Wickham and Dr George Williams.

We express our gratitude to Karen Cornish for her major contribution to the production of this text, in particular her patient collation of materials from a range of sources, her attention to editing detail and her assistance in developing a common voice and style for the book. We could not have done without her persistence, her patience and her amazing capacity to keep focused on the tasks at hand, despite our regular inability to meet agreed deadlines. Thank you, Karen.

Thanks are also extended to Jo Goldsworthy at ACER Press for providing an experienced and essential guiding hand as the book was being drafted. We would also like to acknowledge ACER Press for their patient commitment to the project and for continuing to publish books in the mental health field. Thanks also to

ACKNOWLEDGEMENTS

Alison Mahoney for her meticulous research of references for the final draft, Helen Baker for providing reference material for Chapter 17, Adelia Fuller for proofreading an earlier draft and the administration staff of the NSWIOP for the many and varied tasks they carried out while this book was in development. This book would not have been possible without the support of NSWIOP administration and Board who allowed us the time required and provided the necessary encouragement to write and develop the project.

While all authors collaborated to write the entire book, primary responsibility for particular chapters was allocated to specific authors: Chapter 1 was written by Dr Sarah Mares, Dr Louise Newman and Beulah Warren; Chapter 2 was written by Dr Louise Newman and Dr Sarah Mares; Chapter 3 was written by Dr Sarah Mares and Beulah Warren; Chapters 4 and 5 were written by Dr Sarah Mares; and Chapters 6 and 7 were written by Beulah Warren. Chapter 8 was written by Helen Hardy as a guest contributing author. Helen's expertise in the highly medical area of neonatal care, and feeding issues in particular, has enabled us to include a unique discussion of this specialty focus for infant mental health. We would like to thank Helen for her invaluable contribution. Chapter 9 was written by Beulah Warren; Chapters 10 and 11 were written by Dr Louise Newman; Chapters 12 and 13 were written by Dr Sarah Mares; Chapter 14 and 15 were written by Dr Louise Newman; Chapter 16 was written by Dr Sarah Mares; and Chapter 17 was written by Beulah Warren and Dr Sarah Mares.

Parts of Chapter 2 were adapted from material originally prepared and written by Dr Ron Spielman and Dr Sarah Mares for the Post Graduate Course in Psychiatry, Advanced Topics in the Psychotherapies. A section of Chapter 6 was adapted from material prepared by Dr Jacqueline Small for the Graduate Diploma in Infant Mental Health by Distance Education. The discussion of self-regulation in Chapter 1 was originally developed by Beulah Warren and Jan Heath for a prematurity workshop. We would like to thank these authors for permission to include their work.

Finally, we would like to thank the many infants and parents we have had the privilege to work with. We acknowledge how much we have learned from parents sharing their experiences and the unique ways infants communicate within therapeutic settings. We are also grateful for the contribution that students in the Graduate Diploma and Masters of Infant Mental Health program have made to our understanding of the clinical issues faced by a wide range of professionals in many different workplaces. We hope that this book will contribute to the development of the skills and expertise of these and many other professionals who work with infants and their families.

SM, LN & BW
March 2005

Note to readers

There has been a recent shift in emphasis from the mother–infant focus that characterised earlier writing and research, to a focus on infant–caregiver relationships. This acknowledges the other caregivers who may take a significant role with infants such as fathers, foster parents or grandparents. Referring primarily to the infant–mother relationship contributes to societal ambivalence about mothers and the maternal role. Motherhood is idealised; the mother's capacity to nurture the happy, satisfied infant is portrayed regularly in popular culture. At the same time, despite changing expectations within developed western cultures about women in the workforce and shared parenting, mothers continue to carry the bulk of responsibility for infant and child development.

In attempting to acknowledge both the predominant role mothers continue to play, as well as the other caregivers who may take primary responsibility for the care and upbringing of an infant, we have most frequently used the term 'infant–parent' to refer to the main caregiving relationship. At other times 'mother', 'carer' or 'caregiver' has been used interchangeably with the term 'parent'. We hope that readers will find the use of a variety of terms acceptable given the range of family constellations that exist and are encountered clinically. In this book the infant is referred to as 'he' in some chapters and 'she' in others. Regardless of the terms used, an appreciation of the sociocultural context(s) within which the infant and caregivers live and develop is an essential element of understanding infant–parent interaction and development.

Clinical Skills in Infant Mental Health provides a general introductory approach to clinical practice in the field of infant mental health rather than specific clinical guidelines. This book does not attempt to address issues arising in clinical work with all groups of parents and infants with particular needs and attributes, such as Indigenous families. The authors welcome feedback and the opportunity to build on what we hope is a useful introductory text. Case examples in this book are drawn from the clinical experience of the authors and have been altered to protect privacy. All care has been taken to provide accurate, current information, but this book should not be used as the sole basis for clinical decision making as every family situation is unique and requires individualised assessment. The authors and publisher cannot be held responsible for any problems arising out of the contents of this book.

Authors

Dr Louise Newman is the Director of the New South Wales Institute of Psychiatry and a Child and Adolescent Psychiatrist with expertise in the area of infancy and early childhood. She is undertaking research into the prevention of child maltreatment and interventions for parents who have experienced early abuse.

Prior to studying medicine, Dr Newman completed undergraduate degrees in Psychology, Philosophy and Gender Studies and she has a longstanding commitment to the promotion of women's mental health.

Dr Newman is currently the Chair of the New South Wales Branch of the Royal Australian and New Zealand College of Psychiatrists (RANZCP). She also Chairs the RANZCP Faculty of Child and Adolescent Psychiatry and is the spokesperson on asylum seekers and child mental health issues.

Dr Newman is involved in a review of the training of psychiatrists and child psychiatrists in NSW and the development of innovative approaches to psychiatric and mental health education. In her RANZCP roles she is involved in workforce development and promoting collaborative work practices between psychiatrists and other mental health professionals. Her clinical focus is on the prevention of child maltreatment and development of interventions for early parenting difficulties.

Beulah Warren MA Hons is a psychologist in private practice whose focus is on families and infants. Beulah's clinical emphasis is to help parents see the unique qualities of their child and to better understand their crucial role as parents. She currently coordinates the Master of Infant Mental Health program at the NSW Institute of Psychiatry and provides supervision and consultation to agencies and practitioners in the area of infant mental health.

As a psychologist, Beulah's work began 27 years ago with premature infants and their families. At an early point she achieved reliability on the Brazelton Neonatal Behavioral Assessment Scale and subsequently became a trainer.

Beulah Warren has worked clinically in hospitals and as foundation coordinator of the Benevolent Society of NSW Early Intervention Program, based at the Royal Hospital for Women, Sydney. She is a founding member of the Australian Association for Infant Mental Health.

AUTHORS

Dr Sarah Mares is a Child and Family Psychiatrist with a particular interest in infancy and the early childhood period. She is currently Director of the Clinical Teaching and Research Unit at the NSW Institute of Psychiatry, and Chair of the NSW Faculty of Child and Adolescent Psychiatry of the RANZCP.

She is involved in the development and teaching of the Masters of Infant Mental Health, the Postgraduate Course in Psychiatry and the Child, Adolescent and Family Psychiatry teaching program at the NSW Institute of Psychiatry. Dr Mares has considerable experience in direct clinical work with families with infants and young children and has provided consultation and supervision to multiple agencies and individuals involved in provision of care to this population. Her particular interests include transgenerational issues in parenting and attachment, assessment of risk, parenting capacity and child protection, professional ethics and advocacy, and postgraduate medical education.

Karen Cornish is a writer and editor, with a specialty in the mental health field. Trained originally as an occupational therapist, she has worked in mental health services as a clinician and manager, and in administrative services as a senior policy analyst. Since completing studies in editing, Karen has collaborated to write and edit teaching and training manuals, clinical guidelines and resource books. Her other professional interests include children's literature and learning aids, and health and nutrition.

'There is no such thing as a baby…if you set out to describe a baby, you will find you are describing a baby and someone. A baby cannot exist alone, but is essentially part of a relationship'
(Winnicott, 1964/1978, p. 88).

Winnicott, D. W. (1978). *The child, the family and the outside world*. Harmondsworth, Middlesex: Penguin Books. (Original work published 1964.)

'Sympathy and shared pleasure in the trials and risks of experience are companions to adventure in meaning. The infant hero can suffer shame if submitted to the dull gaze and tuneless voice of indifference, even if kept warm and well fed'
(Trevarthen, 2001, p.119).

Trevarthen, C. (2001). Intrinsic motives for companionship in understanding: Their origin, development, and significance for infant mental health. *Infant Mental Health Journal*, 22(1–2), 95–131.

Clinical framework

PART A

CHAPTER 1

Introduction to infant mental health

KEY CONCEPTS

- Multidisciplinary contributions to infant mental health
- Normal emotional development during infancy and early childhood
- Attachment relationships as the context for development
- Infant competencies and developmental milestones
- Developmental psychopathology
- The biopsychosocial framework for development

PRINCIPLES

- Infancy lays the foundation for later development
- Emotional and psychological development is significantly influenced by the quality of the infant–carer attachment relationship
- Early therapeutic intervention can mediate against risks and positively influence development

Infancy and the field of infant mental health have attracted increasing scientific and clinical interest over the last 25 years. The field has emerged as a result of advances in knowledge of infant development, the development of tools for infant observational research and assessment, and integration of diverse theoretical frameworks that can be used to consider the relationship between infants and carers. There is increasing evidence that the experiences of infants and toddlers in the early years of life have direct and indirect effects on development. Developmental neurobiology and attachment theory provide a complex and integrated understanding of developmental processes, as well as models to look at the interaction of multiple factors affecting infant development. The field of infant mental health reflects this multidisciplinary influence.

There is increasing understanding about infant competencies—the innate skills and abilities they are born with that enable them to attract and maintain the interest, attention and care of their primary caregivers, and the crucial role that early attachment relationships have on development of the individual infant within his social and cultural context.

In this chapter we will look at normal emotional development in infancy and the significance of this for later psychological functioning. In considering why infant mental health is of increasing clinical interest we will review the historical development of ideas that now influence understanding and thinking about infancy. Finally, we will review current models of development and the way that new understandings about emotional development can be incorporated into clinical assessment and intervention.

WHAT IS INFANT MENTAL HEALTH?

Infant mental health is a multidisciplinary field of research and clinical practice. It is an area of rapidly expanding knowledge and of innovation in clinical interventions. At its core is recognition that infancy is a foundational developmental period, physically, psychologically and socially, that infant development occurs within the context of key caregiving relationships, and that infants have abilities, drives, wants and needs but also rights, just as more verbal older children and adults do. Infants communicate in many ways and despite their obvious vulnerability have an extraordinary capacity to adapt and to make the best of what is provided to them. Infant mental health as a field of clinical research and practice is concerned with understanding those factors that allow and facilitate optimal development, and with developing the range of interventions that mitigate against the physical, emotional and social risks experienced by some infants and their families.

Why is infant mental health important?

The relationship between any particular early experience and later infant outcome is not a simple linear one (Zeanah, Boris & Larrieu, 1997). Development proceeds as a complex series of interactions between the innate qualities of infants, their experiences in interaction with their physical and social world, and their capacity to influence and change their environment. There is increasing evidence that those infants and children most at risk of adverse developmental outcomes are those who experience an accumulation of risk factors (Ferguson & Horwood, 2003). There is also evidence from attachment research that the quality of infant–caregiver relationships can act both as a protective and a risk factor, in combination with or as a result of other adversities (Goldberg, 2000).

Clinicians are increasingly aware that paying more attention to the quality of the relationship between infants and parents can have a positive effect on both the presenting problem and their longer term relationship. Infants are not passive recipients of care, but active agents influencing their own lives and environments. This does not rule out the need to acknowledge the very particular physical and emotional vulnerability of the human infant and their absolute dependence upon their caregivers for adequate care and protection. The inclusion of mental health as a core aspect of assessment in all situations involving infants and their parents acknowledges the centrality of relationships and psychosocial factors in human development and well-being.

Influences on the field of infant mental health

Understanding of early childhood development has been influenced by psychoanalytic theory, object relations theory, attachment theory and developmental psychology. Infant research has contributed to an understanding of the capacities of the newborn to interact with the environment and to organise the self and experiences in an active way. Daniel Stern (1985) has described infants as having a 'pre-wired knowledge of the world' or an innate interactive capacity, which from birth promotes the development of an affective relationship with the caregiver, and which is the basis of the sense of self. Stern argues against more traditional psychoanalytic theories (such as Mahler, Pine & Bergman, 1975) who have described infancy as a period of unawareness or 'autism'. Neurobiology and brain research demonstrate that the attachment context of development, or the quality of the emotional relationship an infant has with his primary caregivers directly influences brain growth and development. Infants with 'secure' attachment relationships are more likely than 'insecure' infants to show optimal neuropsychological and social development. (Patterns of attachment are described in Chapter 2.)

It is also clear that a facilitating caregiving environment that is sensitive and responsive to the infant's needs promotes optimal neurological and psychological development, such as learning, memory and self-regulation. Systems theory and population mental health describe the effect of the family system, and social and cultural factors on infant development through their influence on the caregiving environment. (For an overall summary of influences on infant mental health, refer to Table 1.1.)

Psychoanalytic theory

Classical psychoanalytic theory provides an account of the development of the structure of the mind (that is, the id, ego and super-ego) and of infant developments through a series of psychosexual stages over the first five years of life. In Sigmund Freud's (1922) original drive theory, the development of relationships to others (object relations) is motivated by the need for tension reduction and the infant is pictured as having little awareness or capacity to interact with his carer or social environment.

Freud describes three psychosexual stages of development:

Oral stage (birth–18 months)—tension and hunger motivate interaction with the world and the mother is the source of gratification and the first love object.

Anal stage (18–36 months)—the infant is involved in a series of struggles for autonomy and experiences conflicts over aggression and dependency.

Phallic/Genital stage (3 years)—this is the period of oedipal development with the emergence of sexual attachment towards the opposite sex parent. This stage culminates in the development of the super-ego.

Psychoanalytic theories of object relations describe the way in which early relationship experiences influence the development of the sense of self or identity. The infant needs a sensitive caregiver to begin the process of identity development. This process is sometimes referred to as separation-individuation and occurs during the toddler period (Mahler et al., 1975).

Object relations theory

Object relations theory refers to a group of analytical accounts beginning with the work of Klein and Riviero (1937), which moved away from Freud's emphasis on drives and psychological defences towards an increasing interest in relationships. Later writers, such as Fairbairn (1952), came to see 'object seeking', the need to form social relationships, as a motivation equal to, or of greater importance than, drive discharge or tension reduction. Recent theories of infant development (Stern, 1985) and attachment theory (Bowlby, 1969, 1973) also focus on the infant's earliest interactions with the social world and the mother, and describe relationships as becoming internalised structures or models within the brain and the psyche. The infant builds up models or representations of the self and the carer (the 'other') in relationship, along with associated feeling states. This model (known as the inner working model in attachment theory) acts as a template for the child's expectations, behaviour and perception of future relationships.

Attachment theory

John Bowlby, a British psychoanalyst, is seen as the 'father' of attachment theory. He described the development of an attachment behavioural system that has the aim of maintaining the infant's sense of security and safety. In his initial formulation of attachment theory, Bowlby argued that the innate capacity of infants to form relationships has clear evolutionary or species-survival value. Unlike some other animals, human infants are born in a relative state of prematurity and are dependent on an older species member for survival. Infants cannot obtain food, or maintain body temperature, for example, and need a carer

INTRODUCTION TO INFANT MENTAL HEALTH

to regulate basic and essential physiological processes. The infant begins to form attachment relationships from birth, and Bowlby described attachment as a programmed or 'hard-wired' innate capacity of the infant.

Methods for assessing the security of attachment relationships in infants and children and internal working models of relationships in adults, as well as the clinical implications and applications of attachment theory are discussed in detail in Chapter 2.

Developmental psychology

Developmental psychology (or psychopathology) has emerged as an important field over the last 25 years and takes a multidisciplinary approach to development and the understanding of developmental problems. It focuses on both the effect of development on disorder and the ways in which disorder affects ongoing developmental processes (Cicchetti & Cohen, 1995).

Developmental psychopathology focuses on:
1 The interplay between normal and abnormal development.
2 Risk and protective factors in biological, psychological and social spheres of development.
3 Delineating pathways to the development of mental disorder and psychopathology.
4 Understanding critical periods: the notion that there are periods in development that are optimal for the development of specific skills and that these are also periods of greatest vulnerability to disruption of their acquisition. An example is the capacity to form attachment relationships for which experiences in the first two years of life appear to be critical.
5 Understanding brain/environment interactions: there is increasing interest in the way in which neurological development and organisation are influenced by the social environment and quality of social interaction, particularly during the infant period of rapid brain growth. Current research demonstrates that the optimal growth of the infant brain depends on the quality of the relationship between the primary caregiver and infant (Shore, 1997). The anatomical differentiation of the brain is dependent on appropriate stimulation from the environment and brain function can be altered by experiences at certain sensitive periods of development. An area of research interest is the ongoing effect of brain/environment interaction on development and subsequent functioning.

Infant research

Close study of infant development has provided understanding of the innate capacities of infants and the quality of care needed to promote healthy development. Infant research examines the ability of infants to both perceive and communicate affective states, to differentiate their primary carer from others and to interact with them. Carers and infants establish patterns of interaction in which the carer modulates the infant's overall level of neurophysiological arousal. Providing optimal infant care requires the caregiver to maintain appropriate levels of arousal in the infant and be responsive to the infant's expressions of his internal state. The infant experiences his carer as available, appropriately and consistently responsive, and from these repeated experiences internalises and gradually develops the ability to regulate his own emotional responses and level of arousal. Several areas of infant competence have been described in the field of infant research:

Programmed for social interaction—The infant shows preferential attention to the human face and voice, and can imitate facial expressions. The infant responds to changes in his carer's emotional state. The infant shows unease, aversion to 'mistimed communications' or to non-response.

Ability to communicate emotional experience—Infants show a range of emotional expressions from birth that can be recognised by their carers.

Proto-conversation—Infants and carers develop proto-conversations by eight weeks that embody the characteristics of speech, with turn-taking, modulation of attention and matching or mirroring of gesture and vocalisations.

Social and affective interaction—Infants and carers communicate and play by three months. Infants use motor skills and communication skills to engage their carer in joint attention and communications about objects.

Self-regulation—Infants move towards self-development and self-regulation of affect, over time being able to manage their own internal state through repeated experiences of external support from the primary caregiver to assist in managing feelings and arousal. (The development of self-regulation is described later in this chapter.)

Neurobiology and brain research

This expanding area has lead to an understanding of critical periods of brain development (experiences needed for development during infancy). Lack of crucial experiences during critical periods may result in damage to the development of a particular function.

Significant advances in neuroscience point to the importance of stimulation and early experience in brain development. The development of the brain is 'experience-dependent' and the formation of neuronal connections and delineation of pathways occurs in response to environmental stimulation and use. Infant–caregiver relationships form the basis of the 'environment' and are the means through which optimal brain development occurs.

Rapid development during the infant period involves production of synapses, and repeated activation stabilises and strengthens connections between neurons and brain areas. The later pruning of synapses eliminates connections that are not used and brain pathways are delineated in response to patterns of use and activation. This dynamic model of neurological development sees the brain as a socially responsive organ and stresses that the infant period, due to the rapid rate of growth, is crucial in the development of both brain structure and later brain function.

Systems theory

Systems theory focuses on the way individuals, groups and the environment interact to operate as complete structures or systems. In infant mental health this has influenced thinking about infants as involved in complex social networks and being interactive with the social world.

Population mental health

This is an approach that looks at the mental health needs of whole communities and populations and focuses on social risk and protective factors. Infant development and infant mental health outcomes are influenced by social factors such as economic health, social disadvantage, functioning of communities and families, and access to parenting and family supports. This is an important model in the area of social and family policy, and prevention.

Table 1.1 **Summary of influences on infant mental health**

Area	*Focus*
Psychoanalytic theory	Development of self; separation/individuation and psychological functioning; carer–infant relationships; the influence of transgenerational issues on relationships and development.
Object relations theory	Importance of relationship experiences for development of internal models of self and other.
Attachment theory	Development of primary attachment relationships and the role of secure attachment in optimal development; transgenerational issues in development.
Developmental psychology	Infant formative development: socio-emotional; cognitive; psychological.
Infant research	Capacities of infants for interaction, communication, self-regulation, and modulation of infant–carer interaction.
Neurobiology and brain research	The role of the social environment and attachment relationship in facilitating optimal neurobiological development.
Systems theory	Functioning of the infant-carer dyad and family system; systematic approach to developmental theory; transactions between the infant and environment.
Population mental health	Cultural and social factors affecting infant development and mental health: risk and protective factors, social policy; advocacy and infant mental health.

INFANCY: A FOUNDATIONAL DEVELOPMENTAL PERIOD

Infancy is usually defined as the period from being a newborn until three to four years of age. Within infancy, different stages are described using terms that indicate age and development, such as newborn, baby and toddler. Emotional development in infancy is influenced by the overall passage and process of human development, but particularly by the social interactions and relationships that an infant experiences. Emotional development may also be affected by physiological factors or physical illness. For example, an infant who experiences repeated hospitalisations as a result of contracting HIV in utero will be affected by the direct consequences of the illness, and the effect of the illness on the caregivers and their capacity to provide care as well as by the separations associated with hospital admission. Awareness and management of the effect on the infant–parent relationship can minimise harm.

Infancy is often described as 'foundational' in that many crucial structures, processes and functions needed for physical and mental functioning are set up or established during the early years. It is also a critical period of development in that there are time periods when particular experiences are necessary for specific aspects of neuropsychological development to occur. Experiences during infancy influence the course of all later development.

Human development

Human development has traditionally been regarded as progressing through a series of predetermined phases, usually intrinsically or genetically controlled, towards a state of maturity. Stage theories of development focus on the individual's movement along a series of stages with each being dependent on passage through preceding ones. Examples of stage theories include Freud's psychosexual stages (oral, anal, genital) and Piaget's account of cognitive development (see Miller, 2002, for summaries of these theories).

There are several problems with stage models of development:
- Most give an inadequate account of human development and focus only on particular aspects of the individual.
- Developmental processes are not well described and the individual infant is seen as a passive participant rather than actively interacting with and shaping the environment.
- Little emphasis is given to the interactions between the individual and the social environment (interpersonal relationships, family, culture) in many theories, or to the ways in which biological and neurological development are influenced by social interaction and environment.

INTRODUCTION TO INFANT MENTAL HEALTH

Infants are born with the genetic program or blueprint for developmental processes but these require the right facilitating environmental conditions and input if they are to unfold. For example, infants are born with the ability to engage with another human being and communicate in complex ways from birth. However, this capacity to communicate is influenced by the way an infant is responded to and communicated with by primary caregivers.

Normal infant emotional development

Infant research has provided considerable information about the infant's innate capacities for social and environmental interaction from birth. The newborn baby has an amazing range of communication strategies. For example, newborns turn their heads in response to a familiar parental voice or smell, show a preference for face-shaped patterns over other pictures, express a range of emotions and attempt to imitate facial expressions (Murray & Andrews, 2000).

All of these strategies have one primary focus—to ensure that an adult will respond and prioritise the infant's survival. The newborn has an inbuilt capacity to act in a way that promotes the development of a caring, loving relationship with an adult. Normal emotional development in an infant occurs within this relationship, and developmental stages and challenges are responded to within the relationship context.

Several psychological and emotional processes are established in infancy. Rapid neuropsychological development occurs at the same time as physical and cognitive developmental tasks are achieved. Psychosocial development and the development of self-regulation also occur within the infant period and influence later psychological and interpersonal functioning. Developmental and psychological processes are often interlinked; for example, the development of secure base behaviour and exploration in the second year corresponds with the development of crawling and walking. The infant who is mobile becomes interested in exploring the environment more actively and can use the primary caregiver as a secure base from which to begin exploring and learning. (Attachment is discussed in detail in Chapter 2.)

Neuropsychological development

During infancy, brain development is more rapid than at any other time of life, with the development of multiple pathways needed for:
- processing of social and emotional information
- memory and learning processes
- communicating and language
- affective interaction and regulation.

It is easiest to understand this development in the context of the physical, social and emotional development that occurs during the early years and is discussed below. Brain development in the early years is well outlined in Shore (1997).

Developmental tasks of infancy

Emotional development in infancy is linked to and occurs alongside other motor and cognitive developmental tasks or milestones. (For a discussion of emotional development specific to toddlers see Chapter 9.)

THE FIRST YEAR

During the first year of life the infant will grow and develop more rapidly, physically, emotionally and socially than during any other life period. The foundation is laid for language development and mobility that enables infants increasing independence as they explore the world and share their new experiences with key adults. While there is great variation in the speed at which infants develop and the week or month at which particular milestones are attained, it is possible to identify key developmental shifts in the first year, where, providing the environment has been adequate, advances in brain development are marked by developmental shifts in behaviour (Sroufe, 1996). These periods also indicate changes in the role of caregivers, who are required to constantly adapt themselves to the rapidly developing infant in their care (see Sroufe, 1996, p. 161).

For example, the first three months can be thought of as a time when the primary goal is the development of physiological regulation. This includes the routines of settling, sleeping, feeding and alertness. The infant is adjusting to being outside the womb and in the world and the parent is assisting the development of cycles and patterns that mark the infant's day and lay the foundation for later development of self-regulation. In the following three months the infant is less overwhelmed by bodily sensations and has more time for social interaction. This is a time when ideally parent and infant have more time to enjoy each other. The baby develops physical control of his body and upper limbs, enabling him to view and interact with the world in a new way.

Between 6 and 12 months the stage is set for the further development of attachment relationships. Through repeated interactions with caregivers, the infant begins to internalise representations of themselves and the world that form the basis of the security or otherwise of their attachments to their primary caregivers. Mobility also develops and as the infant is able to crawl and then walk away, to explore independently, he increasingly exhibits attachment-related behaviours that link him to his caregiver. During this time separation protest is likely to be present and the infant begins to show a clear preference for certain adults.

The last three months of the first year have been described as a period of 'initiative and internalization' (Lieberman & Slade, 1997a). Infants seek to share

INTRODUCTION TO INFANT MENTAL HEALTH

their experiences with key others and language is added to gesture and vocalisation as ways to communicate. Trevarthen (2001) has called this 'intersubjectivity', the desire to share experience and emotional state with significant others.

In the following example, Netta, mother of Kyle (aged 10 months) describes his increasing physical mobility and exploration and his need to check in with or stay connected to her with voice or visual cues before further exploration.

> *Kyle has been crawling for a few weeks now. Usually I sit in the lounge room while he crawls around and he seems to feel safe to just cruise the room while I am there. If I get up and walk away, he cries and needs to be picked up and carried to where I am, or sometimes he'll settle if I call out to him to let him know I'm still there. He doesn't seem to want to follow after me though. Today, when I was sitting watching him crawl, I noticed him heading off further than usual, down the hall. He got about half way down and then turned around and looked back at me. I smiled and encouraged him for making such a big effort and he crawled a bit further. Then he really seemed like he had got to the end of a 'rope', I guess it was his comfort zone, and he needed to turn around and head back to base.*
> (Netta, mother of Kyle, 10 months.)

THE SECOND YEAR

The second year of life is marked by two major developmental achievements: the development of language and symbolic play, and increased mobility and independence. There is a consolidation of secure base behaviour and exploration seen towards the end of the first year and as the infant, now toddler, experiments with independence the foundation is laid for regulation of affect and aggression and the development of self-awareness as an individual. Language development is rapid during this year and indicates the developing capacity to use symbols and imagination. This is linked to the development of imaginative play, and there is great interest in their own bodies including bodily excretions. Between 14 and 18 months toddlers begin to show recognition of themselves in the mirror and to include the personal pronouns 'I', 'me' and 'mine' in their speech. Along with this goes the ability to say 'no' and to experiment with the degree of control they have over events and other people. The role of the caregivers changes in this period as they are required to set limits and ensure safety while also remaining responsive and available, continuing to provide a 'secure base' while managing what at times is their inevitable frustration with an increasingly independent and unpredictable small person in their care (Lieberman & Slade, 1997b). In the following example the development of language and imaginative play combined with the increasing desire to be 'in control' are shown:

> *Today Mia used a rubber ring as a pretend car. She said 'Go work! Bye' and 'drove off' to the next room. I go to work three days a week and I got the sense*

> *that she was pretending to be me and perhaps also dealing with the fact that we are separate and that going to work is something I do. We needed to go out so I told her it was time to get out of the 'car' and come with me. She didn't want to and said 'no no!' before crying and throwing herself on the floor.* (Mary, mother of Mia, one year and 11 months.)

THE THIRD YEAR

By the beginning of the third year the foundation is laid for the unique thinking and feeling individual that the toddler will become. Language is established, as are physical competence and mobility. Over this year children further develop a sense of themselves and their place within a network of relationships. They develop a range of words for their own emotions, and as Fonagy, Steele, Steele, Moran and Higgitt (1991) put it, 'children in their third year are evidently capable of understanding that other people have feelings and intentions different from their own' (p. 204). Children begin to be able to manage their interaction with others, including peers. Memory and language enable them to tolerate longer separations and to begin to predict events. Their emerging sense of self is evident in what is sometimes called the 'terrible twos', wilfulness and possessiveness. As they continue to experiment with their own power or lack of it, they may become ritualistic or picky about food or clothes and unpredictably oppositional. They are now also able to be fully collaborative partners in activities and in anticipation of events.

> *I notice Lara's individuality when I take her to child care and see the enormous range of kids there and the ways they relate to each other. Some appear to be always cheerful, greeting others at the door and running around in a pack, while others like Lara are more cautious and take a little longer to connect with the group. Lara seems to need a 'link' in to other people—an activity, a shared experience such as a story, or identifying something in common with another person. I think this reflects her nature as a great observer of life, and one who participates after careful assessment and reflection. I used to try to encourage her to 'leap in' a bit more, but lately I have found that helping her find her connection with the group by staying alongside her for a while helps much more.* (Freya, mother of Lara, two years and nine months.)

The fourth year is a period of dramatic integration and reorganisation that prepares the child for the school years. Language becomes more elaborate, as does symbolic and imaginative play. Children become increasingly aware of social expectations and responsibilities and their friendships strengthen and develop. In parallel with this, there is further development of what is known as 'theory of mind': the capacity to know that others have thoughts and feelings that are separate from our own (Fonagy & Target, 1996). This is intimately linked to the later capacity for empathy and self-reflection.

Psychosocial development

The infant develops an attachment relationship and internal representations or working models of relationships. The capacity for empathy also develops during infancy as well as the development of self-representation or sense of self-identity.

THE ATTACHMENT RELATIONSHIP

An attachment relationship is an enduring affective relationship with a particular preferred individual, usually the person who provides most of the primary caregiving, and from whom the infant seeks security and comfort. A major developmental task for an infant in the first year of life is the establishment of an affective interaction with his caregiver and the development of an attachment relationship. First attachments are usually formed by seven months of age and secure attachment is linked to later social and emotional competence.

To foster a secure attachment relationship, the role of the caregiver is to:
- be responsively available to signals from the infant
- encourage appropriate exploration by the infant
- be a 'secure base', that is, be appropriately responsive and available for comfort and shared enjoyment
- support autonomy and self-control
- internalise the parent function, that is, accept the role of parent to the child, being available and responsive and giving priority to the needs of the child.

Attachment behaviours are those behaviours that promote proximity to the attachment figure (crying, approaching and following) with the aim of producing feelings of safety and security. These behaviours are more evident when the child is tired or unwell, or stressed, for example, by an unfamiliar situation. The development of secure attachment involves a balance between proximity-seeking and exploratory behaviours. For the secure infant it is safe to explore because there is someone reliably available to return to.

Attachment patterns or classifications can be assessed and can influence later mental health and adjustment. Classifications of attachment relationships are described in Chapter 2.

DEVELOPMENT OF INTERNAL REPRESENTATIONS

Importantly, the infant begins to develop a sense of self, and an understanding of the emotions of other people and relationships (empathy), through his early experiences with his caregiver. These understandings or models of relationships are known as internal representations or internal working models in attachment theory.

Internal working models are crucial in development as they set the template or basis for later relationships. Ideally, internal working models allow humans the adaptability to form and maintain relationships over the lifespan and to deal with the range of emotions that go hand in hand with living.

Internal working models developed through experiencing a secure attachment relationship enable the infant to develop empathy, a crucial aspect of effective relationships. As in the example of Judy and Bess below, an infant's developing ability to respond to the pain experienced by another person shows the beginnings of empathy.

> *Today Bess looked at me when I bumped my head on the cupboard door and said, 'Hurt mummy? Ouch?' I knew for the first time that she was expressing concern for me! It was a magical moment.* (Judy, 27, mother of Bess, three.)

SELF-REPRESENTATION

The development of self-representation occurs around 12 to 18 months of age after the infant comes to distinguish himself from others and begins to develop an idea of 'me' and 'you'. Bowlby (1969, 1973) proposed that from infancy we construct models of the world, of ourselves and of significant others based on our experiences. These models then guide and focus our subsequent experience and behaviour in relationships. It is presumed that these 'models' or representations are incorporated at a neurobiological level into neural networks and pathways linked to regulation of affect and arousal.

Self-regulation

Self-regulation is the process of the infant gaining regulation of his behaviour—physiological, social, sensory–motor and emotional—to achieve functional goals such as settling to sleep, effective interaction, holding the body still so attention can be focused on a toy, task or person, and satisfactory and satisfying food intake (Siegel, 1999; Sroufe, 1996). This occurs through the integration of social interaction experiences (infant–parent relationships) with the infant's maturing systems. Emerging self-regulation is affected by sensory motor experiences and infant maturation.

THE DEVELOPMENT OF SELF-REGULATION

All newborns are dependent on a consistently available carer to respond to a range of needs including tiredness, hunger, temperature variations, discomfort, and fear and anxiety at separations. Predictable and responsive caring interactions between the infant and carer form the basis of the infant's capacity to self-regulate biologically and socially (Anders, Goodlin-Jones & Sadeh, 2000). The aim of these interactions is to help the infant achieve physical and, eventually, emotional regulation. Routine caregiving activities, such as feeding, holding, comforting, settling and adjusting temperature, help the infant begin to regulate intense feelings, as the parent feels for the infant and responds to his perceived emotions and needs. Repeated interactions that assist the infant to

INTRODUCTION TO INFANT MENTAL HEALTH

relieve feelings of distress are believed to affect the development of neuronal pathways, with those circuits that are repeatedly stimulated during infancy being enhanced and consolidated (Schore, 1994).

Parenting strategies that alleviate discomfort are internalised by the infant over time. If distressed, an infant of only a few weeks of age will quieten to a familiar, positive, warm voice. The infant has learnt that the voice indicates that he will be responded to. This repeated pattern of having needs met means the infant anticipates the parent's responsiveness, and cries less. Gradually, characteristic patterns of behaviour in the child emerge that have their basis in the caregiving environment—infant constitutional factors, parenting responses and repeated interactions between the infant and parent. (See Figure 1.1.)

SENSORY MOTOR EXPERIENCES

Part of self-regulation is the infant's capacity to process sensory input. Sensory input may be from the internal (the infant's body and mind) or external environment. Initially, parents filter and modify the sensory input to avoid the infant becoming overwhelmed, for example, by wrapping, using a soothing voice or darkening the room. Infants vary in their capacity to control their motor movements and be still. Initially, parents assist the infant by holding or wrapping until the infant is still and able to go to sleep.

Figure 1.1 **The caregiving environment and regulation**

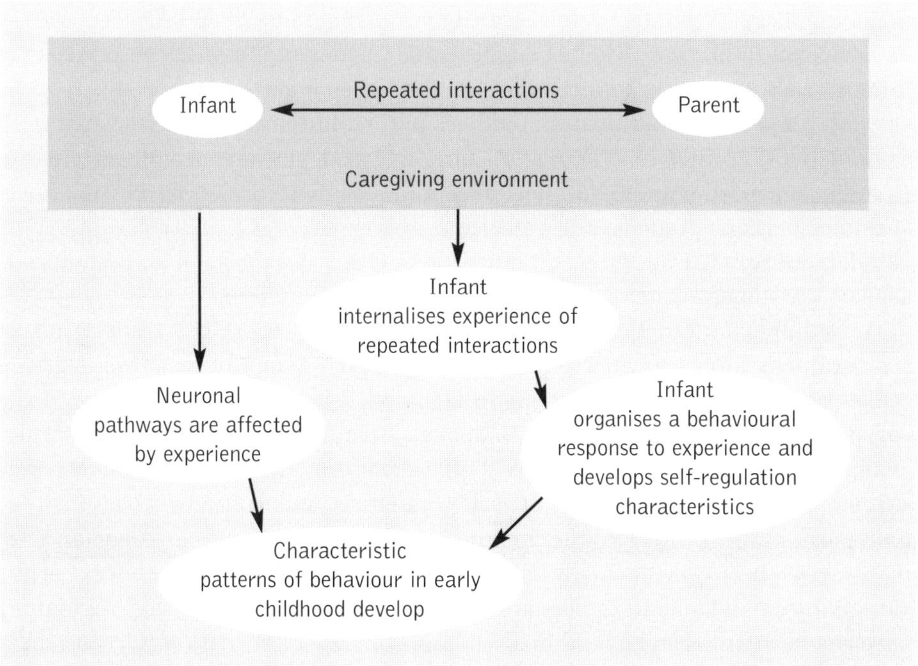

Adapted from Barton and Robins (2000).

MATURATION

An infant's neurological development determines his innate capacity to process sensory stimuli. Less neurologically mature infants (such as those born prematurely) require more assistance from the caregiving environment to filter and integrate stimuli, and more easily become overwhelmed and distressed.

TEMPERAMENT

Temperament has been defined as 'a behavioural and physiological profile that is under some genetic control…a changing, but coherent, profile of behaviour and emotion linked to an inherited physiology' (Kagan, 1997, p. 269). Thomas and Chess (1977) originally suggested three temperamental or behavioural categories (easy, slow to warm up and difficult), defined by a profile of dimensions (activity, regularity, approach or withdrawal to unfamiliarity, adaptation to new situations, responsiveness, energy, a happy or irritable mood, distractibility and attention span).

Temperament is a controversial construct because of the lack of correlation between parental and observer ratings. It covers several dimensions of infant behaviour including self-regulation, sociability (ranging from shy to extroverted behaviour) and emotionality (ranging from positive to negative responses) (Kohnstamm, Bates & Rothbart, 1989). Temperament may also include qualities such as persistence, reactivity and rhythmicity. One dimension of temperament for which there is increasing evidence is the shy–extroverted continuum, including a characteristic first described by Kagan, Snidman and Arcus (1998) as 'behavioural inhibition'. Studies suggest that at four months, 15–20 per cent of infants react negatively to a novel stimulus. These infants are more likely to be shy, inhibited and withdrawn as toddlers and children. This is associated with asymmetrical frontal lobe activation on EEG and indicates a vulnerability to shyness and social withdrawal. In contrast, other infants are excited by the novel stimulus, perhaps predisposing them to extroversion and novelty seeking (Fox, Henderson, Rubin, Calkins & Schmidt, 2001). Other dimensional and categorical aspects of temperament require further empirical validation.

It is important to be cautious about explaining behaviour as a result of temperament alone, as it may result in underlying family or developmental issues being overlooked, and fails to acknowledge the important role of the caregiving environment—the primary caregiver's responsiveness and availability to the infant—in shaping characteristic patterns of behaviour. The contemporary understanding of self-regulation incorporates the effect of biological vulnerability in the infant, but also considers the importance of interactions between the infant and the caregiver, and the overall context of the caregiving environment. It appears from preliminary research that regulatory patterns in infants can be modified with appropriate intervention (Greenspan & Wieder, 1993; Maldonado-Duran & Sauceda-Garcia, 1996).

The significance of early experience

Debate about the significance of the infant experience has been going on for some time and is referred to as the 'continuity debate'. Some theorists see infant experience as crucial in setting lifelong, relatively unchanging patterns. Discontinuity theorists argue that later life experience can change early patterns and that infancy does not necessarily determine later outcomes. The basis of the argument is the extent of 'hard-wiring' that occurs as a result of infant experience, and the extent of adaptation and flexibility that is possible in later development.

Current developmental models argue that experiences in the foundational period of infancy set up models or templates for neurological and social functioning, and these are then shaped and influenced by changing environmental factors and life events. Infancy sets up core vulnerabilities and strengths, which are modified by experience. Early experiences appear to have both direct and indirect long-term effects on development. Adverse early experiences, for example, may cause damage to some infant capacities if severe, but will also produce a greater vulnerability to stress as the infant matures. For example, severe stress in infancy will affect the developing stress-regulation mechanisms of the brain and hormonal systems, influencing the capacity to deal with and respond to stressful events throughout life (see Chapter 10).

CURRENT MODELS OF EARLY DEVELOPMENT AND INTERVENTION

Current accounts of early development describe the infant's move towards self-regulation and self-organisation in the context of the relationship with his mother or the primary carer. The attachment relationship and the quality of infant–carer interaction have a major influence on early neurobiological and psychosocial developmental processes. Contemporary models of infancy also emphasise infant competencies (or innate abilities) and the ability of the infant to elicit responses from the caregiving environment. Current thinking about development also looks at the complex interaction between the individual and environment and the ways in which the infant or child engages with the social world and influences environmental responses.

For example, the transactional view of development proposed by Sameroff and Fiese (2000) points out that each child and parent brings specific characteristics to their relationship. These mutually interact and influence each other. Experiences in infancy influence multiple processes of development and are also mediated by the differential response of parents. Assessment and understanding of the infant has to include the caregiving context, as the joint characteristics of parent and infant are important and interacting.

A biopsychosocial model of development, discussed below, emphasises the equal and co-existing contribution of biological, psychological and social contributing factors in the issues and concerns of parents about their infants. Using the biopsychosocial model, disturbances to early development are seen as arising from an interplay of factors in the infant, parent and their environment. Infant mental health interventions using this framework are similarly comprehensive.

The biopsychosocial model

Clinicians working with infants and their parents are often called upon to consider a range of issues from both the infant's and the parents' points of view. Many concerns that are presented in a clinical setting may be described in a linear way, as a straightforward problem such as 'He won't eat' or 'I can't get her to sleep'. There are multiple factors that may contribute to descriptions of problems such as these, and some parents may be further worried about existing physical or developmental concerns about their child.

A comprehensive account of infant development needs to look at biological, psychological and sociocultural factors and the manner in which these interact and contribute to overall developmental outcome. This is called the biopsychosocial model and is an important framework for understanding developmental problems and for approaching intervention and prevention. Many clinical interventions and preventive programs aim to identify risk factors and enhance protective factors. It also follows from this model that developmental problems are multifactorial—that is, several factors usually interact to result in a particular problem and numerous different clusters of factors may interact to result in the same clinical presentation.

The framework allows clinicians to consider a range of factors in formulating an approach to a problem that includes information from many sources, such as medical tests, observations, talking with the parents and understanding their observations. These concepts are discussed in more detail in Chapters 3 and 4.

Disturbances to early development

Developmental problems in infancy result from the complex interaction of factors in the infant, factors in the carer, factors in the infant–carer interaction and factors in the broader social environment. Risk and protective factors may be biological and/or psychosocial. They may also be acute or longstanding and vary in intensity. Understanding the clinical presentation involves an assessment of the functioning of the infant–carer system on each level and balancing risk and protective factors. (The assessment process is discussed in detail in Chapters 3 and 4.)

Early developmental problems, such as failure to attain normative milestones, or atypical development, usually reflect an interaction between intrinsic vulnerability (factors in the infant) and environmental risk (factors in the infant–caregiver relationship and social environment). Given the interdependence of neurobiological and psychosocial development, severe disturbances in infancy frequently involve impaired functioning in both domains. For example, emotional neglect can have effects on brain development and physical growth, as well as on emotional development and social functioning.

Approaches to intervention in infant mental health

Interventions in the infant period have the core aim of promoting infant development and motivating infant potential. Interventions may occur or be targeted at multiple levels of the individual, family and social system. For example the focus may be the infant individually, the infant–parent relationship, the family, the social group or community, or broad-based population approaches that support infants and families. Interventions may be preventive and aimed at reducing potential developmental problems in high-risk situations, or may be focused on infants already experiencing developmental difficulties. A comprehensive program for infant mental health involves support across the community for parenting and early childhood, preventive interventions and targeted services for high-risk infants and parents.

Interventions focused on the infant

Clearly when an infant has specific developmental or medical problems, aspects of any clinical intervention with the infant and family need to acknowledge and address these issues, while also supporting the caregivers in their interactions with the health system and helping them adapt to the particular needs of their baby. As quoted at the start of this book, the paediatrician and psychoanalyst Donald Winnicott is famously reported to have said, 'There is no such thing as a baby…if you set out to describe a baby, you will find you are describing a baby and someone. A baby cannot exist alone, but is essentially part of a relationship' (1964/1978, p. 88). His contemporaries and subsequent writers have not always agreed with him, in that there is more ready acknowledgement of the infant as an active participant in his own destiny from the first moments after birth.

Approaches to intervention based on the transactional model (Sameroff & Fiese, 2000) suggest the 'three Rs' of early intervention—remediation, redefinition and re-education. Remediation is an approach to intervention focused primarily on facilitating changes in the child with the aim of improving the infant–caregiver relationship. It can form part of an overall intervention strategy. For example, infants who have had repeated intrusive medical procedures may benefit from gentle touch and interactions that provide them with a new experience of physical contact and 'being with' another, enabling the infant to be more responsive to parental touch and interaction. This allows parents who may have become anxious, or felt incompetent in interaction with a sick or easily overstimulated baby, to see their infant behaving in a different way, and to approach him in a new way (Field et al., 1986; Als, 1992).

Abused babies and toddlers may also benefit from individual therapy as part of supporting their transition to a new caregiving environment. As children get older and develop their own inner world and more established patterns of behaviour, the argument for individual intervention increases, as individual therapy to address maladaptive behaviours may support the development of new relationships with foster or alternative caregivers. Therapeutic support at an interactional or family level may also be indicated. Whatever therapeutic interventions are provided for an infant and his caregivers, the overall focus must be developmentally informed and sensitive to the young child's need for continuity in his relationships with sensitive, responsive adults.

Interventions for the infant–parent relationship

There are a range of approaches to therapeutic intervention in the infant–parent relationship (Sameraff, McDonough & Rosenblum, 2004). Infant–parent therapies can be understood as working across both the domains of observed behaviours and interactions between infant and parent, and their existing and developing internal representation of relationships. A number of these therapies used video-taped interactions of infant and parent, then replayed and examined them to enable the parents to reflect on and gain new knowledge about themselves and their infant. Approaches to infant–parent or parent–infant therapy are discussed further in Chapter 2.

Interventions for the family

Family approaches to intervention acknowledge the interconnectedness of family members and their inevitable impact on each other. The arrival of a new infant in a family requires adjustment by everyone, including existing siblings and extended family. Critiques of dyadic approaches to infant–parent work suggest that exclusion of the father or other siblings, for example, denies the significance of the wider family context, with excessive focus on parent (usually mother) and infant alone. The nature of the presenting problem and the family structure and constellation should inform decisions about who is involved in therapeutic interventions.

Group therapies

Group work can be undertaken with infants and parents, either with a psycho-educational or a more experiential and therapeutic focus. This enables new parents to learn from each other and from other infants in the group about themselves, their own infant and approaches to parenting. New parents groups are an example of community–based groups, but group programs are also offered to higher risk groups such as families with infants with prematurity or other medical problems or parents who have suffered perinatal mental illness.

Population-based and targeted interventions

Some services and programs are offered to all new parents independent of their particular needs or risk factors. Sometimes they include a screening or identification process of families with risk factors, which may indicate they would benefit from more targeted or intensive intervention. Examples include universal home-visiting programs, sometimes staffed by trained volunteers, with extra visits or professional supports offered to families and infants at risk.

Clinicians working with infants and families need to be aware of the range of services and facilities in their area, and to advocate for the provision of trained staff with specialist expertise if an adequate range of interventions and supports is not available.

SUMMARY

Infancy is increasingly recognised as a crucial period for the development of a range of emotional and psychological capacities. Our understanding of the importance of the infant period has been influenced by research and clinical practice over a number of years. The contemporary view of infancy incorporates the following principles:
- infancy is a critical period for brain development and a range of abilities including the capacity to form intimate relationships, empathy and cognition
- infant development is complex and involves a process of mutual interaction between the infant and the environment
- biological, psychological and sociocultural factors affect infant development
- adverse developmental experiences in infancy are risk factors for developmental problems and later psychopathology
- intervention in infancy aims to prevent the emergence of infant mental health disorders
- promotion of optimal development and positive mental health in infancy involves interventions with parents, carers and infants who are identified as being at risk.

ADDITIONAL READING

Cicchetti, D., & Carlson, V. (Eds.). (1989). *Child maltreatment: Theory and research on the causes and consequences of child abuse and neglect.* Cambridge: Cambridge University Press.

Field, T. (1990). *Infancy.* Cambridge, MA: Harvard University Press.

Fonagy, P. (2003). The development of psychopathology from infancy to adulthood: The mysterious unfolding of disturbance in time. *Infant Mental Health Journal, 24*(3), 212–239.

Kowalenko, N., Barnett, B., Fowler, C., & Matthey, S. (2000). The perinatal period: Early interventions for mental health. In R. Kosky, A. O'Hanlon, G. Martin & C. Davis (Eds.), *Clinical approaches to early intervention in child and adolescent mental health* (Vol. 4). Adelaide: Australian Early Intervention Network for Mental Health in Young People.

Lewis, M., & Miller, S. (Eds.). (1990). *Handbook of developmental psychopathology.* New York: Plenum Press.

Osofsky, J. (1998). On the outside: Interventions with infants and families at risk. *Infant Mental Health Journal, 19*(2), 101–110.

Thomson-Salo, F., & Paul, C. (Eds.). (2004). *The baby as subject: New directions in infant–parent psychotherapy.* Melbourne: Stonnington Press.

Zeanah, C., Anders, T. F., Seifer, R., & Stern, D. N. (1989). Implications of research on infant development for psychodynamic theory and practice. *Journal of the American Academy of Child and Adolescent Psychiatry, 28*(5), 657–668.

CHAPTER 2

Attachment: theory, disruptions and disorders

KEY CONCEPTS

- Importance of attachment theory in infant mental health
- Secure and insecure attachment relationships
- Primary attachments and interpersonal functioning
- Implications of early attachment disruption and attachment trauma

PRINCIPLES

- Attachment quality influences infant development
- Attachment history affects parenting capacity
- Attachment theory can be applied to a range of clinical situations

In Chapter 1, the emergence of an attachment relationship as one of the core aspects of psychological and emotional development in infancy was discussed. Understanding the nature of attachment relationships provides information about how the infant–parent relationship develops, what factors influence this development, and how this relationship goes on to affect later psychological and social functioning. Assessment of the attachment status of adults, that is, their experiences during childhood and the effects on their psychological development into adulthood, also leads to an understanding of interactions between these adults and their own infants. Studies have shown a correlation between the attachment status of adults and that of their infants.

A grounding in attachment theory allows clinicians to assess presenting problems from a relationship perspective. This is not to say that all infant mental health interventions require an assessment of attachment status in the infant, but given that the emotional relationship between the infant and primary caregiver has an effect on brain development, then the fundamental process of attachment, the building block of psychological functioning, is crucial to all aspects of infant development. It is not possible to easily separate aspects of physical, emotional, behavioural and neurobiological development.

This chapter will review the history of attachment theory, classifications of attachment and the current understanding of attachment disorders—their origin in disturbed relationships, relationship to attachment disorganisation, and links to ongoing mental health and personality problems. The chapter will also provide intervention principles based on attachment theory that can be applied to a range of clinical situations and settings.

ATTACHMENT THEORY

Attachment can be defined as an enduring emotional bond characterised by a tendency to seek and maintain proximity to a specific figure(s) particularly when under stress. As we have seen in Chapter 1, parental protection acts as a provider of vital support and external emotional regulation for the young child. Caregiver sensitivity and attachment are linked to subsequent social competence in infants.

Attachment theory understands the nature of the infant's attachment to her caregivers, as a primarily biologically determined phenomenon, upon which the infant's survival depends. The infant develops internal working models of relationships from the quality and nature of early experience with caregivers, and this influences ongoing social and emotional development.

Attachment theory holds that there is an innate system that has evolved within the brain that is activated by separation and which strives to re-unite the infant with her caregiver (usually the mother).

Attachment theory has its origins in ethological studies of animal mother–infant behaviours, meticulous observational studies of human mothers and their infants, and psychoanalytic theory. It potentially bridges the gap between theories of human development and behaviour arising out of psychological research, developmental observation and clinically based theories, including psychoanalysis.

The origins of attachment theory

The key historical figure in the field of attachment theory is John Bowlby. Dr John Bowlby (1907–90) was a British child psychiatrist who trained as a psychoanalyst. The work that was to become attachment theory had its origins in Bowlby's interest in ethology (the study of the behaviour of animals in relation to their natural environments), his experience with deprived and affectionless children and a report he prepared for the World Health

Organization on the mental health of homeless children in post-war Europe (Bowlby, 1951). He was profoundly influenced by work with deprived children, and out of this developed his conviction that maladjustment follows early maternal deprivation and loss.

Bowlby was considerably aided by his working relationship with two other researchers. In the late 1940s he hired James Robertson, a social worker, to assist in observation of hospitalised children, and Mary Ainsworth, who conducted the first empirical study of attachment on a group of mothers and babies in Uganda in the mid-1950s.

It is likely that Bowlby reacted strongly against what he perceived to be too strong a psychoanalytic emphasis on the inner world of the infant and a neglect of the realities of the external world. Regrettably, this was in turn reacted to by psychoanalysts of that time, with an equal and opposite criticism of Bowlby's alleged neglect of the infant's inner world.

The result was an unfortunate schism between a talented researcher and theorist and the psychoanalytic orthodoxy of the time. This is being repaired by the significant work of Peter Fonagy (2001), Mary Target (Fonagy & Target, 2000), Jeremy Holmes (2001) and others.

The Strange Situation Procedure

The next major impetus to the development of attachment theory was the design and implementation, by Ainsworth, Blehar, Waters and Wall (1978), of the Strange Situation Procedure (SSP): an observation of the phenomena that occur when infants are separated and then re-united with their caregivers.

By careful observation of video-tape of the infants' behaviours on separation and reunion with their primary carer, a number of 'styles' of reunion behaviour were categorised, which have become the basis of a highly fruitful body of infant development research over the past 25 years.

Initially, three categories of attachment were identified by Ainsworth: the secure, the avoidant and the ambivalent. Subsequently, a group of difficult-to-classify behaviours was recognised as representing a further style, now called disorganised/disoriented.

The securely attached child has experienced predictable and consistent emotional availability of the attachment figure, while the insecurely attached child is anxious about the availability of the 'other' and attempts to deal with this in various ways. The disorganised infant is understood to have been faced with an insoluble conflict, that is, the source of comfort and protection, the caregiver, is also the source of distress and fear. Disorganised attachment is most often seen in infants exposed to abuse or neglect, or to caregivers preoccupied with their own trauma or loss. This is discussed further below.

PATTERNS OF ATTACHMENT

The attachment patterns identified at 12 to 18 months of age in the Strange Situation Procedure are:

B: Secure—the infant knows how to signal her needs and the parent is able and happy to meet her in a relatively consistent way. The secure pattern is characterised by a balance between attachment and exploration, and by openness in emotional expression.

A: Insecure/Avoidant—the parent rewards independence and exploration and is relatively intolerant of the infant's dependency needs, and the apparently independent infant learns to focus more on 'doing' than on 'being with' and minimises expression of emotional cues. This pattern is characterised by a dominance of exploration over attachment and by hiding feelings.

C: Insecure/Ambivalent—the parent is inconsistent, and a fussy, dissatisfied infant maximises expression of emotional cues. This pattern is characterised by a dominance of attachment behaviours over exploration and by heightening or exaggerating emotional expression.

D: Disorganised—The frightened or frightening parent who is the source of distress as well as comfort for the infant results in contradictory infant behaviours. This pattern is characterised by mixed and disorganised attachment behaviours, including showing signs of fear of the parent, withdrawal, or a mixture of avoidant and ambivalent behaviours.

In community samples (there is some minor cultural variation), infant attachment classifications show the following approximate distribution:

- Secure—55–65 per cent
- Insecure/Avoidant—20–30 per cent
- Insecure/Ambivalent—5–15 per cent
- Disorganised—10–18 per cent.

The avoidant and ambivalent patterns are part of the normal population distribution and represent the infant's adaptation and response to the parent's caregiving style. They are not pathological patterns. Nevertheless, longitudinal studies show that attachment security conveys a selective advantage in the development of:

- social intelligence
- regulation of emotions and regulation of stress
- self-reflective functioning.

It is important to note that there was not an intention to 'pathologise' any of these attachment categories. However, further research suggests that infants showing 'disorganised' behaviour on the SSP are over-represented in high-risk populations, including infants exposed to neglect and abuse. They are also at high risk of later psychopathology (Lyons-Ruth & Jacobovitz, 1999). The characteristics of each attachment pattern are described in Table 2.1.

Table 2.1 **Patterns of attachment**

Pattern	Characteristics
Secure (B)	Uses the attachment figures as a secure base from which to explore. The infant is distressed by separation but is able to be comforted by the parent and returns to exploratory play. A balance between attachment and exploration, independence.
Insecure/Avoidant (A)	On reunion with the parent, the infant avoids close contact but observes the parent. Associated with some rejection or ignoring by the parent. Independence is rewarded.
Insecure/Ambivalent (C)	On reunion the infant clings to the parent while protesting. Unable to return to exploratory play. Associated with caregivers who are inconsistent or intrusive. An emphasis on seeking proximity.
Disorganised (D)	This is an additional classification given to infants who show fearful, confused or mixed behaviours on reunion. It is associated with trauma, parental bereavement and disturbed parenting.

The Adult Attachment Interview

More recently, Mary Main and co-workers have developed the Adult Attachment Interview (AAI) protocol, a semi-structured interview that includes a series of increasingly targeted questions and prompts designed to elicit memories and representations of early attachment relationships (George, Kaplan & Main, 1996).

This standardised interview undertaken with adults is transcribed and rated, not only on the *content* of what is said, but *how* the adult talks about their early experiences. Interviews are classified as:

- Secure/autonomous or free (F)
- Dismissing (D)
- Preoccupied or enmeshed (E) or
- Unresolved/disorganised (U).

These categories correspond to the infant classifications. (See Adult Attachment Interview classifications and corresponding patterns of infant Strange Situation behaviour in Holmes [2001] and Hesse [1999].)

The significance of the AAI for infant mental health is that it is possible to predict with approximately 70 per cent accuracy from AAIs performed on expectant parents what the attachment classifications of their infants will be 12 months later (van IJzendoorn, 1995).

For more information on the AAI, read Hesse (1999).

SELF-REFLECTIVE CAPACITY

The capacity to talk cogently and coherently about one's self and one's difficulties (called the 'reflexive function' on the AAI) is linked with security of attachment. Fonagy and Target (1997) emphasise the importance of 'Reflective

Self Function' and the parents' capacity to 'mentalise' their inner world and the inner world of their infant. They demonstrate this as central to the child's developing 'theory of mind', security of attachment and sense of self. This function is absent or limited in people with personality disorder, particularly of the borderline classification.

Attachment theory—hypotheses

Holmes (2001, p. 6) lists several hypotheses arising from attachment theory. To paraphrase here:

- Universality hypothesis: In all known cultures, human infants become attached to one or more specific caregivers.
- Normality hypothesis: About 70 per cent of infants become securely attached. Secure attachment is numerically and physiologically normal.
- Sensitivity hypothesis: Attachment security is dependent on sensitive and responsive caregiving.
- Competence hypothesis: Social and emotional competence is predicted by attachment security.
- Continuity hypothesis: Attachment patterns in childhood persist and have an impact over the lifespan.
- Mentalisation hypothesis: Secure attachment is based on and leads to capacity for reflection on states of mind of self and other (Fonagy & Target, 1997).
- Narrative competence hypothesis: Secure attachment in childhood is reflected in adult life by the ways in which people talk about their lives (as reflected in the Adult Attachment Interview, Main & Goldwyn, 1994).

Attachment theory then, developed initially by John Bowlby from the integration of information from a range of previously separate and diverse areas of knowledge, remains an integrative body of theory and practice that enables links to be made between outer behaviour and inner representations of relationships and between the experiences of one generation and the care they will provide to the next, that is, the transgenerational aspects of parenting. It provides an explanatory link between observed parenting behaviour, the quality of parent and infant relationships and the later functioning of the child socially and emotionally. Most importantly, attachment theorists have developed established scientific methods to elicit and evaluate aspects of the inner representational world of the infant, child and adult.

Initially, Bowlby's work was taken up by researchers on child development and not by clinicians. Recently, this has changed, with the increasing application of the understanding and knowledge that comes from attachment theory and research being applied to therapeutic interventions with parents and infants, and also informing a range of other therapies with adults, children and families. This is discussed further below.

DEFINING DISORDERS OF ATTACHMENT

It has long been recognised that infants and children exposed to disturbed and traumatising early care may have long-term difficulties in emotional interaction and relationships. Only recently, however, have there been attempts to describe the mechanisms involved in some of the observed longer term difficulties, or to describe and classify types of attachment disorders. One of the ongoing discussions in the theoretical literature relates to the nature of these proposed disorders and at what point an infant or child can be said to have an individual disorder that lies within, particularly when the origins of the problem can be identified in the attachment relationship itself. Also, it is unclear how attachment disorders relate to the classification of insecure attachment, given that insecure attachment occurs in 'normal' populations and is not seen as a disorder, nor does it usually result in an attachment disorder. Recent work on the developmental implications of early disorganised attachment may help clarify this question, as it suggests that attachment disorganisation rather than attachment insecurity can disrupt relationship and personality development, and is related to psychological disorder in later life.

Early studies of attachment difficulties resulting from traumatic early care included the descriptions of indiscriminate sociability in institutionalised children during the Second World War (such as the studies of Burlington & Freud, 1944). Bowlby (1944) was also interested in the effects of early deprivation of care and described a form of emotional detachment and avoidance of interaction in children who had experienced separation from attachment figures. These two varieties of attachment abnormality are sometimes described as disinhibited and inhibited patterns and this is reflected in the current DSM classification system, which first included attachment disorder in the 1980 DSM-III (American Psychiatric Association [APA], 1980).

Organised and disorganised attachment patterns

As discussed previously, attachment theory describes three types of 'organised' attachment and a pattern of disorganised or disoriented attachment. Organised attachment refers to strategies the child develops in response to the relationship with her caregiver. These are classified as secure, insecure/ambivalent or insecure/avoidant. Disorganised attachment refers to the child who fails to develop coherent or effective strategies to deal with attachment anxiety, usually where the caregiver is simultaneously the source of comfort as well as distress or anxiety. A modified approach to the classification of attachment patterns, in particular the disorganised pattern of preschoolers, older children and adults, has been developed by Crittenden (1992).

Insecure attachment

Recall from earlier in this chapter that securely attached infants ('B' pattern) experience the carer as consistent, available and sensitive and that they are able to use the carer as a secure base from which to explore the environment. Insecurely attached infants may have experienced insensitive and/or inconsistent care and remain anxious about the availability of their attachment figure. Some insecure infants will show heightened attachment behaviours such as clinging and separation distress and are described as 'ambivalent or resistant' ('C' pattern) in attachment classifications. Others may appear distant or unemotional with the carer as a way of managing anxiety and are classified as 'avoidant' ('A' pattern). These are styles or strategies for managing anxiety about the parent and are not 'disorders' but refer to potential personality vulnerabilities as they become incorporated into the child's characteristic interpersonal style.

Disorganised/disoriented attachment

Infants who have experienced maltreatment or abuse at the hands of an attachment figure or whose parent is preoccupied with loss or trauma, will show signs of disturbed attachment behaviour and chronic stress. These infants may be classified as 'disorganised' ('D' pattern) in their attachment behaviours, as they do not develop an effective strategy for coping with a dangerous and unpredictable attachment figure. The disorganised pattern is the only one directly linked to the development of emotional and behavioural disturbance and externalising disorders in early childhood. This pattern occurs when the child is faced with the insoluble dilemma that the one she must turn to for comfort is also the source of her distress. Disorganised attachment behaviours may be confused and contradictory, and strategies may at times resemble other attachment patterns.

Attachment disorders

Attachment disorders are seen as generalised difficulties in relationships that may emerge from disturbed interactional patterns in the child's primary caretaking experiences. In other words, the patterns observed reflect the infant's current issues with attachment relationships and the way in which past relationship experiences have influenced current relationship models. Attachment disorders are not directly related to the attachment categories identified by the Strange Situation Procedure; however, many infants diagnosed with an attachment disorder will also have a disorganised pattern of attachment.

Assessment of attachment disorders is made on both observation of relationship behaviour and a comprehensive history of the child's previous

ATTACHMENT: THEORY, DISRUPTIONS AND DISORDERS

relationship experiences. Looked on in isolation, the attachment difficulties may be difficult to understand. For example, an attachment disorder begins in disturbance of the infant's relationship with her primary carer or attachment figure and then, if persistent, will generalise and affect other relationships, such as those with peers or other adults.

Attachment disorders develop when there is a persistent disturbance in the relationship between the child and her attachment figure. If ongoing, this will then influence the child's perceptions and behaviour outside of the primary relationship and become incorporated as part of the developing child's style of attachment or personality.

Serious early adverse experiences such as abuse and neglect are associated with long-term difficulties in relationships and attachment behaviour. These children may show a variety of disturbed attachment behaviour but all experience insecurity and anxiety in close relationships and difficulties in trust.

Children who have been institutionalised pose specific challenges for foster-carers and may be provocative and 'test' the commitment of carers.

Attachment disorders are clearly detrimental to interpersonal functioning and are associated with ongoing difficulties in development and relationships.

Classification of attachment disorders is complex, as these conditions are essentially referring to a relationship construct as opposed to any 'disorder' of an individual. The issue raises several questions:

- What is the distinction between normal and abnormal attachment?
- Are attachment disorders psychological and behavioural disorders in their own right?
- When does an infant's attachment disturbance constitute a clinical disorder as opposed to a risk factor for later disorder?

These questions are being discussed in an ongoing way in the theoretical and empirical literature. The current classification systems, ICD-10 and DSM-IV, offer limited descriptions of attachment disorders.

REACTIVE ATTACHMENT DISORDER (DSM-IV)

Reactive Attachment Disorder (RAD) was first introduced in 1980 in DSM-III (APA, 1980) and modified in DSM-IIIR (APA, 1987) and DSM-IV (APA, 1994). DSM describes pathogenic care by primary carer as the underlying cause of the disorder and described two subtypes, 'inhibited' and 'disinhibited'.

RAD is characterised by disturbed social relatedness in most contexts. The inhibited pattern is characterised by inhibition of normal attachment seeking. Children appear withdrawn or 'unattached'. This pattern has been observed in neglected children. The indiscriminate pattern is characterised by diffuse and unselective attachments. Children may show 'indiscriminate sociability' and over-friendliness. This has been observed in children in foster-care who have experienced multiple placements.

ALTERNATIVE CRITERIA

Zeanah and colleagues are developing and refining descriptions of a wide variety of attachment disorders (Lieberman & Zeanah, 1995; Zeanah, 1996; Zeanah & Boris, 2000). They distinguish between a group of disorders in which there is no preferred attachment figure and a group characterised by disturbed attachment to a preferred figure (Zeanah, Boris, Bakshi & Lieberman, 2000).

Disorders of non-attachment

In these disorders the infant has not developed a clear preference for a specific attachment figure. This may occur in situations where infants have been seriously neglected or had multiple changes or carers. Two types of non-attachment are described:

1. With emotional withdrawal—In this situation the infant is emotionally withdrawn and unreactive and avoids social interaction or comfort-seeking.
2. With indiscriminate sociability—These infants seek interaction and comfort from available adults, including strangers, and show no preference for any particular figure. They may protest when separated from a stranger and be inappropriately close and show comfort-seeking behaviours. These behaviours have been observed in groups of institutionalised children (Hodges & Tizard, 1989).

Secure base distortions

In this group of disorders children have developed a clear preference for a particular attachment figure but the quality of the relationship is disturbed. Four types are described by Zeanah et al. (2000):

1. Attachment disorder (AD) with self-endangerment—In this condition the infant prioritises exploration and does not check with the attachment figure or maintain normal proximity. Behaviour can be reckless or dangerous and include running away from the carer repeatedly.
2. Clinging/Inhibited exploration—In this condition the infant inhibits normal exploratory behaviour and is clingy with the attachment figure, evidencing insecurity.
3. AD with vigilance/hypercompliance—Infants are highly attuned to the requests and needs of the attachment figure and are fearful of displeasing them. This may result from the caregiver being angry or hostile towards the child and in cases of abuse.
4. AD with role reversal—In this situation the infant takes emotional responsibility for the caregiver to a developmentally inappropriate degree, with adverse effects on her overall development. This may develop when the parent is isolated, depressed or in other ways dependent on the child for comfort and intimacy.

Disrupted attachment disorder

An additional group known as 'disrupted attachment disorder' refers to cases in which the child experiences the sudden loss of an attachment figure such as following death or acute separation. The child may show features of mourning, anger and rage, and be clingy towards the alternative caregiver.

CLINICAL APPLICATIONS OF ATTACHMENT THEORY

Attachment theory can be applied to a range of clinical situations as a way of understanding and formulating the presenting concerns. Specific types of infant–parent intervention have been developed as the body of knowledge has grown. Principles of intervention for attachment disorders are discussed below.

Application to infant–parent interventions

Attachment theory grew and developed out of ideas and observations arising from both the internal world (psychoanalytic theory) and what can be observed and measured (developmental psychology, ethology). Similarly, infant–parent therapies can be understood as working across both the domains of observed behaviours and interactions between infant and parent, and their existing and developing 'internal representation of relationships'.

Fraiberg, Adelson and Shapiro's (1975) seminal paper 'Ghosts in the Nursery' outlined an approach to disturbances in early relationships based on the assumption that such difficulties are manifestations in the present of unresolved parental conflicts, usually with their caregivers. To protect herself from experiencing or re-experiencing distress or trauma, the caregiver restricts her attention and reflection both on her own inner state and on that of her infant. This leads to restrictions in responsiveness to the infant, which Fraiberg (1980) proposed were amenable to interventions focused on what was observed between, but going on inside, both members of the dyad.

Attachment-based, infant–parent therapy has been significantly developed and researched by Alicia Lieberman and her colleagues (Lieberman & Zeanah, 1999).

Another significant approach to work with the infant–parent dyad, and informed by both psychoanalytic ideas and attachment theory, is the 'Watch, Wait and Wonder' program. This intervention emphasises the infant as an active participant in the interaction, current difficulties and the process of change, moving away from Fraiberg's original notion of the infant as a stimulus or catalyst for psychological change in the parent.

The therapy 'allows the infant his own therapeutic space through enabling him, in the presence of his mother, to play and/or act out his own concerns' (Muir, Lojkasek & Cohen, 1999, p. 16). The parent is asked to sit with and 'follow' the infant's lead in interaction and play. This is a way of instructing the parent in aspects of providing a secure, responsive base for the child. The structure of the therapy sessions provides time for the parent and therapist to reflect on what has happened during the session and potentially to make links between the behaviour of the infant with the parent, the parents' responses and their own inner world of feelings and memories (Muir et al., 1999).

Daniel Stern (1985, 1995) has elaborated a theory of self-development based on data from infant research rather than clinical observation. His work includes the notion of 'internal working models' of relationships and schemata to describe 'ways of being with' that begin and are encoded in our earliest relationships. This overlaps with and expands ideas emerging from attachment theory and research.

In his book *The motherhood constellation: A unified view of parent–infant psychotherapy*, Stern (1995) articulates a range of approaches to infant–parent intervention, variously focusing primarily on behaviour (McDonough's Interaction Guidance) or on internal working models of relationships (Parent Infant Psychotherapy). He concludes that at this highly fluid life stage (infancy and early parenthood), interventions with a focus on either observed behaviour between infant and parent or internal representations and the parental past will be effective in changing experience and behaviour. He also summarises commonalities in approaches to parent–infant work.

Further examination of a range of approaches to parent–infant relationship problems, all informed to some extent by attachment theory, is provided in Sameroff, McDonough and Rosenblum (2004).

Application to attachment disorders

Where an attachment disorder is evident, specialist intervention is required from an experienced clinician. There is relatively scant evidence on effective treatment for established attachment disorders. Issues of intervention are frequently raised in situations where children with adverse early attachment experiences are placed with alternative carers and continue to have difficulties with basic trust and intimacy. Carers often describe these children as avoidant, provocative and sometimes behaving in ways that undermine the relationship. Some children and adolescents with histories of severe abuse and attachment disruption have been seen as unable to tolerate close relationships and to be 'unplaceable' within alternate family settings. These children may respond well to more structured and less emotionally intensive care as in group or residential facilities. In all situations of persistent attachment disturbance the issue of parenting capacity and risk to the child must be considered (see Chapter 4).

Assessment and formulation principles

General principles of assessment include:
1. History of the child's attachments—It is important to focus on a chronological account of the significant attachment figures available to the child since birth and particularly any disruptions in care, abandonment or losses, alternative carers, neglect of care or abuse. Availability of the current primary carer and contact with other carers should be noted, as well as the child's behaviour with each and responses to changes of carer. In older children relationships with peers and siblings should be described.
2. History and details of the infant and child's current emotional and behavioural problems.

    Of particular interest in relation to attachment disruptions or disorder are:
    - help or comfort-seeking behaviour
    - response to pain or distress
    - ability to use caregiver or another adult for comfort
    - response to limit-setting
    - responses to physical proximity.
3. Assessment of attachment behaviours, including:
    - observations of attachment-related behaviours
    - quality of interaction with interviewer
    - interaction with current caregiver
    - ability to organise self in a new setting
    - ability to play and explore.

Intervention principles

The central principles of intervention for children with attachment disorders are based on the need to allow these children to develop an alternative, more secure, attachment relationship to their current carer, a clinician or therapeutic setting. Any attempt to do this should only proceed if the child's current safety is assured and if there has been a thorough assessment of the child's psychological and emotional capacity to form relationships, cognitive development and overall level of ongoing disturbance related to early trauma. Extremely traumatised children with ongoing symptoms of Post-Traumatic Stress Disorder may need specific interventions for anxiety prior to looking at longer term interpersonal issues. Interventions all focus on improving the child's understanding of interpersonal interaction—improving emotional regulation and building the ability to use a safe person as a secure base. Children who have experienced abuse will have fundamental difficulties in socio-emotional processing, basic trust and maintenance of reciprocal relationships.

A decision based on clinical assessment needs to be made about whether individual work with the child or relationship-based work with the current carers or both is best indicated.

Early intervention in the infant period may be particularly important in the prevention of ongoing interpersonal difficulties. This type of intervention with high-risk carers and infants aims to improve the carer's capacity to provide a consistent attachment experience and sensitive care. Many carers in this group will have had early experiences of abandonment and neglect themselves and will find the emotional tasks of parenting particularly difficult. Interactions should involve the carer and child together and focus on the quality of the relationship, maximising positive interaction and giving the child an experience of being with an adult who is safe and consistently available.

PSYCHOLOGICAL INTERVENTIONS

Various psychological interventions have been used, ranging from individual psychodynamic approaches to group therapies to behavioural programs. The choice of intervention should be based on the capacity and needs of the individual child, the child's family/care situation and the developmental age of the child.

PSYCHOLOGICAL THEMES OF TREATMENT

Many children with histories of trauma and attachment disruption have been in a series of disturbed caretaking relationships and have adapted to or accommodated to this in a psychological sense as a matter of survival.

Several key psychological themes can emerge for these children and will need to be addressed during a course of treatment.

Common issues include:
- self-blame
- powerlessness—ongoing vulnerability, anxiety, victimisation
- loss and betrayal—avoidance, lack of trust
- stigmatisation—feelings of shame, guilt
- the need to mourn and rebuild relationships.

SUMMARY

Since Bowlby's initial attempts to integrate observations of the impact of early deprivation with psychoanalytic ideas and ethological research, attachment theory has been enthusiastically embraced and developed, particularly by developmental psychologists and infant researchers. The last decade has seen developing rapprochement between psychoanalytic theory and attachment theory and research, and the increasing application of attachment theory to psychotherapeutic and psychiatric work in a range of settings. An understanding of attachment theory can assist clinicians in a wide range of settings as the crucial infant–parent relationship can influence the nature of the presenting problem and the effectiveness of interventions.

Attachment disorders should be considered in children with histories that involve neglect, abuse, instability of the primary caregiver or loss of a caregiver through death or separation. Specialist psychological approaches to children with attachment disorders must be based on an understanding of the particular psychological themes for the child given her previous experiences.

Interventions may be long term and require consistent responsiveness and respect for the child's anxiety.

ADDITIONAL READING

Adshead, G. (1998). Psychiatric staff as attachment figures: Understanding management problems in psychiatric services in light of attachment theory. *British Journal of Psychiatry, 172*(1), 64–69.

Brisch, K. H. (1999). *Treating attachment disorders: From theory to therapy.* New York: Guilford Press.

Fonagy, P. (1998). An attachment theory approach to treatment of the difficult patient. *Bulletin of the Menninger Clinic, 62*(2), 147–169.

CHAPTER 3

Principles of assessment in infant mental health

KEY CONCEPTS

- Development occurs in the context of relationships
- Biopsychosocial approach
- Developmental perspective

PRINCIPLES

Comprehensive assessment includes:
- Consideration of infant, family and contextual factors
- The interaction or 'fit' between the needs and abilities of each family member
- The assumption that parents want the best for their children

This chapter outlines a framework for assessing infants and their families and understanding or 'formulating' their difficulties. No matter what the presenting problem, a comprehensive assessment always includes consideration of factors in the infant, parents and social and cultural context that contribute to vulnerability and resilience. These factors are used to inform and focus interventions. Assessment of risk is an aspect of all infant mental health assessments. This is explored in Chapter 4, including notions of developmental risk in infancy, and assessment of parenting capacity.

As outlined in Chapter 1, the developmental significance of infancy and the capacities and vulnerabilities of infants and young children are increasingly recognised and understood. Health professionals encounter families with infants and young children in a broad variety of settings and circumstances. Consideration of mental health, social or emotional issues should be a necessary part of all health and welfare assessments. The extent to which mental health is the focus will be determined by the setting and the purpose of contact with the family.

PRINCIPLES OF ASSESSMENT IN INFANT MENTAL HEALTH

This chapter will provide a framework that can be adapted to a range of clinical settings. The aim is to enhance the interest and ability of health professionals to consider mental health and developmental issues in all their dealings with families who present during this exciting period of rapid developmental change.

THE CONTEXT OF ASSESSMENT

Infants are born ready to relate and not just to anyone but to specific caregiving individuals. Infants organise their development in the context of these relationships. They bring their individuality to this, and so does each parent or caregiver. Because the human baby is born extremely vulnerable and remains dependent for longer than the young of any other species, the parent or caregiver's role is intense and prolonged. The parents have a crucial role in facilitating and supporting the infant's development throughout the early years, and their capacity to do this affects the strengths and vulnerabilities that the infant will carry for his lifetime. The family (infant, caregivers and siblings) also exists within a network of relationships. This network includes the social and physical circumstances that either enhance and support the family's quality of life and relationships, or undermine them.

Principles of assessment

There are a number of core principles and issues that need consideration in any assessment of a family with an infant or young child, independent of the setting within which the assessment occurs or the background of the clinician. These principles are drawn from clinical experience, and are informed by research and theoretical understandings of infancy, early childhood and family processes. An approach informed by these core principles enables the clinician to develop an understanding of the presenting problem, how and why it has developed and where intervention and assistance are best targeted.

Principles

1 ASSESSMENT OF RISK

Assessment of the immediate and longer term safety or risks to the infant and other family members is a necessary and inevitable aspect of all assessments. This focus may or may not be clear to the family, but is an unavoidable and core component of the clinician's responsibilities and obligations.

2   PARENTS WANT THE BEST FOR THEIR CHILDREN

Parents want the best for their children and family. The clinician's role is to assist them in providing this.

3   BIOPSYCHOSOCIAL FRAMEWORK

A biopsychosocial approach ensures a focus on the physical, psychological or interpersonal, and social and cultural factors that contribute to the presentation of the family and infant at this time.

4   DEVELOPMENTAL CONTEXT

The perinatal and early childhood period is a time of enormous transition and growth for infant and family, and difficulties need to be understood in a 'developmental' context. Problems presenting in infancy can have lifelong consequences, but, equally, some presentations represent difficulties in negotiating normal developmental transitions.

5   A RELATIONAL APPROACH

A relational approach is essential. Infant development can only be understood within the caregiving context. Although individual factors in the infant or parent may contribute to current difficulties, it is the interaction or 'fit' between the needs and abilities of each family member, and the sources of stress and support in the family context, that determine outcome.

6   VULNERABILITIES AND STRENGTHS

Identifying vulnerabilities and strengths helps shape and target interventions. These are also called risk and protective factors.

7   THE TRANSACTIONAL MODEL OF DEVELOPMENT

The transactional model of development (Sameroff & Fiese, 1990) emphasises the interaction between genetic and environmental factors over time and 'the development of the child is seen as a product of the continuous dynamic interactions of the child and the experience provided by his or her family and social context' (Sameroff & Fiese, 2000, p. 10).

THE PROCESS OF ASSESSMENT

Assessment of infants and their families is undertaken in a number of ways, and occurs in a wide range of settings and circumstances. Visiting a family at home provides very different information from that obtained in an outpatient setting. Where a family is seen depends on the clinician's professional role and practice and the aims of the assessment process.

For example, a family may present only once to their local emergency department late at night when the parents come in concerned their baby is unwell and won't sleep. If seen at home, the practical and financial difficulties (for example, a one-room house and noisy neighbours) that affect their ability to focus on and settle their baby might become more evident, but this would alter the focus of the assessment and require a very different use of the clinician's time. There are no right or wrong ways to undertake assessments but every clinician needs to think about the benefits and limitations of the approach they take, and the information obtained as a result.

Assessment may occur in a mental health setting, over two or three sessions, because there is concern about parental depression; or a family may be seen regularly in an early childhood clinic or centre, allowing observations over time as their relationships develop and the infant grows.

Concerns about abuse or neglect require evaluation and inevitably involve the clinician in the difficult task of establishing rapport and cooperation with parents who feel threatened, afraid or criticised. A developmental assessment or follow-up of a family with an infant with medical or developmental problems may have a more directly medical or biological focus but nonetheless needs to include consideration of the family and social context.

In summary, the approach to assessment of infants and their families will vary depending on the clinician's role, the purpose of the assessment, the setting and the professional relationship with the family. All assessments are greatly enhanced when a biopsychosocial approach is taken, to enable the integration of information from a range of sources. Infant physical and mental health are not separable, just as infant well-being and safety cannot be considered outside the context of primary caregiving relationships and the family context. The focus of an assessment will vary but the clinician's obligation is to keep in mind the bigger picture in order to work with the family and other professionals to optimally facilitate infant development and potential, and the quality of family life and relationships.

EXAMPLE: SALLY AND HARRY

At a routine post-natal check up at the Early Childhood Centre, Sally mentioned that her baby Harry wasn't sleeping as much as she had expected during the day and was crying a lot. Harry had gained little weight since discharge from hospital where he had a three-week admission after a difficult caesarean birth. He was fussy and irritable during the examination, but also had slightly floppy motor tone. Sally looked tired and anxious.

In this situation the clinician needs to make a number of decisions about what to do next. Will reassurance and information about feeding and settling be enough? Does Harry need to be seen soon by his paediatrician? Has Sally become depressed or physically unwell post-partum? What supports are available to the family? Is there any immediate risk to the safety of family members? Does the service undertake research or routinely use standardised assessments and scales? The assessment process will vary depending on information obtained at each stage of the initial interview, and the clinician's experience and judgement inform this decision-making process.

Aims of the clinical assessment

The essential aim of the assessment process, whatever the context or setting, is to identify and understand the problems facing the family, their strengths and vulnerabilities, in order to assist them in maximising their parenting capacity and the developmental potential of their infant (parenting capacity is discussed in Chapter 4). Information obtained during assessment may also be used for other activities, such as research into clinical or social conditions that affect parenting and infant development.

A thorough assessment is necessary:
- for accurate diagnosis and/or formulation (discussed later in this chapter)
- to help the family maximise their infant's developmental potential
- for appropriate, targeted intervention and management planning
- to collect data for research and statistical purposes.

Sources of information

During the assessment process a range of information is obtained from a number of sources, again determined in part by the clinical setting and purpose of the assessment.

Direct sources of information include:
- clinical history provided by the referring agent and the family
- observations of family members and their interactions
- tests and investigations
- other sources (for example, the referring agency or other services involved with the family).

Other information that informs and is incorporated into the assessment and formulation may include:
- written documentation of past history and interventions
- emotional or 'affective' information—including the clinician's responses to and feelings about the family and their presentation
- information (knowledge, skills and attitudes) drawn from the clinician's professional experience.

Formulation

At the end of any assessment the aim is to have an understanding of why *this* family is presenting with *this* problem at *this* time, and what the impediments or obstacles are that have prevented them from resolving their difficulties without professional help. This information forms the basis of making what is called a 'formulation'. Formulation is an integrative statement that provides an aetiological understanding of factors contributing to the presentation. It can take different forms, but ideally includes consideration of biopsychosocial factors. This multilevel summary informs the development of a comprehensive intervention plan.

Formulation differs from diagnosis in that it enables identification and integration of a broad range of factors across several domains that interact and contribute to the presenting problems. This allows the clinician to shape interventions appropriately. Another way of thinking about this is to identify, or organise the information obtained in an assessment into what can be called 'the 4 Ps'.

These can be identified as factors that are:
- **Predisposing**—what made this family vulnerable?
- **Precipitating**—why have they come now?
- **Perpetuating**—what makes it hard for things to get better?
- **Protective**—what strengths and resilience can we identify and build on in our intervention in the infant, the family, and the social and cultural context?

Ideally, during the process of assessment, the family and clinician come over time to a new, shared understanding—a story—about the meaning and nature of the presenting difficulties, and also the way forward.

EXAMPLE: SALLY AND HARRY, CONTINUED

> *Returning to Sally and Harry: You obtain a history that Sally had a long period of infertility before Harry was born. She also miscarried during the second trimester of a previous pregnancy. Harry's birth was difficult and occurred three weeks premature. Because he had breathing difficulties he required a period in hospital before he was discharged home to Sally and her partner Michael's care. Sally's mother had died in the preceding year. Michael had recently been promoted to a job that required them to move from interstate. He was currently required to travel overnight at least once a week. When Harry was observed during a breastfeed he was seen to latch on poorly and to be fussy and unsettled. Sally was unsure how to help him and rapidly became upset.*

A diagnosis of depression or unresolved grief might be appropriate for Sally, and Harry may have physiological problems contributing to his 'poor suck'. A formulation could integrate this information. Thus, Sally is a woman with a past history of infertility and obstetric loss, recently bereaved, who gave birth to Harry three weeks prematurely. While Harry has no evident serious medical or developmental problems, his poor motor tone is contributing to feeding problems and low weight gain. This perpetuates Sally's sense of incompetence and fuels her anxiety and depression, making it harder for her to settle and respond to Harry's irritability. The family is new to the city and Michael is away a lot, perhaps responding to the situation by focusing on his role as breadwinner. The result is an isolated parent with unresolved losses having trouble meeting the needs of her new baby.

Thinking about this example in terms of the 4 Ps mentioned above:

Although they present for a routine check up, the *precipitant* for a more thorough assessment is Harry's poor weight gain. *Predisposing* factors include his early birth and low motor tone and his mother's unresolved grief. *Perpetuating* factors include social isolation, Michael's absence and preoccupation with work, and Sally's high expectations of herself, making it hard for her to seek help or to let Michael know how hard she is finding things. Her isolation maintains her depression and sense of inadequacy.

This formulation does not yet include consideration of strengths or *protective* factors for this family. Developing an intervention and anticipating prognosis requires the clinician to think about and identify protective factors and resources that can be built on.

In this case, Sally and Michael are committed to each other and their baby and their marital stresses are temporary. They are financially secure, educated people who are able to use the information you provide. Sally has a good relationship with her general practitioner and there are local resources, including a lactation service that helps her to get Harry's feeding on track. She also connects with local resources that reduce her isolation. As part of this, she attends a support group for women with previous perinatal loss as well as a new mother's group that brings her into contact with other new parents in the local area. Michael is able to renegotiate his work schedule and in the process develops a better relationship with his new boss.

This may seem like a 'too good to be true' story—an able and willing family in an area with adequate resources. The aim is to show that formulation gives a broader and more comprehensive picture of the family's difficulties and the possible targets of any intervention, even if not everything can be addressed or resolved. Whatever the role of the clinician in this scenario, she has considered multiple aspects of the family's functioning, identified a range of interacting difficulties as well as other services, agencies and resources to involve. Formulation is more than diagnosis and enables interventions to be appropriately targeted. In families with complex multiproblem circumstances and presentations, a comprehensive assessment and formulation allows the family and clinician to identify and prioritise problems and difficulties and to develop realistic interventions and treatment goals.

EFFECTIVE CLINICAL ASSESSMENT

In clinical work with infants and their parents or caregivers, the assessment process is central to an overall understanding of the presenting problem and to formulation and intervention. The interview takes on a significant meaning for caregivers in this context as they reveal concerns, fears and sometimes disturbing thoughts that they have about themselves or their infants. Enabling parents and caregivers to explore the complex emotions related to parenting and identify obstacles that may impede their best parenting efforts requires clinicians to acknowledge the difficulties of exposing inner feelings related to parenting. Effective assessment enables observation of more than what is spoken, through an understanding of the rich and essential information conveyed in interactions between infants and their caregivers, in the context of the assessment process.

EXAMPLE: ANN AND JAY

> *A paediatric physiotherapist undertaking a developmental assessment of Jay, a nine-month-old boy who is slow in developing motor skills, noticed the negative way his young mother, Ann, spoke about her son, her sense of frustration that he was so dependent on her, and her boredom and isolation. This enabled the clinician to ask in a sensitive way about Ann's supports. The clinician found that Ann had very little information about normal infant development and was spending most days walking with Jay in the stroller around the local shopping centre, resulting in few opportunities for essential floor time and play. Appropriate referrals and suggestions were then included along with a program of exercises for Jay, which the clinician realised were unlikely to succeed if the social and psychological issues weren't taken into account.*

A comprehensive approach to assessment includes:
1. the clinical assessment interview
2. assessment of parent–infant interaction
3. infant developmental assessment.

The clinical assessment interview

Whether a family is seen only once or the initial meeting is the first in a series of ongoing contacts, the process of developing a 'therapeutic alliance' runs parallel to and determines success in eliciting the 'facts' of the history. Just as parenting is primarily about significant relationships, so contact with distressed families needs to be understood as a professional relationship within which the family can feel heard and understood, and therefore better able to care for their baby. Even when assessing concerns about child abuse or neglect, or providing a medico-legal report, it is important to be aware of the crucial importance of the therapeutic alliance while also being clear and direct about the purpose of the interview, professional role and responsibilities, and any limits to confidentiality. Equally central is the importance of listening to the family. Why have they come, what are their concerns, what do they want help with?

A unique aspect of assessing families with infants is that frequently the 'patient' has no words to tell their part of the story. In this case what is observed about the infant, his behaviour, his responses and the interaction between family members is crucial in helping the clinician and family to understand the infant's experience and his part in the current difficulties.

Establishing an alliance

The first contact is a time to join with family members, letting them talk about life with this infant—their joys, fears, hopes, disappointments, pleasures, worries—in their own words. It is a time when the clinician can clarify expectations and roles, begin to defuse fears, support parental concerns, demonstrate a genuine interest in them and their infant, and begin to develop an alliance, or working relationship.

Understanding the core of the problem

The process of assessment, of listening and observing, and of asking questions, allows the clinician and the parents to begin to develop a clear and focused understanding of the core of the problem—or problems—underlying the family's presentation.

Information gained helps the clinician and parents together to organise and understand the experience of the family in order to construct a narrative or 'story', an account of the family's experience with the baby. This is constantly updated and modified through the duration of assessment and intervention as development and change occur.

Sometimes a particular instance or event may demonstrate the core dynamic or problem. The Jewish aphorism, 'The Lord God dwells in detail', usefully contains the sense that the essence of the whole resides in the smallest part. Exploration of a particular situation or event in detail may provide an understanding of the whole, or of an aspect of the family's difficulties.

EXAMPLE: MARIA AND TONY

Maria presented with feelings of depression, saying she was not enjoying parenting in the way she had expected. She spoke self-critically about feeling disorganised, not managing to return to work yet, and not living up to the expectations she felt her family had for her. Her parents had migrated when she was a baby. They were busy, successful people. She said that as children she and her siblings had been required to fit in a lot with their parents' agenda and activities. She had been expected to manage and achieve. She had high self-expectations, and attempted to be compliant. While she talked, her baby, Tony, aged five months, became increasingly restless and distressed. She tried a number of things to settle him, continuing to talk as his cries increased.

Maria's situation, above, presents an opportunity to wonder whether what you are observing is a small example of both some of the difficulties between Maria and her baby and of her own experience growing up. She is struggling for time to talk and think about herself, and to meet what she perceives as your expectation that she answer your questions. Meanwhile, Tony needs more of her attention than he is getting. Perhaps this is a bit like what she describes about her own experience of growing up. She feels unable to get it right with Tony, perpetuating her sense of inadequacy, but also at that moment not able to sort out what is most important. Can Tony's need for attention be the most important thing for a moment, or are both he and she having to 'fit in' with the agenda of the interview? A core issue may be how to reconcile her own sense that she wants to give Tony more attention and time than she received, with her conflict about how to do that without again having little time for herself.

During the interview a decision needs to be made about how to use this kind of observation. Sometimes a simple empathic comment about how hard it is to know what he needs at times may be enough to help her feel understood. This may help her to focus on him and sort out why he is unsettled. Sometimes it may be appropriate to make a more detailed link between what she is saying and what is happening in the room. Selma Fraiberg (1980) was referring to the same phenomenon in her work with disadvantaged, high-risk families, when she commented that parents often repeat with their infants their own childhood traumas 'in terrible and exacting detail' (p. 165).

The goal of the interview process then is not only to gather objective data but to form a therapeutic relationship within which the problem can be understood and progress made towards resolving it.

The relationship between the clinician and the family is crucial:
- to develop trust
- to facilitate engagement in the treatment plan
- to support and enhance the infant–parent relationship: parents who feel their experience has been understood in the process of information gathering are more likely to be able to think about and understand their infant's experience.

Taking the history

During the interview at which the infant and, where possible, both parents and other significant caregivers are present, the clinician will explore with the family their hopes and fears, their expectations of themselves and this infant, as well as their experience, if any, with medical and psychological services in the past. Information is obtained about the following:

1 THE CURRENT PROBLEM

- How do the family understand and describe what is concerning them?
- Where do they locate the problem, and has it happened before?
- Was there a precipitant? Why have they sought help now?
- What have they tried?
- What has been helpful?
- What made them decide to seek help from you and your service?
- What do they want help with? What are their priorities?

2 THE BACKGROUND HISTORY

This includes information about the:
- individual parent's history of his or her own family, and relationships
- parents as a couple
- conception, pregnancy, labour and delivery
- infant's development since birth.

The information obtained will include risk and protective factors in the:
- infant
- parent(s) and their relationship
- social and cultural context.

This material will include consideration of biological, psychological and social factors.

The biopsychosocial framework

Information will be obtained about biological, psychological and social factors that have helped or hindered the family now and in the past.

Biological factors—This includes genetic vulnerability, and past and current health, and any significant family history of illness. In the infant it includes intra-uterine exposure to drugs or other toxins, and other factors affecting development and physical health.

Psychological factors—This includes intra-psychic and interpersonal factors. *Intra-psychic factors* include current psychiatric illness, personality factors and attachment style. *Interpersonal factors* include the history and quality of current relationships.

Social/cultural factors—Includes factors in the social context, the degree of cultural and social isolation or support, financial security and parental employment. Socioeconomic status is a powerful predictor of infant developmental outcome (Zeanah, Boris & Larrieu, 1997). Assessment of social and cultural factors includes:
- the extended networks that support or abandon the family at this time of rapid developmental change
- the social and cultural factors that impinge on the family
- relationship quality and interactions

- family violence
- practical issues, circumstances—the practical reality of the family situation, including housing, poverty, and employment and educational opportunities.

Infant and parent factors can be considered within the biopsychosocial framework.

INFANT FACTORS

Infants are born with a genetic endowment, including what is sometimes called temperament, and is already at birth affected by their environment in utero (for example, the adequacy of nutrition, drug or alcohol exposure, prematurity or medical illness). These are biological contributions to the presentation. The quality of parenting may alleviate or exacerbate an infant's constitutional difficulties. This is described as 'goodness of fit' between parental expectations and capabilities and infant capabilities and needs. It includes psychosocial and interpersonal factors as well as perhaps biological aspects of the parents' and infant's health that affect their ability to meet their baby's needs. The place of the baby in the family, including gender and birth order, and the meaning of this baby to these parents at this time in their lives, and their place in the sociocultural context should also be considered.

PARENTAL FACTORS

In considering what each parent brings to the relationship with their baby, we need to take into account:
1. Biological factors:
   - medical and psychiatric history
   - current physical health
   - family and genetic background.
2. Psychological factors:
   - their psychological and social strengths and resources
   - their imagination of what and who the infant will be for them
   - the history for each parent and the parents as a couple that precedes conception and birth, including their experiences in their own family, and their experiences of being parented
   - their expectations of themselves as parents, which are enormously influenced by their own experiences of family life
   - parental psychopathology—each parent's past and family psychiatric history and any current difficulties (aspects of parental psychopathology are discussed in Chapters 12–14)
   - parental substance abuse, current or past (see Chapter 15)
   - parental age and life stage (see Chapter 16 for issues related to adolescent parents).

3 Parent's family background:
   Having a baby to care for is a powerful trigger for feelings, thoughts and memories about one's own upbringing. Many aspects of parenting are determined by how we were parented, who held us, how we were comforted, how our needs were met. This information is stored in procedural memory, memory for actions, not in verbal memory. Obviously, the earliest experiences with our parents occurred long before we were able to put things in words. Winnicott (1987) puts it: '… she was a baby once, and she has in her the memories of being a baby; she also has memories of being cared for, and these memories either help or hinder her in her own experience as a mother' (p. 6).

Assessment of infant–parent interaction

Even in a brief interview with a family, many useful observations can be made that provide information about the 'quality' of the interaction and relationship.

Relationship factors

The interaction between parent and infant and, where possible, between the parents while they are with the baby, needs to be observed. This provides information about:
- parental sensitivity to the infant
- infant responsiveness to parental care and attention
- the 'fit' between them
- infant and parent safety
- the parents' capacity to work together to care for the infant and the quality of their relationship.

The relationship and interaction with the infant is affected by:
- immediate contextual factors
- individual aspects and characteristics of the caregiver and infant
- events in the past, especially the parents' experience of being parented.

The behaviour of the parents and infant while they are with you is as important as what is said. It is recommended that the clinician pay as much attention to what the parents and infants are *doing* as to what they are telling you. With the infant in the room you will see how easily the infant settles, how responsive the infant is to parental voice and touch, how the infant indicates his needs and how these are responded to. With a toddler present, you will learn a great deal about how free he feels to explore the room, how much proximity he seeks from his parent and the behaviours that gain parental attention.

That said, the language used by parents, the way they talk to and about their baby also provides a great deal of information. You may notice, for example:

PRINCIPLES OF ASSESSMENT IN INFANT MENTAL HEALTH

1. offhand remarks and nicknames
2. stories, when a parent may consciously or unconsciously be talking about other people or situations but describing something about the infant or their interactions with the infant
3. non-verbal communication between parents, and between parent and infant, particularly facial expression and touch
4. what the parents say to the infant, what they say about the infant and how these compare.

EXAMPLES

The following examples illustrate how offhand remarks and comments need to be taken in the context of the overall assessment process.

> 1. *Karen had a severe post-partum haemorrhage after delivery of her first child. Her mother had died early in her own life. She presented with anxiety and depression, having difficulty caring for her baby. She described her daughter a couple of times as 'to die for', conveying an aspect of her own sense of almost dying during labour but also some uncertainty about whether mother and child could both survive. Would she also have to die in some way for her daughter, replicating her own loss?*
>
> 2. *Observed in a supermarket queue: Two young women with an infant of about 18 months were talking. The mother called her daughter a 'pest' a couple of times. They began talking about going home for lunch. One turned to the infant and said, 'And what shall I give you for lunch Christie? Dog food I reckon'. Now if asked about this, the parent may have said it was a joke and that her daughter had tried eating the dog food, but unmistakable hostility to the infant is conveyed in these offhand remarks and generates concern, which in this context cannot be addressed—but could be, in a sensitive clinical interview.*
>
> 3. *During a clinical interview, Jane described how she has been depressed, and was still having difficult days when she would spend a lot of time lying on the couch and crying, with her little girl of 12 months just beginning to take steps. During the clinical interview the infant was a little shy but then began to play. Sitting most of the time, she played independently, apparently ignoring the conversation. However, when her mother took a tissue out and blew her nose, the little girl's head shot around to look at her and her fingers went to her mouth. The mother apologised, explaining she had a cold and that her little girl heard a lot of that noise. The clinician asked if perhaps the little girl was sensitive to her mother's emotional state and was fearful of her mother crying. The mother confirmed this sensitivity and talked about how her toddler tries to comfort her when she cries.*

Observation of the quality of the relationship with the infant is also a central part of assessing risk. The interaction reflects the caregiver's current nurturing capacity and the infant's ability to accept nurture. Daily routines (feeding, sleeping, changing) are the setting for important social exchanges and also times of increased risk for the infant if the caregiving system is stressed or inadequate. The parent's sensitivity to the infant's communications is central to the development of the relationship. This could be called the parent's central task and is clearly predictive of the kind of attachment relationship that the infant develops with each parent.

EXAMPLE

A woman recovering from post-partum psychosis responded appropriately to her baby's cry saying, 'she's hungry'. She talked to her fondly as she lifted her to her breast. Unfortunately, she forgot to lift her shirt or open her bra, and the infant was frustrated and became distressed attempting to latch onto her mother's shirt. This observation showed both the extent and limitations of the mother's recovery and her current capacity to recognise her baby's needs and respond appropriately.

Ideally, communication between infant and parent is:
- **contingent**—the parent is able to be responsive to the infant's cues, rather than intrusive and insensitive
- **collaborative**—both parties are active participants in the interaction and build or 'repair' their communication together to restore optimal and comfortable levels of arousal
- **emotionally attuned**—the parent is able to identify and 'tune into' the infant's emotional state and to organise their response appropriately.

This depends on the capacity of the caregiver to be empathic, and to *perceive the mind of the child*. It requires the caregiver to reflect on her own experience and inner state and to acknowledge her infant as an 'experiencing being': to *be with* rather than *do things* to her infant.

Infant developmental assessment

Developmental assessment can be included, when appropriate, as part of the therapeutic intervention. There are many different kinds of developmental assessment undertaken, depending on the purpose of the assessment, the clinician's skills and abilities, and the family's needs and concerns. Involving parents in the assessment process can provide them with useful information about their infant's abilities and needs and also allows the clinician to see what use they are able to make of this information.

Conducting a developmental assessment

Some general principles apply:
- First, as in any assessment, ask what information the parents want to receive. This helps build rapport and indicates to the family that the process is for the benefit of the infant and family. Respecting parents' requests at this stage may enable more sensitive or difficult information to be discussed at a later stage.
- Provide a safe, comfortable environment for the infant.
- Assess the infant's optimal level of functioning and/or what he can do with support.
- Involve one or both parents (in the room for infants, or behind a one-way mirror for older children) in the process of assessing their infant's skills, interests, behaviour and adaptive capacities.
- Be aware of and sensitive to cultural differences, respecting and appreciating these when interacting with and assessing infants and their families.

What should a developmental assessment include?

Conducting a developmental assessment involves:
- obtaining information about the infant's developmental, health and family/social history
- engaging with the infant or toddler in order to assess his developmental skills and emerging capacities across a range of areas (for example, motor, sensory and social)
- assessment of the infant's behaviour and coping abilities during the testing and play sessions
- observation of the infant in different settings (that is, home, clinician's office and day care)
- evaluation of the quality of parent–infant relationships/interactions, including strengths and areas of concern.

Video replay of parts of the assessment can be used to engage parents in understanding their infant's needs and abilities.

THE NEONATAL BEHAVIOURAL ASSESSMENT SCALE

The Neonatal Behavioural Assessment Scale (NBAS) (Brazelton & Nugent, 1995) was designed to capture the early behavioural responses of the infant to his new environment before that behaviour is shaped by the parental care. Brazelton and Nugent's assumption is that a baby is both competent and complexly organised and an active participant in interaction with caregivers. Thus, the assessment helps to understand the infant's side of the interaction. The NBAS scale:
- *is an interactive examination*. The infant is not assessed alone, but as an active participant in a dynamic situation. The skilled examiner observes the infant's

response to her handling, bearing in mind how much effort the examiner has to put in to enable the infant to give his best performance.
- *is an assessment of the infant's best performance*, not an assessment of deficits.
- *gives information about the infant's adaptation to his new environment.* The stimuli used in the NBAS include the kind of experiences—touch, rocking, voice and facial expressiveness—that parents use in handling and caring for their infant. There is a graded series of procedures used by the examiner—talking, placing a firm hand on the newborn's tummy, holding and rocking—which are all used by parents and designed to soothe or alert the infant.
- *is not a formal neurological assessment*, although there are some neurological measures.
- gives a better indication of the coping capacities of the infant in the process of adaptation to environmental stimuli with repeated examinations.

EXAMPLE: SUE, MIKE AND PATRICK

Patrick was born the third child to Sue and Mike. The older children were two girls. In the maternity hospital Patrick's loud cries were heard frequently. His birth had been difficult for Sue, but Patrick was checked by the paediatrician and found to be healthy. The hospital staff decided to offer Sue and Mike the opportunity to have Patrick assessed using the NBAS. Patrick was asleep when he was picked up by the examiner. He adjusted or 'habituated' well to this but once moved onto his back he began to wake and was quickly crying intensely (a state 6 arousal on the NBAS), and needing to be consoled. It was not until Patrick was wrapped, held and given a dummy that he quietened and it was possible for the assessment to continue. Once settled Patrick could focus and follow a face and a rattle from side to side, he could turn to each side in response to a voice, he could focus his attention and interact.

Each time he was unwrapped to examine other responses Patrick quickly escalated to intense crying. His limbs and muscle tone were tight and his movements jerky. Because his body felt tense, he did not cuddle in when being held and he showed no strategies for self-soothing.

Used therapeutically, the NBAS allowed Sue and Mike, above, to observe how their son responded to someone else's handling. The observation reassured them that Patrick's behaviour was not because they were inadequate. They could see that when wrapped and held Patrick's body relaxed and he was able to be responsive to interaction. The assessment served a number of purposes—reassuring the parents of their ability to assist their baby, providing an opportunity for the parents to see and understand the effect of stimulus on their baby, and providing a framework for discussion of ways to manage their baby's particular needs.

Through the assessment, the clinician had the opportunity to discuss with

Sue and Mike the importance of respecting Patrick's needs for wrapping and being held. Once Patrick's body was relaxed he was available for brief periods of interaction and also better able to drop into sleep and sleep well.

SUMMARY

Assessment of families with infants and young children occurs in a variety of contexts and for many different clinical reasons. Nonetheless, a comprehensive assessment always includes a relational and developmental focus, with consideration of both strengths and vulnerabilities that the parents and infant bring to their current circumstance, and attention to biopsychosocial factors that help or hinder the family at this time of rapid developmental change.

It is not always possible to follow through with treatment as a consequence of the assessment. There needs to be recognition of the collaborative effort between the clinician and the family in understanding and addressing the problems. If a successful alliance has been formed between the family and the clinician, this supports proposed interventions. When this is not the case, it is important to 'finish' with the family and infant in a manner that is respectful. A follow-up contact may be helpful to aid the family in their transition to a new clinician. Concerns about the immediate or long-term safety of the infant or caregivers need to be addressed openly and directly with the caregivers and referring agency. Appropriate intervention must follow, and processes put in place for monitoring the ongoing safety and well-being of family members. Risk assessment is discussed in Chapter 4.

ADDITIONAL READING

Hoghughi, M. (1997). Parenting at the margins: Some consequences of inequality. In K. N. Dwivedi (Ed.), *Enhancing parenting skills: A guide book for professionals working with parents* (pp. 21–41). Chichester: Wiley.

Jones, D. (2001). The assessment of parental capacity. In J. Horwath (Ed.), *The child's world: Assessing children in need* (pp. 255–272). London: Jessica Kingsley.

Reder, P., Duncan, S., & Lucey, C. (2003). What principles guide parenting assessments? In P. Reder, S. Duncan & C. Lucey (Eds.), *Studies in the assessment of parenting* (pp. 3–26). New York: Brunner-Routledge.

CHAPTER 4

Assessing risk in infancy

KEY CONCEPTS

- Definitions of risk
- The cumulative effect of risk factors
- Developmental impact of risk
- Uncertainty in predicting risk
- Transgenerational issues in risk assessment

PRINCIPLES

- Risk occurs within the caregiving relationship and social context
- Assessment involves weighing up risk and protective factors
- The greatest development risks are those that are present over time
- The presence of multiple risk factors has a cumulative effect on development

Assessment of risk is an aspect, implicit and sometimes explicit, of all assessments of infants and their caregivers. Most health workers in Australia now have a mandatory responsibility to report infants and children who are considered to be at risk. Risk to the infant or to the relationship with the infant occurs whenever the caregiver's resources are overstretched. In considering risk in infancy and early childhood we are considering risk *within a relationship*. Infants can be at risk developmentally or physically because of medical illness or prematurity, but the caregiving relationship and the social context of that relationship are major determinants of the psychological outcome for the infant developmentally.

There are various degrees and types of risk that range from physical illness or disability in the infant, to those associated with child abuse and neglect. As well as prematurity and medical illness, factors that contribute to developmental risk listed by Zeanah, Boris and Larrieu (1997) include infant temperament, attachment, parental mental illness, marriage quality and interactions including violence, socioeconomic status, poverty and adolescent parenthood.

In this chapter we will focus particularly on the assessment of risk to the infant within the caregiving relationship. At times when one or both parents have psychiatric illness or are in unsafe domestic situations, it is also necessary to assess the risk (of self-harm or violence) to the infant's caregivers. When the caregiver is at risk, the infant is also at indirect risk, because of the centrality of the caregiving relationship to the infant's well-being. Therefore domestic violence, even in the absence of violence directed towards the infant or child, represents a significant developmental risk.

DEFINITIONS OF RISK

Risk can be defined as the probability of an event occurring, including the consideration of the losses and gains associated with it. In this context (infant development and child protection) it is not free of moral and emotional overtones. There is a high degree of uncertainty in prediction of risk in child-protection matters and inevitably this contributes to the anxiety felt by even very experienced clinicians working in this area.

A number of different risks can be identified. These are:
- risk to the infant's immediate physical or emotional safety.
- risk to the infant's optimal development. This acknowledges the importance of early experience in contributing to later outcome.
- indirect risk, such as repeated separation from a parent hospitalised with a psychiatric or medical illness.
- cumulative risk. This occurs when an infant and family are exposed to multiple risk factors. For example, a premature infant born to a young single mother with a narcotic addiction with little family support is clearly at greater risk than a premature infant with similar medical and biological risk factors, born to a couple with adequate financial and practical support.

The greatest developmental risks are those that operate long term, for example:
- chronic neglect
- chronic instability in the family's personal and social circumstances
- exposure to:
  - parental personality disorder or dysfunction
  - ongoing hostility towards the child
  - chronic marital disharmony or domestic violence.

FACTORS TO CONSIDER IN RISK ASSESSMENT

Assessing risk of neglect, abuse or significant developmental disadvantage needs to include:
- what each partner (caregivers and infant) brings to the relationship—their *strengths and vulnerabilities*
- the *parenting capacity* of the caregivers
- the quality of the *interaction* between the caregiver and infant
- the *social context*—sources of support, stress and practical issues such as housing
- the *capacity for change* in the infant, caretaker, relationship and environment.

Strengths and vulnerabilities

The infant is born with a particular genetic endowment (sometimes called temperament) and is at birth already affected by her environment in utero (for example, the adequacy of nutrition, drug or alcohol exposure, or prematurity). Some infants are harder to care for, less rewarding and more difficult to read. These include sick, disabled and premature infants who may be delayed in social responsiveness, and those with a 'difficult temperament'. The quality of parenting may alleviate or exacerbate an infant's constitutional difficulties. A healthy infant may also have qualities or characteristics that do not conform to parental expectations, described as the 'goodness of fit' between parental expectations and capabilities and infant capabilities and needs. Therefore the meaning of the infant to the parent and the quality of their interaction and relationship also need to be considered. This is contributed to by, for example, the infant's gender, birth order and circumstances of conception.

Consequences of maltreatment

Infants and children who have been abused or neglected may have developed physical, emotional and behavioural consequences of that maltreatment. These characteristics and behaviours may make caring for them more difficult. For example, traumatised infants may continue to show avoidant or disruptive behaviour even when placed in safe fostering environments. Infants with brain damage after head trauma may have long-term physical and emotional symptoms, meaning that their care is particularly difficult and challenging. This presents parents (including foster and adoptive parents) with challenges that they may not have anticipated, requiring them to demonstrate more patience or perseverance than with less traumatised infants.

Parenting and parenting capacity

Many definitions of parenting and parenting capacity have been suggested over time (Jones, 2001; Reder, Duncan & Lucey, 2003b). The core elements of parenting as defined by Hoghughi (1997) are: *Care* (meeting the child's needs for physical, emotional and social well-being, and protecting the child from avoidable illness, harm, accident or abuse); *Control* (setting and enforcing appropriate boundaries); and *Development* (realising the child's potential in various domains). In order to be an effective parent, knowledge, motivation, resources and opportunity are necessary.

Parenting capacity

Parenting capacity can be briefly summarised as the capacity to recognise and meet the infant's changing physical, social and emotional needs in a developmentally appropriate way, and to accept responsibility for this. It is determined by:
- parental factors (and the infant–parent relationship)
- infant factors (and the infant–parent relationship)
- contextual sources of stress and support (and the family-context interaction) (Reder, Duncan & Lucey, 2003b).

Recently, there has been consideration of the relative weight or emphasis to be given to each of the above factors in considering risk to infants and children. Donald and Juriedini (2004) argue that parenting-capacity assessment should centre primarily on the parent's ability or potential to provide empathic, child-focused parenting, in other words, on the 'adequacy of the emotional relationship between parent and child', specifically 'on the parental capacity for empathy' (p. 7). They describe factors in the child or the relational and social context as 'modulating effects' upon the primary domain of parenting capacity. While their approach is recent and untested in practice, it has the advantage of focusing the clinician upon the quality of the relationship and the parent's potential for an adequate emotional relationship with his or her child.

Parental factors

What each parent brings to the relationship with his or her infant includes:
- personal strengths and resources
- the history for each parent and the parents as a couple that precedes conception and birth—this includes their experiences in their own families, and their experiences of being parented
- their expectations of themselves as parents—this is enormously influenced by their own experiences of family life
- their imagination of what and who the infant will be for them and their capacity to empathise with their infant

- parental psychopathology—past and family medical and psychiatric history and personality functioning, including the capacity for intimate relationships
- parental substance abuse
- parental age (for example, adolescent parents)
- their capacity to use support and willingness to do so.

Transgenerational issues in parenting

Parents with a history of abuse or neglect in their own backgrounds enter parenthood at a disadvantage. This is because of the inadequate internal models they have to draw on, the effect of early neglect or abuse on their own capacity for self-regulation and reflection, and often limited current family and social support. Studies estimate that only about a third of children who have been abused go on to be abusive parents (Kaufman & Zigler, 1987), but this is clearly a risk factor for difficulties in parenting. (These issues are discussed in more detail in Chapter 13.)

Infant–parent interaction

Observation of the quality of the relationship with the infant is a central part of assessing risk. The interaction reflects the parent's current nurturing capacity and ability to respond sensitively and appropriately to the infant's cues, as well as the infant's ability to accept and respond to parental care.

The daily routines of feeding, sleeping and changing are the setting for important social exchanges and also times of increased risk for the infant if the caregiving system is stressed or inadequate. What parents do is more important than what they say or think they do, and invaluable information is obtained from observation of their interaction with their infant.

The parent's sensitivity to the infant's communications is central to the development of the relationship between them and is predictive of the kind of attachment relationship that the infant develops with each parent. Developmentally, infants who form secure attachment relationships are at an advantage socially and emotionally as they grow up (Thompson, 1999).

Infants in high-risk situations are more likely to develop insecure or disorganised attachment relationships with their caregivers. There is evidence that disorganised attachment during infancy is linked to emotional and behavioural difficulties in childhood and adolescence. Therefore, although an infant may not be at an immediate physical risk, an erratic, neglectful or unstable caregiving environment is a threat to her social and emotional development and has significant long-term implications.

In child neglect, which has profound developmental implications, abnormal behaviour is persistent rather than an impulsive outburst that leads to abuse. Unfortunately, many infants at risk suffer both neglect and abuse, and neglect—particularly emotional neglect—can be difficult to detect.

Social context

Socioeconomic status is a powerful predictor of infant developmental outcome (Zeanah, Boris & Larrieu, 1997), but it is also the family's willingness and ability to access and use support that is crucial. Factors to be considered here, identified by Reder, Duncan and Lucey (2003a), include:
- the context and the interaction between the family and the social environment
- family functioning, for example, poverty, unemployment, responses to stress, social or cultural isolation
- potential for stability in relationships and social circumstances
- relationships with others and the ability to use interventions and community support.

EXAMPLE: LISA

Some infant–parent relationships can be identified as at risk ante-natally.

> *Lisa was 3 months pregnant with her second child when her husband, Tom, left. Their marriage had been difficult since the birth of their daughter Hilary 12 months earlier. Lisa had been working to support the family with her mother helping to care for Hilary, while Tom studied. Lisa suffered hypothyroidism after Hilary's birth but this had not been diagnosed for several months and she had felt very tired and depressed. She had no past psychiatric history. When her husband left, she had to move into rental accommodation and had financial difficulties because of legal action by her husband. Her parents offered financial and practical help.*
>
> *She presented saying that she did not want another baby, but also could not consider termination or adoption of her current pregnancy.*

There are identifiable risk and protective factors evident in even this brief vignette. Clearly, the foetus is at risk as Lisa is considering termination. If the pregnancy proceeds we do not yet know what this infant will be like once delivered. Hilary, currently 12 months old, may also be at risk if her mother is depressed and preoccupied with the marriage break up and ambivalence about the current pregnancy. Also, Lisa suffered depression post-natally and despite the contribution of hyperthyroidism to her mood disturbance she is at risk of recurrence of depression with a subsequent pregnancy. The family has strengths as well, including Lisa's insight and willingness to seek help, her parents' practical and emotional support, and relative financial stability.

Capacity for change

Assessing the capacity for change in situations where risk to the infant or caregiving system has been identified, or abuse and/or neglect has occurred, is a necessary but difficult task.

For example, an adolescent mother has been unable to help her infant into organised patterns of sleeping, waking, eating and playing. The infant is failing to gain adequate weight and is fussy and restless. This parent may lack adequate information about infant development but is otherwise motivated and has just enough resources to meet the infant's needs. Support and education may reduce the risk to this infant, allowing her to get on with her development. However, if there is a lack of motivation from the parent, then provision of resources and information will not be enough to protect the infant from the consequences of neglect.

Repetition of abuse

Repetition of abuse occurs in 25–50 per cent of families where children are returned to their parents after removal following abuse or neglect (Reder, 2003). Care and control conflicts are common in parents with histories of maltreatment. This can affect their capacity to parent, and to use available resources and support services.

Care issues include tensions about being cared for and caring for, arising out of early experiences of abandonment or neglect. Parents with care conflicts may present with excessive clinging or dependence, inability to use and accept help, and intolerance of others' needs.

Control issues include tensions about self-control, desire to control and fear of being controlled possibly stemming from experiences of helplessness in the face of abuse or coercion. Parents with control conflicts are prone to violence and controlling behaviour and see others as controlling of or attempting to control them.

RISK FACTORS FOR REPETITION OF ABUSE

Risk factors for repetition of abuse include (Reder, 2003; Sturge & Glasser, 2000):
- the parent's inability to give a coherent and emotionally appropriate account of their own childhood abuse, or their abusive behaviour towards their own children
- significant use of dissociation, denial and minimisation as psychological defence mechanisms, which reduce their capacity to empathise with and meet the needs of their infant
- denial of responsibility for abusive behaviour in the past
- an external locus of control, that is, a tendency to blame others for what happens in their life
- a limited capacity for self-reflection
- current instability in housing and relationships, chaos and lack of support
- continuing or recent parental substance misuse.

PROTECTIVE FACTORS AGAINST REPETITION OF ABUSE

For the parent, protective factors include (Egeland, Bosquet & Chung, 2002):
- availability of support (social, cultural and professional)
- a stable, safe social and personal situation
- willingness to ask for help and use it
- acceptance of responsibility for the parenting role and their past and present behaviours
- minimal current mental illness or substance misuse.

Factors that promote resilience in the infant and child long term include (Ferguson & Horwood, 2003; Sameroff, Gutman & Peck, 2003):
- a well parent or other involved adult
- social supports
- professional intervention
- consistency in other relationships and activities
- being good at something.

There is an interaction between individual characteristics of children and the environment in which they develop that enhances or mitigates against resilience, but as Luthar and Zelazo (2003) put it, 'resilience based interventions must address the quality of parent–child relationships and, more generally, the well-being of caregivers' (p. 533).

EXAMPLE: LISA, CONTINUED

Lisa decided to proceed with the pregnancy, and, before the birth of the second child, moved in with her parents. She began seeing a psychiatrist regularly and was referred to the social worker at the maternity hospital. After a period of great hostility, relations with her husband improved enough for her financial situation to stabilise and for him to express an interest in seeing his children. The second child, a boy was born uneventfully and Lisa felt immediately very fond of him. He was an easy and settled baby. Despite this, about six weeks after his birth, Lisa became troubled by intrusive thoughts that the children would be better off without her. She had intense mood swings and frequent thoughts of suicide. She was admitted to a psychiatric hospital for six weeks with the new baby. Her daughter Hilary, now aged 21 months, stayed with her grandparents.

Despite intervention and support, Lisa suffered a severe recurrence of post-natal psychiatric illness. Her intrusive thoughts were of harming herself, not her children, but clearly the well-being of the children was linked to her recovery. The stability and quality of caregiving provided to the children by grandparents and hospital staff during Lisa's illness contributed to the long-term effect of this period on their development. Concerns about immediate risk to their safety would increase if she had delusional or preoccupying depressive ideas that included the children, or if she did not seek or refused medical and parenting assistance while she was unwell.

Concerns about the immediate or long-term safety of an infant or a caregiver need to be addressed openly and directly with the caregivers and referral agency. Appropriate intervention must follow, and processes put in place for monitoring the ongoing safety and well-being of family members.

SUMMARY

All assessments involving infants and parents, including infant mental health assessments, involve consideration of risk. The notion of risk in infancy and early childhood is complex and multifactorial. It includes a spectrum ranging from consideration of immediate risks to physical safety to the notion of developmental risk and psychopathology following early adversity. The vulnerability and dependence of infants on the availability of their caregivers means that threats to the safety of either or both parents inevitably impacts on the infant's well-being.

The infant and the caregiving context are at increased risk whenever the infant's needs outweigh the capacity of the carers and their supports to meet these needs. As described, this can occur because of factors in the infant, the caregiving system (parents) and/or the social context, and many at risk infants and families have vulnerabilities in all three areas.

When considering risk in infancy:
- remember that there are degrees of risk
- risk factors may be cumulative—there is rarely a linear correlation between any one risk factor and later developmental outcome
- risk may be direct or indirect
- risk may be to immediate physical safety or long-term development.

Situations of high risk are distressing for all concerned, particularly when the clinician is required to recommend the removal of an infant. A comprehensive assessment ensures that these decisions are based on sound information, obtained from a variety of sources, and are made in the best interests of the infant and her family.

PART B

The early infant–parent relationship

CHAPTER 5

Pregnancy, labour and birth

KEY CONCEPTS

- Transition to parenthood
- Psychological adjustment and maturation
- Parenting alliance
- The imagined baby
- Experience of labour and delivery

FACTORS IN ASSESSMENT AND FORMULATION

- Health problems for mother and/or foetus
- Obstetric and psychiatric history
- Parental background and family of origin
- Quality of family relationships
- Contextual sources of stress and support

Pregnant women, their partners and relationships with extended family and friends undergo changes during pregnancy that influence their capacity to include a new baby in their lives. The most obvious transition to parenthood for the mother is physical, and the physical safety and health of mother and infant are a priority at this time. These physical, including hormonal, changes are accompanied by social and psychological adjustments that come more easily for some parents than for others.

There are situations where these psychological, social or interpersonal adjustments can lead to difficulties in the transition process. These difficulties can contribute to relationship problems between the parent and infant and therefore potentially have an influence on infant development. The dramatic transition from foetus in utero to infant in parents' arms illustrates for all family members the enormity and significance of what is both a very common but also profoundly unique life process.

The extent to which the actual infant who arrives in a family can be welcomed and cared for is influenced by the network of relationships, supports and stressors that impact on the adjustment and coping of the parents during pregnancy and after delivery. It is well known that maternal physical health affects foetal well-being but there is increasing evidence that maternal stress and anxiety may also influence foetal development.

This chapter will explore difficulties in this transition process. We will look at the processes of change that occur during pregnancy, the adjustments to existing relationships and the range of difficulties that may arise during this period. We will consider how the quality and nature of the relationship that develops between the parent and infant is affected by expectations and wishes about the baby, and experiences before and during pregnancy and delivery. This chapter will also consider how early intervention for transitional problems during the ante-natal period can support the development of the infant–parent relationship, maximising the infant's developmental potential and family well-being, leading to better infant mental health.

TRANSITION TO PARENTHOOD

> In the transition to parenthood, a pregnant woman must not only carry the baby through safely, but square up to the sacrifices that motherhood demands. She must ensure the acceptance of the child by the family, develop an attachment to the baby within, and prepare for the birth. She must adjust to the alteration in her physical appearance, and develop a somewhat different relationship with the father of the child (Brockington, 1996, p. 63).

The transition to parenthood begins during the ante-natal period, as each new pregnancy is affected by, and affects, the family's current situation. The early relationship with the unborn child (and even with the imagined child before conception) is influenced by the nature of the conception, the life circumstances of the parents and their support system, and the social and environmental world the infant is born into.

Factors that influence and contribute to adjustment in pregnancy include:
- current level of support and/or stress, including the relationship with the woman's partner
- physical well-being of the mother and the unborn infant
- parental personality structure, including defence and coping mechanisms
- past experiences in family of origin
- past psychiatric history
- current or unresolved conflict, loss or trauma.

The transition to parenthood involves adjustment and change at a number of interconnecting levels:

PREGNANCY, LABOUR AND BIRTH

- physical and emotional changes
- psychological adjustment
- interpersonal changes
- social changes.

There is more information about the transition process for women than for men. Condon and Corkindale (1997) in a series of Australian studies have found that expectant men also go through a series of changes, but usually take longer than their pregnant partners to focus on the reality of the coming baby. There is little information about the transition process for the non-pregnant woman in same-sex female partnerships. Rapid changes in artificial reproductive technology (ART) may also affect the psychological processes that go with becoming a parent.

Adoptive parents often have a long period of loss, then waiting, before the arrival of their child. The process is less predictable, more public and more vulnerable to legal and practical complications. There can be a greater sense of powerlessness and uncertainty for adoptive parents, but similar processes of anticipation, fantasy and practical preparation occur, without the physical and hormonal changes that accompany pregnancy, labour and delivery.

Physical and emotional changes

For the newly pregnant woman, months of physical and emotional change are ahead. The three distinct stages in pregnancy are described as trimesters. The first trimester runs from conception to about 12 weeks' gestation, before any foetal movement is felt. The second trimester is from the end of the fourth to about the eighth month—most growth occurs during this time and foetal movement can be felt. During the third trimester the parents have a physical and emotional orientation towards the baby's birth and arrival in the world.

The first trimester

For many women the first trimester is associated with fatigue and nausea as their body adjusts to carrying and nurturing another life. In this early stage of pregnancy a range of emotions are common, including excitement and anxiety, elation and fear.

> *I very much wanted to be pregnant, but I hadn't expected how up and down I would feel. Sometimes I felt so tired and sick. I woke up at night, so anxious about the changes ahead. Other times, I couldn't be happier.* (Celia, 37.)

The range of normal transient emotions, driven by hormonal and psychological changes, affects thoughts and feelings about the pregnancy. Parents may feel ambivalent, even with a wanted pregnancy, and may have difficulty accepting that these feelings are a common experience. Prolonged or intense mood disturbance indicates the need for mental health assessment.

The second trimester

For most women, the second trimester is associated with an increase in energy levels without the physical discomfort that occurs in the later stages of pregnancy. Feeling the baby's movements occurs around fourteenth to sixteenth week. Tests to determine foetal health and well-being are usually completed in the early months of this trimester and bring reassurance to most parents. Inconclusive or abnormal test results can herald a difficult period of uncertainty as the process of clarification occurs. Concerns about maternal or foetal health, or issues such as previous obstetric loss, may have a negative effect on the usual enjoyment of this phase of the pregnancy.

> *I felt so well once I got to about 15 weeks, I felt fantastic, physically and mentally, really full of life! I loved feeling the baby move and my husband and I both shared a lot of excitement then.* (Celia, 37.)

During the second trimester the foetus gains about 285 grams in weight and 12.5 centimetres in length. The mother feels the first flutter, called 'quickening', in her abdomen and by the fifth and sixth months a pregnant woman and her partner can feel her baby kicking and moving about.

The third trimester

In the last trimester expectant parents, especially the woman, begin to think and worry about how the baby is going to be delivered. The realities of parenting an infant are often hard to anticipate as energy goes into planning and preparing for delivery. As the reality of the birth approaches, it is common for fears of foetal abnormality or illness to resurface. The mother to be may also experience a conscious or unconscious anxiety that she or her infant may not survive the labour intact. This state of emotional confusion gives the impetus to and prepares for a woman's emotional birth as a mother when her baby is born.

> *I got very physically uncomfortable towards the end, and focused on the delivery. I also felt very happy and complete at times, the baby and I felt so close and connected. I also felt more dependent and needy—vulnerable really. I needed reassurance. It was a time of contradictions again—happiness a powerful feeling, but lots of worries too.* (Celia, 37.)

Women, including those with a previous difficult or complex labour, may become very anxious and fearful about labour and delivery. A clear discussion of options for pain and obstetric management during labour can be very helpful, allowing the woman and her partner to anticipate and make choices about how labour and delivery will be managed. Few women want to repeat an experience of pain, powerlessness and anxiety, and discussion of interventions that enable parents to make informed choices (including for example, elective caesarean delivery) is often appropriate.

Labour and birth

The experiences of labour and birth contribute to the development of the relationship between parents and infant, and to the meaning of this particular infant to this family. For example, what may be considered a medically successful outcome of a healthy infant and mother may have been experienced by the woman as a frightening, painful loss of control, something that didn't go the way she had imagined. For another woman, the same sequence of events would have different connotations, depending on her expectations of herself and her partner, the medical personnel and the labour process.

Birth can feel like a shared experience or an ordeal for the woman and those with her at the time. She may feel closely connected to the baby during stages of the labour but it is also common for women at times to feel alone, surviving each contraction, focused only on getting through the next few moments.

At the start I knew Andrew and Talia (birth support people) were with me, I could talk to them, tell them what I needed. Later, as it got more intense I was shouting at them sometimes I think. I didn't care about anything except surviving, me and Sam (the baby). The labour went on and on and I got so tired. I had an epidural and got a bit of sleep. Afterwards I thought about Sam, he didn't get a break like I did. I wondered if I had let him down. That didn't last, once I held him and got to know him a bit, I didn't care how hard it had been or how it hadn't gone the way we had planned, I was just happy that he had arrived, and I kept thinking, 'he's so beautiful', even though he was all squashed and funny looking at first. (Celia, 37.)

Psychological adjustment

Psychological factors that may affect infant mental health include imaginings about the unborn baby and changes to the parent's identity. This requires a reworking of experiences and attitudes about one's family of origin experiences. It involves intra-psychic changes as well as actual changes in the relationships with parents and other family members.

One aspect of the transition to parenthood can be thought of as involving a change in identity from that of a child (to one's own parents), to that of a parent (to one's own child) (Stern, 1995).

During pregnancy, many women become increasingly introspective, and emotions may be more intense. This can create problems as old conflicts (with parents, for example) are reactivated. The pregnant woman is likely to feel sensitive and psychologically vulnerable as she moves towards the birth of herself as mother and the birth of her infant. Similarly, expectant men experience a less obvious transition, a reworking and thinking through of the kind of parent they want to be. This is inevitably influenced by their own experiences in their family of origin.

The imagined baby

Babies carry powerful wishes, hopes and dreams for their parents and, to a lesser extent, for the extended family. The infant may have existed in the imagination of parents, grandparents, siblings and others long before conception. However, the baby that arrives is rarely the baby who was imagined and wished for. The relationship that develops between the parent and infant is affected by the nature of expectations and wishes about the baby, the experience of pregnancy and birth, and the capacity of the family to accept and welcome the infant who does arrive.

Daniel Stern (1995) wrote:

> between the fourth and seventh months of gestation there is a rapid growth in the richness, quantity, and specificity [of the imaginings] about the baby to be…The elaboration…peaks at about the seventh month…Between the seventh and ninth month…representations about the baby decrease and become progressively less clearly delineated, less specific, and less rich…After all, birth is the meeting place for the baby now in her arms and the one in her mind. As far as possible, she needs to keep the real situation unburdened with the past so that she and her real baby can start to connect, with a minimum of interfering baggage (p. 23).

As Stern indicates, the histories of each parent, and of their relationship before conception, influence imaginings about who the baby will be. The imagined baby is also affected by the circumstances of conception, the obstetric history, and other factors in the parents' lives.

For example, a couple, pleased to be pregnant for the first time, may tell family and friends as soon as the pregnancy is confirmed. They are keen to include others in their excitement. A couple who have had difficulty conceiving or have experienced a past obstetric loss may find it hard to let themselves imagine the baby, wonder if the infant is a boy or a girl or discuss names, because of the intensity of past disappointment and loss. Where the pregnancy is unplanned, and the parents are uncertain whether to continue the pregnancy, it is unlikely that much imagining about the infant will occur, and this may be psychologically necessary until a decision is made about whether to continue the pregnancy.

The physical experience of pregnancy can influence how the baby is imagined and talked about. This may give clues to how the parent experienced her infant even before he or she was born. Some quotes illustrate the range of experiences women may have:

I vomited for nine months, and spent three months in hospital on my back. I was so depressed, I didn't want him. (Kate, 29.)

She used to get her feet up there under my ribs and really have a go at me. (Theresa, 31.)

I loved being pregnant, I felt so close to her then. Both of us had everything we needed. (Desi, 35.)

Changes to the woman's identity

During pregnancy a woman struggles to answer the question 'What kind of mother will I be?' This may be a conscious or unconscious process and feelings and thoughts may be confusing, bemusing, surprising or frightening. Past unresolved conflicts and present traumas can affect a woman's fantasy life and attitude to her pregnancy. For example, she may identify with characteristics she liked and admired in her own mother and others she does not want to repeat. She may be anxious, with high expectations, wanting to do things very differently from her own parents.

I knew all the things I didn't want to do and be. I just didn't know what was realistic. I think I set myself unrealistic goals to be perfect almost, and when I wasn't, that was hard. (Roxanne, 29.)

Interpersonal changes

Just as each expectant parent experiences psychological and emotional changes and challenges during pregnancy, so intimate relationships also undergo a transition in preparation for the baby's arrival. The ability of a couple, their extended family and social network to adjust affects the amount of support the new parent receives. Lack of support from a partner or spouse, especially when combined with high levels of stress, increases vulnerability to post-natal difficulties (O'Hara, 1997).

Relationship with partner

In most cases the transition to parenthood involves the entry of a third individual into an established dyad. Of significance is the development of a parenting relationship distinct from the pre-existing couple relationship.

This can be called the parenting alliance and it develops after a child is born (Van Egeren, 1998). It is not the same as marital satisfaction and involves:
- shared investment in the child
- valuing the other parent's involvement with the child
- respect for the judgement of the other parent
- desire to communicate regarding parenting issues.

The function of this alliance is to provide support and affirmation to each other in a stressful period of transition. This alliance is likely to be fairly stable within each developmental stage of the child, but as each stage brings new challenges to parents individually, their alliance is also stressed. Some individuals and some couples find one developmental stage much easier than another.

Van Egeren found that a positive parenting alliance was correlated with parental confidence and a warm authoritative style. The frequency of disputes over child rearing is a better predictor of behaviour problems in the child than marital adjustment or satisfaction. Marital satisfaction peaked at one month post-partum followed by a steep decline at six months. The realities of parenting an infant, the sleep disturbance and other influences on life as a couple contributed to this.

Preparation for first-time parenting also requires a change in role definition for most couples, including a renegotiation of financial and domestic responsibilities. For some couples this comes more easily than for others.

Social changes

Becoming a parent affects how one is perceived and related to in the world. Motherhood is a state or occupation that carries high expectations and paradoxically, in our society, a low status. Many women in our culture parent in isolated, unsupported situations, becoming parents with little or no experience of infants or of life undefined by paid work. For many women the physical and emotional demands of pregnancy increase their sense of vulnerability and dependence on others.

For most women, there is an inevitable impact on their place in the world of work and their working or professional identity. Most women take some paid or unpaid leave from employment when they have a baby and there can be losses and anxieties about what this will mean for their careers and jobs. For a couple, roles may become more traditionally defined for a while, with the woman at home with the infant and the man providing financial support. These are big adjustments that do not necessarily come easily. Combined with changes to their personal, financial and social lives, these contribute to the losses associated with adjustment to parenthood.

DISRUPTIONS TO TRANSITION

Distress may be prolonged or intense in the ante-natal period if there are significant threats to maternal or infant well-being, or if relationship conflict or past events (for example, past obstetric loss or trauma) become preoccupying. Prolonged or intense emotional distress during pregnancy may indicate a need for more thorough mental health assessment, as significant depression and anxiety during pregnancy indicate a high risk of ongoing psychiatric disorders post-partum. (This is discussed further in Chapter 12.)

Effect of ante-natal mental health problems

Stressful life events in the ante-natal period affect parental physical and mental well-being. This can impact on foetal and therefore infant development and mental health in a number of ways. There are the possible effects of maternal mental health on obstetric outcomes, and potentially on the neurobiological development of the foetus (Orr & Miller, 1995; Sacker, Done & Crowe, 1996). Stressful life events during pregnancy increase the risk of post-partum psychiatric disorders (O'Hara, 1997), and during this period of enormous transition can affect the quality of subsequent infant–parent interaction, and, as a consequence, infant development.

Foetal development

> There is no such thing as a baby—meaning that if you set out to describe a baby, you will find you are describing a *baby and someone* (Winnicott, 1964, p. 88).

It is conceptually and methodologically difficult to study the psychological interconnectedness of mother and baby during the ante-natal period. How the maternal state of mind might affect, through mediating mechanisms, foetal development, and conversely how foetal mental functioning might affect the maternal state of mind, is a relatively recent area of study.

There is growing empirical evidence to suggest that the foetus has sensory and cognitive abilities, including the capacity to learn in utero (Glover & O'Conner, 2002; Hepper, 1989). Current research suggests that the infant at birth is already primed in emotional and behavioural ways that shape responses to interpersonal and environmental interactions. Some research suggests that maternal psychosocial distress may affect foetal development and neonatal outcome. For example, Glover (1997) proposes that ante-natal maternal anxiety could possibly alter the foetus's neurophysiological responses in lifelong ways.

Though the evidence is inconclusive and at times speculative it is worth consideration. Maternal distress in pregnancy traditionally has been viewed as subjectively unpleasant, but unless psychiatrically severe, as transient and benign for most women (Hrasky & Morice, 1986). These assumptions may require reassessment if emerging evidence about the effect of maternal stress on the developing foetus is confirmed. Research in this area is complex and runs the risk, if not thoughtfully undertaken and reported, of contributing to another area where women are made to feel guilty and responsible for many things beyond their control.

Infant–parent interaction

Characteristics of the infant–parent relationship demonstrated to affect infant development include parental sensitivity and responsiveness to infant cues and what is known as the 'fit' between parental resources and abilities and infant needs. The security of the attachment relationship that develops between infant and parent shows a correlation with the infant's capacity for self-regulation and his subsequent social and emotional development (see Chapters 1 and 2). The implications of this are far-reaching in terms of both individual and social well-being.

Risk factors for psychological disturbance during pregnancy and birth

Women experiencing mental health or relationship problems increasingly are identified during routine ante-natal screening. Ideally, this enables referral for appropriate assessment and intervention. A range of screening tools and processes have been developed to suit the needs of obstetric services. Questions about past psychiatric history, and current levels of social support and stress have become a more standard aspect of obstetric history taking.

Risk factors for psychiatric disturbance during pregnancy and birth include:
- threats to maternal or foetal health
- past obstetric trauma or loss
- current or unresolved conflict, trauma and loss
- social isolation and/or adversity
- past psychiatric or psychological difficulties
- experience of trauma during labour and delivery.

Threats to maternal or foetal health

Many potential medical difficulties can occur during pregnancy, and concerns may arise for the physical well-being of the mother and/or the infant. An example of this is when threatened miscarriage occurs. The woman's central focus and preoccupation becomes the survival of the foetus. She may feel powerless to ward off danger and damage to her baby and may feel guilt or imagine she has caused it by something she did, something she ate, a cold she had or even a walk she took. The normal fears every pregnant woman experiences may develop out of proportion as she attempts to find an explanation for the threatened loss. Her partner and extended family may unwittingly contribute to this sense of guilt and search for an explanation, in comments made as a result of their anxiety and concern.

A woman or couple with a threatened miscarriage need a great deal of support, and the medical details need to be explained several times if necessary.

Threatened miscarriage interrupts the process of preparation for parenthood, and depending on the circumstances and individuals concerned, may delay the imagining and psychological preparation for the infant's arrival.

Maternal ill health carries with it concerns about the foetus. Women with diabetes in pregnancy or pre-eclampsia, for example, require extra monitoring of their own and foetal health during pregnancy and while some women and their partners take this in their stride, for others it colours anticipation and preparation for the baby with anxiety. Alternatively, women who manage to deliver a healthy infant after a medically complicated pregnancy may feel particularly fortunate or grateful. It is important to explore the particular meaning of events to any individual or family, rather than to make assumptions about how an experience has been and what it has meant for them. Listening carefully to the way events are discussed and the language used about experiences and about the infant help the clinician to make an accurate formulation.

Past obstetric trauma or loss

This includes previous miscarriage, termination, adoption or stillbirth, a history of traumatic labour and delivery, infants born with a disability or deformity, and, for some couples, prolonged infertility prior to conception.

The loss of a baby, a miscarriage, abortion or infant relinquished for adoption or removed by child-protection services may leave grief for the rest of a parent's life. When a woman becomes pregnant again this previous emotional trauma is reawakened in a powerful way. The trauma is not just remembered, but relived as the physical changes and landmarks associated with the progression of pregnancy are reached. Unless there has been some resolution of the previous loss, it can be hard to make space psychologically for the new baby. Some individuals or couples will need an opportunity to discuss and work through a previous loss if it becomes too preoccupying.

Pregnancy is also a time when old wounds can begin to heal. A lost baby cannot be replaced by having another one but previous psychic pain can be relieved by the experience of a new baby surviving and thriving. For some couples the experience of death and loss is eased by the practical and emotional realities of parenting the new baby.

Previous obstetric difficulties, including prolonged infertility or an infant born with a hereditary disorder, may also affect the transition process. It may be more difficult to enjoy and anticipate the pregnancy and the infant and, as with other obstetric losses, feelings of grief and anger may be reactivated.

A woman and her partner who already have an infant with a hereditary disorder may suffer apprehension and fear of repetition in a new pregnancy. Every couple has a right to thorough investigation and discussion of genetic determinants and risks so that becoming pregnant again is an educated choice.

There are some cases where the answers and prognosis for subsequent infants are not so clear or obvious and this makes the choice harder for these couples.

For the individual or couple who have chosen to become pregnant again after a prior loss or trauma it can be an emotionally difficult time. For either parent, feelings of guilt and shame may accompany loss, anger and anxiety. Depending on the circumstances of past events and the meaning that has been made of them, support from professionals, family and friends may be needed during the pregnancy.

Current or unresolved conflict, trauma and loss

There are implications for the infant–parent relationship if trauma and loss for the parent are not adequately resolved. This can include current circumstances, for example, intimate relationships characterised by conflict and violence or bereavement during pregnancy. Unresolved childhood or adolescent trauma or ongoing conflict with family members can also preoccupy expectant parents in ways that interfere with their ability to anticipate and imagine the baby to be. Feelings about and a preoccupation with these events may intrude on present relationships and the mother or father to be may require psychological support and intervention. Parents with unresolved loss and trauma may have difficulty providing sensitive, responsive caregiving to their infant if aspects of the pregnancy or caring for an infant reactivate traumatic past experiences and memories. (See Chapter 13.)

PREVIOUS HISTORY OF ABUSE

How we were parented affects how we are as parents (van IJzendoorn, 1992). If the experience of being parented was abusive or inadequate, there may be difficulties in adjusting to parenthood and parenting. All expectant and new parents reconsider their experience of being parented and growing up in their family of origin and sometimes make a clear and conscious decision to do it differently. Couples also have to negotiate their different family experiences and expectations.

Some anxieties about parenting or the changes that becoming a parent will bring are based on unconscious experiences from the past. Conflict can be stored in implicit or procedural memory and may manifest as depression or anxiety.

Most of us cannot consciously remember much before three years of age, but the early years have a profound effect on our development and our later capacity for relationships. Much of what we cannot recall in a narrative sense is stored in procedural memory and comes into play when we have children of our own. Not all that is reactivated from our own past is conscious or immediately available to recall or discussion. Winnicott (1987) puts it this way: 'After all she was a baby once and she has in her the memories of being a baby; she also has memories of being cared for, and these memories either help or hinder her in her own experience as a mother' (p. 6).

Practical and emotional support from extended family can help the adjustment to parenting. But for some families, the extended family is a source of stress or conflict, either by absence or intrusive involvement that is experienced as critical or because of ongoing conflicted or abusive relationships. At such a vulnerable time, it can be hard for the parents and in-laws to get the balance of support and independence quite right.

RELATIONSHIP CONFLICT

A lack of practical and emotional support, particularly from her partner, puts a woman at higher risk of psychiatric difficulties post-natally. Equally, the partner of a woman who becomes depressed in the post-partum period is at higher risk of becoming depressed himself (O'Hara, 1997).

Couples where one partner is very keen to parent and the other less so, may have difficulty negotiating parenting roles and the changes in financial and domestic responsibilities. Sometimes this aspect of the transition to becoming parents, the renegotiation of roles and responsibilities, remains a problem long after the child or children have arrived.

BEREAVEMENT

Because of the increased importance of support from partner and family during pregnancy, the loss of a partner (through separation or death) or other important person during pregnancy is particularly difficult. If relationship breakdown has even in part been related to ambivalence or conflict about the pregnancy, this may complicate feelings and imaginings about the baby.

Attempting to mourn cuts across the process of imagining and preparing for a new relationship with the baby. In attachment terms these are contradictory processes. For some parents this can contribute to depression during pregnancy or a sense of emotional numbness and difficulty imagining and preparing for a relationship with the new baby. The pregnancy may complicate or prolong the process of grieving because of the 'psychological space' that both preparing for a new infant and grieving require.

Social isolation and/or adversity

Because pregnancy is a time of increased emotional vulnerability, and preparing to parent an infant has multiple practical and emotional consequences, lack of social and emotional support increase the risk of post-partum psychological difficulties and therefore can affect the infant.

Many women parent in isolation, some by choice, others by circumstance. Some choose motherhood before it is 'too late', deciding to have a baby without the support of a partner rather than miss the opportunity.

Pregnant single women may experience themselves as disadvantaged during pregnancy and unless well supported by family and friends may find the transition to parenthood difficult. The practical reality of caring for a young infant on your own, the lack of sleep and the sense of social isolation can be very hard.

Recent immigration or even relocation within a country during pregnancy can heighten a sense of vulnerability. Migration involves adjustment on multiple levels, as does the preparation for parenthood. At a practical level, language and cultural factors may make access to services and supports more difficult. At an emotional level, loss of family, friends and familiarity may affect the preparedness to welcome a new life. Alternatively, new migrants coming from situations of ongoing conflict may feel hopeful that their infant will be born into a better world.

Past psychiatric or psychological difficulties

A history of mental illness or ongoing personal difficulties increases the risk of a recurrence of these problems during the ante- and post-partum period. This is due to the interaction of physical, hormonal, psychological and social factors involved in the process of transition to becoming a parent. At this time of huge adjustment, women with previous vulnerabilities may become unwell or experience in a particularly intense way the fluctuating emotions associated with pregnancy.

Also, women and their treating doctors may decide to cease psychotropic medication for all or part of the pregnancy to protect the foetus. Women with a past history of psychiatric or ongoing personality difficulties require close monitoring and support during pregnancy, and rapid referral for assessment and intervention if difficulties arise. A past history of psychosis, bipolar illness or severe depression must not be ignored. (Parental mental illness is discussed in Chapters 12 and 14.)

Experience of trauma during labour and delivery

When labour and delivery are experienced as traumatic this can affect the initial interaction between mother and infant, particularly if the baby becomes associated with trauma and pain in the mother's mind. Women with a past history of trauma or abuse are at risk of having these feelings and experiences reactivated during labour and birth if they are not adequately supported emotionally and provided with the pain relief that they require and request. Also, when interventions, for example, rupture of membranes or epidural anaesthetic, occur without a sense of adequate information or time to consent, this can be a disempowering experience, leaving a woman feeling cheated or angry.

Most women benefit from the opportunity to talk about their labour after having a baby, and one function of this is to assist the woman to psychologically process and begin to make sense of what has occurred for her in the hours prior to meeting her baby for the first time. Mothers often have this chance in new parent groups and in meetings with early childhood staff. There are fewer opportunities for partners to talk through these experiences. Partners also may be traumatised after attending their baby's delivery. The most common difficulty is a feeling of helplessness or anxiety about their partner during labour and delivery, especially when unanticipated interventions such as caesareans have occurred (Boyce & Condon, 2000).

ASSESSMENT, FORMULATION AND INTERVENTION

Women, couples or families suffering psychological difficulties in the ante-natal period will be seen in a range of inpatient and outpatient settings in obstetric, psychiatric and community-based services. They may be assessed by a variety of medical and allied health clinicians, referred from a variety of sources with the range of issues and difficulties described previously.

The details of a comprehensive assessment and formulation will be guided by the presenting problem, the referral information, the setting in which the family is seen and the skills and resources of the clinician. The following principles can be used to guide an assessment, in whatever setting and capacity it is being undertaken.

The developmental progression that occurs during the nine months of gestation and knowledge of the inevitable end to the pregnancy, usually with delivery of the baby, can increase the pressure on the woman, the family and the clinician for resolution of difficulties and appropriate adaptation and change. At the same time the physical progression of the pregnancy adds to the impetus for change and resolution of psychological and interpersonal difficulties.

Weighing up risk and protective factors

Assessment of an individual or family at this time involves consideration of:
- biological factors—for example, medical concerns for the mother or foetus such as genetic risk
- psychological and interpersonal factors—adaptive and coping mechanisms, past psychiatric and obstetric history, resolution of trauma and loss, and relationship quality
- social factors—extent of social support, stress and isolation.

Important protective factors include adequate personal and material support and a collaborative obstetric, allied and mental health team who will work together to integrate care of the pregnant woman, the foetus and the extended family.

Principles of intervention

For most of this chapter we have thought about assessment and intervention of individuals and families referred for assessment during pregnancy. It is important to remember that preventive interventions also occur during this time of regular contact with medical services. Most expectant parents are highly motivated during pregnancy to 'get things right' in preparation for their baby's coming. It is a time when timely intervention and professional help can save later pain, conflict and heartache. It can help the couple develop a more healthy relationship for the future. The momentum associated with the transition to parenthood supports therapeutic interventions and change. Interventions can be:
- *population based*—that is, provision of psycho-educational material about pregnancy, childbirth and the challenges of early parenting to all women or couples presenting to hospital obstetric services in a particular area
- *targeted*—for example, women identified during routine intake interviews or screening in ante-natal clinics as being at high risk of mental health problems may be referred for assessment, support and intervention
- *indicated*—those that are provided to women and families already identified as having mental health problems.

In this last group (those identified as having mental health problems and referred for assessment and intervention), intervention and treatment planning:
- must be based on a thorough assessment and formulation of the family's problems and resources
- needs to include consideration of maternal and foetal well-being and the quality of the support networks around them
- must be based on a biopsychosocial formulation and address relevant factors in all these domains
- must be responsive to and based on the physiological and psychological changes occurring over the nine months of pregnancy
- needs to anticipate the potential medical, psychological and practical complications that may occur following labour and delivery
- must involve collaboration between obstetric, mental health and paediatric staff and services and the community-based practitioners who will provide follow-up
- needs to be based on awareness that while pregnancy lasts nine months, parenthood is for life.

For example, intervention with a woman with a past history of significant depression who presents with a recurrence during pregnancy needs to include consideration of risks to the physical and mental health of mother and baby, including:

- current physical health of mother and foetus
- stage of pregnancy
- factors in the relationship and social circumstances that are supportive or stressful.

If medication is indicated as part of treatment, a woman and her partner need to be able to provide informed consent about their decision based on the provision of accessible and accurate information. The decision to prescribe any medications during pregnancy needs to be made by weighing up:

- potential benefits to maternal (and infant) health against potential risks to the mother or foetus of prescribing medications
- the risks of an illness remaining untreated, as women with untreated or inadequately treated mental illness in pregnancy are at higher risk of obstetric complications than women without this diagnosis or who are adequately treated (Newport, Wilcox & Stowe, 2001; Sacker et al., 1996).

Collaboration with the obstetrician in planning and implementing mental health interventions is essential if integrated and therefore adequate care is to be provided to the woman and her family.

EXAMPLE

Toula was referred by her obstetrician for psychiatric assessment when she was three months pregnant with her second child. She was depressed and ambivalent about continuing the pregnancy and she and the obstetrician were requesting an assessment prior to a decision about a mid-trimester termination. The obstetric history was very significant. Toula and her husband Theo had their first child, a baby boy, almost exactly 12 months prior to the date this new baby was due. Their son had been stillborn after an apparently uncomplicated pregnancy. The foetal heart rate had disappeared just before he was delivered. Despite resuscitation he suffered severe anoxia and after two weeks in NICU, was removed from the respirator and died a few hours later in their arms. Despite this Toula and Theo continued to trust their obstetrician, who had also been very distressed by Alex's death, and had returned to see her when Toula discovered she was unexpectedly pregnant again. Initially, they were seen together as a couple and their different ways of expressing their grief about Alex were explored. Toula had kept the room she had prepared for him unchanged since she went to hospital in labour. Theo had begun renovating other parts of the house, was drinking more heavily and had taken on extra shifts at work. They were angry with each other, feeling distant and unable to talk together about Alex's birth and death. Termination of the current pregnancy ceased to be the primary issue as discussion turned to anxiety about risking another loss so soon. Unresolved grief and trauma for both parents and the obstetrician became the focus of sessions and telephone conversations. Toula was preoccupied with anger towards parents with healthy babies and with sadness and guilt about Alex. She had no room at all to think about the developing baby inside her and little time for Theo.

A gentle process of grief work was commenced, with the parents eventually bringing in their photos of Alex after his birth, in the NICU and as he was dying. As this work progressed they both began to talk more about the new baby who had been virtually ignored until then. Once it was clear that the new baby would always be their second child, a space opened up for the new baby, a sibling who sadly would never know her brother. Because they had a good relationship with the obstetrician, a clear plan was developed for delivery. Labour and delivery proceeded uneventfully and a baby girl, Tina, was delivered and went home with her parents. When seen three months later, mother, father and baby girl appeared to be doing well, with continuing acknowledgement of the sadness associated with loss of Alex, but increasing enjoyment of Tina as well as the normal adjustment to the realities of new parenthood.

SUMMARY

A pregnant woman and/or her partner may need psychological assessment and intervention during the pregnancy. Problems of a previous miscarriage, a previous baby born with genetic or other physical impairments, migrating to a new country or having a close family member die during the pregnancy will make the pregnant woman or couple vulnerable. A difficult childhood and adolescence, or other areas of unresolved conflicts, make this time of transition difficult. It is a time when old conflicts are awakened, and when unconscious feelings are near the surface. For both partners emotional strains are increased by changes in their external world and their emotional inner world as they make the transition to parenthood. Pregnancy is not only about producing a healthy baby, it is about producing a healthy mother and father and a supportive network of family and social relationships.

CHAPTER 6

Biomedical problems in infancy

KEY CONCEPTS

- Synactive theory of development
- Disturbances to neurobehavioural development

FACTORS IN ASSESSMENT AND FORMULATION

- Support needs
- Hospital ecology
- Events surrounding the birth
- Effect of parents' past experiences

Where biomedical problems affect infant health and development the consequences for the infant and family are profound. Infants may be born prematurely, with illnesses, defects, syndromes and disorders, and there may be developmental delay as a result of these conditions, ranging from mild to severe. Many infants born with a biomedical problem require immediate and ongoing hospitalisation, and the effects of their condition may be lifelong.

There is some evidence available in infant mental health literature that explores the relationship between infant illness and psychological development. Most research has been conducted with premature infants and their families. Illness in infants often occurs with prematurity so it is possible to draw parallels between the experiences of premature infants and those with an illness. Repeated hospitalisations and the effects on the developing attachment relationship is one area of concern to mental health clinicians working with premature and/or ill infants. The experience of infants with a birth defect, disorder or syndrome is not so well understood, in terms of effects on attachment and mental health outcome.

In this chapter we will explore infant mental health issues when the presenting condition is medical, either prematurity or a chronic medical condition. We will discuss risk to the infant's development and the possible effect on the developing relationship between parents and infant. The importance of the infant–parent relationship as a key aspect in the development of self-regulation will be explored. We will also discuss the effect of a premature birth or a sick infant on parents, and what factors need to be taken into account to assess and manage the mental health needs of these infants and their parents.

NEWBORN NEUROBEHAVIOURAL DEVELOPMENT

The importance of the infancy period has been clearly established and emphasised in earlier chapters of this book. The infant's genetic make-up, constitutional factors and birth experience will influence early behaviour and the caregiving received. The capacity of the parents and other caregivers to sensitively respond to the subtle cues of the infant will in turn influence the infant's attempts at self-regulation and subsequent development. An explanation of early development within this approach has been detailed by Dr Heidelese Als (1982).

In the Synactive Theory of Development (Als, 1982; Brazelton, Als, Tronick & Lester, 1979), Als proposed a method of conceptualising the biological basis of newborn behaviour and a framework for organising observations of newborn infants. Newborn behaviour is the expression of five hierarchical, sequentially maturing and interdependent areas of function, which are: the autonomic system, the motor system, the state organisational system, the attentional and interaction system within the state system, and a self-regulatory and balancing system. Autonomic homeostasis is seen as forming the core, in terms of being the earliest system to achieve stability, and as being required as the foundation for other behaviour. All of the systems are an integration of physiological adaptation and maturation and the caregiving environment. For example, when a baby is born, respiration, nutrition and temperature control are dependent on particular physiological adaptations and also appropriate caregiving. The baby needs maximum support to maintain homeostasis and to avoid excessive stress. Thus, those caring for the baby modulate the timing, intensity, duration and appropriateness of stimulation.

Infants born premature, or compromised in some anatomical manner, will require greater assistance from the caregiving environment to establish and maintain homeostasis and establish circadian rhythms.

Als has identified within each subsystem behaviours displayed by infants that indicate approaching or engaging behaviours, or withdrawal from stimulation, that is, stress and defensive behaviours. In balancing these behaviours to achieve self-regulation, infant signals range from mild and subtle to more dramatic expressions, and are generally understood by caregivers. Under ordinary circumstances, loving parents either intuitively or quickly learn their baby's signals that indicate availability and interest, or withdrawal, and respond accordingly. When subsystems are disturbed by medical and biological conditions, this process becomes more difficult.

PREMATURITY, ILLNESS AND EARLY DEVELOPMENTAL PROBLEMS

Normal infant neurobehavioural development is disturbed or interrupted by prematurity, perinatal illness and developmental delay.

Disturbances such as prematurity and illness influence the infant's:
- ability to manage stress and modulate response to stimulation
- quality of relationship with caregivers.

Developmental delay varies widely in cause and origin, but, regardless, has the potential to affect infant mental health.

Premature birth

A premature birth is likely to be a traumatic event for both the parents and their baby. For the mother, the process of holding her baby within is interrupted, often with no prior warning and no explanation as to why. Sometimes it is a life-threatening experience for the mother as well as the baby.

A premature birth occurs when a baby arrives at less than 37 weeks' gestation. In general, the earlier the baby's birth, the greater the risk to the infant of developmental problems. The terms, 'small for dates' or 'small for gestational age' are used to indicate that a baby is not only premature but also underweight. (These terms also apply to full-term babies—that is, you can have a 'small for dates' baby who is full-term.) A baby born very early but of a reasonable weight usually has a less problematic medical path through the intensive-care nursery.

Premature births in Australia

The incidence of prematurity, that is, infants born at less than 37 weeks' gestation, is about 10 per cent of all live births. However, about 1.4 per cent of all annual live births in the United States are infants born less than 1500 grams, referred to as very low birthweight (VLBW), while infants born less than 1000 grams are referred to as extremely low birthweight (ELBW) (Browne, 2003). The figure is probably similar for Australia. These infants are usually born at least eight weeks early. Minde (2000) quotes studies indicating that in well-equipped hospitals the survival rate for these infants has improved dramatically over the past 10 years. However, Minde states 'these data, which document the improved overall outcome, also suggest that more premature infants remain in hospitals for a longer time now than ever before' (p. 177).

Why do premature births occur?

Many factors are associated with premature birth but causative mechanisms are little understood (Stratton, 1982). Premature births are more common in situations of 'lower socioeconomic status' with strong association with factors such as poor ante-natal care, inadequate diet, smoking, drug taking and teenage pregnancy. However, premature birth also occurs to women who have good ante-natal care, adequate diet, do not smoke or take drugs and do not experience any more stress than the average woman. For many women the immediate cause of prematurity is unknown. Rates of premature birth are higher in women under 20 and over 35 years of age (American College of Obstetricians and Gynecologists [ACOG], 1999).

Neurological outcomes

Neonatal intensive care has advanced considerably since the late 1980s, with a subsequent decline in mortality but the rate of moderate to severe disability has remained relatively stable at around 8–10 per cent, while other neurodevelopmental conditions continue to be identified, for example, sensory impairment (Browne, 2003).

A recent study by Brisch (2003) of very low birthweight (VLBW) infants found that neurological outcome at 14 months (corrected for prematurity) was highly correlated with the infant's Nursery Neurobiological Risk Score—NBRS (Brazy, Eckerman, Oehler, Goldstein & O'Rand, 1991), measuring biological risk factors (such as birthweight and gestational age) and complications arising from neonatal treatment (for example, cerebral haemorrhage, intubation, infection and number of days in hospital).

In the Brisch (2003) study, at 14 months corrected for prematurity, 40.9 per cent were found to have functional neurological problems, 18.8 per cent were mildly disabled, 7.2 per cent severe and 1.4 per cent very severely disabled with no possibility of locomotion. Thirty-one per cent were healthy.

Psychological outcomes

The information on attachment of premature infants has been contradictory. Initially, it was assumed that the distribution of attachment classifications (see Chapter 2) with premature infants was similar to that found in the normal population. Other studies found that there was a higher incidence of insecurely attached infants in the pre-term group, especially those in the higher risk group of very low birthweight (Mangelsdorf et al., 1996). The situation appears to be more complex. Brisch, Bechringer, Betzler and Heinemann (2003) found that the percentage of secure versus insecure attachment quality in high-risk infants was similar to that found in term infants. However, there was a difference between intervention and control groups of high-risk premature infants in that only in the control group did impaired neurological development correspond significantly with an insecure quality of attachment. The attachment-oriented psychotherapeutic intervention offered appeared to counteract the impact of neurological impairment, protecting such infants from insecure attachment, perhaps by assisting the parents' resolution of past experience of loss or trauma, or the trauma associated with the severity of the impairment. In a population of parents where the child had a diagnosis of cerebral palsy, Marvin and Pianta (1996) found that parental resolution of the child's diagnosis correlated highly with quality of attachment, with parents classified as 'resolved' having securely attached infants.

Usual hospital care of the premature infant

If a woman shows signs of going into premature labour, every effort is made to ensure the best outcome for mother and baby. Effort is made to postpone the labour with bed rest and medication, prepare the foetus for delivery with drugs to strengthen the lungs and/or transport the pregnant woman to a maternity hospital with an intensive care (Level 3) nursery to ensure that the premature newborn will receive appropriate care. When a baby is about to be born prematurely a neonatal team is on hand in the delivery to immediately attend to the baby.

The extent of immediate intervention is dependent on the condition of the newborn—the basics would be temperature control and ensuring oxygen to the lungs. Infants born less than 28 weeks are more likely to have breathing difficulties that will require ventilation. If born before 35 weeks premature infants have difficulty sucking and swallowing and will probably require artificial feeding, either intravenously or via a nasal tube into the stomach. Once again, it depends on the gestational age and health of the newborn as to which method is appropriate.

Conditions that place premature infants at risk are recurrent apnoeic attacks (cessation of breathing), respiratory lung disease, infections, jaundice, intracranial haemorrhage and feeding problems. Apnoeic attacks occur relatively frequently in the first couple of weeks of life in infants born at less than 35 weeks. To avoid negative consequences of this condition, premature infants have their heart rate and breathing constantly monitored.

Hospitalisation experiences

The length of stay in hospital for premature babies varies with the extent of their prematurity with babies born earlier (<28 weeks) and lighter weight

(<1500 grams) more likely to have longer stays. However, the length of stay is also dependent on the quality of the hospitalisation experience, that is, the infant avoiding such experiences as infection, respiratory distress syndrome, necrotising enterocolitis and surgery, intracranial haemorrhage or an extended period on ventilatory support. Length of stay is also influenced by the quality of handling and environmental stress experienced by the infant.

Parental involvement during infant hospitalisation

In recent years efforts have been made to facilitate parents' participation in the care of their infants through the introduction of such programs as the Newborn Individualised Developmental Care and Assessment Program (NIDCAP) (Als, 1982, 1986, 1991) and family-centred neonatal care (Sizun, Ratynski & Boussard, 1999; Symington & Pinelli, 2003). Parents are encouraged to visit frequently, gently touch and talk to their baby, express milk, nurse their baby when the baby is stable enough to be held and assist in care of their baby as their baby matures. As soon as possible, parents are encouraged to feed their babies, usually with a bottle initially and then the breast. In some nurseries, parents are encouraged to hold their baby skin to skin underneath their clothing, known as 'kangaroo care'. This method of care, introduced once the infant is stable for a few hours a day, is believed to help the infant to maintain body temperature, conserve energy (Feldman & Eidelman, 2003) and show less negative affect (Feldman, Weller, Sirota & Eidelman, 2003).

If the nursery has an individualised, family-centred approach to care, then as early as possible the parents are encouraged to observe their baby and identify cues for hunger and comfort, and signs of distress and tiredness. A program that involves the parents in the care of their baby addresses the problem frequently expressed by parents of premature infants, that the baby did not belong to them but to the staff.

Where parents feel that the baby does not belong to them there is a danger that the parents visit less often, believing that the baby is better cared for by the experts, the nurses and doctors. Parents who are supported and involved in the care of their infants in the Neonatal Intensive Care Unit (NICU) have the opportunity to get to know their infants, which facilitates the interaction between the parents and the infant and increases the parents' confidence as they take their baby home. For the premature infant, it is now known that the environmental sensory input affects her development. For the stable premature baby, evidence suggests that the best sensory environment 'is his or her parents' faces, voices and bodies (Als, 1998; Als & Gilkerson, 1997; Glass, 1999). They are familiar, appropriately complex, multimodal, specific to the infant's individual expectations and needs and can readily modify themselves according to the baby's responses' (Browne, 2003, p. 7).

BIOMEDICAL PROBLEMS IN INFANCY

After the birth of a premature infant some women stay in the hospital in a post-natal ward for a few days before moving to other accommodation on the hospital site if the family lives some distance from the hospital. Some tertiary hospitals provide family accommodation. Prior to discharge, most tertiary hospitals provide accommodation on the ward for parents to 'room in' with their baby for one or two nights.

EXAMPLE: LISA, ANDREW AND ROBERT

Lisa and Andrew were very excited, yet apprehensive in anticipation of taking baby Robert home. It had been a long three months with Robert having been born at 27 weeks' gestation. Initially, Robert had difficulty with his breathing and was on a ventilator for five days. He then got an infection, which caused a lot of anxiety until the infection passed and he continued to grow and put on weight. Lisa had been visiting the hospital daily, offering Robert the breast for three feeds a day. In preparation for discharge a plan was made for Lisa to come in to hospital for two nights to give her the opportunity to breastfeed each feed. Given that this would be the first night Lisa would be getting up to Robert through the night, she was concerned about how she and Andrew would cope. The first night neither Lisa nor Andrew slept as Robert's noises kept them awake, although Robert had slept soundly between feeds. Robert had fed well at each feed and Lisa was pleased that Robert had no difficulty doing so. Lisa and Andrew wanted to talk to the staff about Robert's noises and were pleased they had a second night in the hospital.

During the time of the baby's hospitalisation the parents have contact with other parents of premature infants either informally on the ward and around the hospital or formally in a group, conducted by a staff member or sometimes by parents of older premature infants.

Going home with a premature infant

As the time for discharge approaches, parents are encouraged to be more involved in the care of their infant. Most families have had contact with a social worker and their psychosocial needs assessed. At most hospitals there is a discharge planner who assists the family in the transition to home. Sometimes, in the case of sick or frail infants, a home visit from hospital staff is arranged after discharge. Most hospitals with a Level 3 neonatal nursery have some form of follow-up clinic, available to infants born weighing less than 1000 grams. If the infant was born weighing less than 1000 grams the family are given an appointment for follow up in a few weeks or months time. However, for most families, there is no home visit; rather, families are encouraged to link in with their local early childhood centre and other support services in their area and a local paediatrician.

Sometimes, infants are transferred from a hospital with a Level 3 nursery to a feeder hospital where the mother was initially booked to have her baby and which is closer to the family home. However, this transition is sometimes difficult for families as it feels like another wrench, perhaps mirroring the premature birth if it is done suddenly, without appropriate preparation of the parents.

For most families, discharge of their premature baby from hospital is a time of high anxiety. Parents often express it in terms of 'it takes several hospital staff to look after the baby one day and the next it is left to just us'. It is believed that parents who have been involved in their baby's care have more confidence in their ability to care for their infant at home.

EXAMPLE: LISA, ANDREW AND ROBERT, CONTINUED

The second night was much easier for Lisa and Andrew. Robert again slept in between feeds and so did they. The staff had explained that the noises Robert made were normal and would reduce as he matured and he had longer periods of deep sleep. Lisa had been at the hospital every day since Robert was born. She had been expressing milk and spending time by his isolette. In the last few weeks she had been able to hold him and care for him. Lisa was getting to know Robert, how he liked to be stroked, which movement and touch seemed to help him settle. She and Andrew had bathed him twice in the past week. Lisa in particular was beginning to feel more confident in understanding Robert's needs and felt she was ready to take Robert home.

In addition to the initial period premature infants spend in hospital there is a high rate of repeat hospitalisations in their early years, which puts additional psychosocial stress on the families. Using figures from the United States, readmission rates for all VLBW infants vary from 10 to 38 per cent. This is, on average, two and a half times higher than for full-term infants (McCormick, Shapiro & Starfield, 1980). Thus, families of premature infants have ongoing difficulties of separation, anxiety about the well-being and prognosis of their infant, and the psychosocial issues of parenting away from home.

Perinatal illness

Many of the longer term illnesses in infants are associated with prematurity. Low-birthweight infants continue to suffer from more cerebral disorders than do full-term infants (Kopp, 1987). Although there has been an increase in the survival of VLBW and ELBW infants, there has also been an increase in the incidence of neuropsychiatric disorders in this population (Lorenz, Wooliever, Jetton & Paneth, 1998; Volpe, 1998).

A number of full-term infants are hospitalised because of genetic abnormalities such as severe cystic fibrosis. Others suffer from conditions such as orthopaedic or cardiac anomalies, immune deficiencies or chronic respiratory diseases. A small number of infants are hospitalised because of malignancies and congenital abnormalities such as tracheo-oesophageal fistula and biliary atresia, who often require multiple and complicated operations or organ transplants. Although these conditions are not necessarily associated with neurological and intellectual impairments, many of these children suffer from conditions that can mark their future development (Minde, 1993). However, there are few studies that examine the effects of long-term illness or frequent hospitalisations on infants born at term, according to Minde.

Psychological effects

Two studies, Douglas (1975) and Quinton and Rutter (1976), examined the behavioural outcomes of infants who were repeatedly hospitalised during their first three years of life. The authors found that one brief hospital admission of less than a week was not associated with later difficulties but several hospitalisations with at least one between six months and five years were strongly associated with both psychiatric disorder and delinquency in adolescence. However, the data is more complex because Quinton and Rutter point out that those who had multiple admissions were from more disadvantaged homes.

Beavers (cited in Minde, 1993) and Shapiro (cited in Minde, 1993) examined the long-term effects of multiple hospital admissions early in life, where the abnormality could be treated permanently. The first group had undergone surgery for oesophageal atresia as infants and were compared with normal controls on academic and psychological criteria. The clinical group did not differ on academic achievement or intelligence. However, they were found to have lower self-concept and to be more anxious. Similar findings were found in the Shapiro study with infants who had undergone heart surgery.

EFFECTS OF FREQUENT HOSPITALISATION

Frequent hospitalisations create stress on the infant–parent relationship in a number of ways, independently of the condition of the child. Whatever the condition, the infant is unable to function at the expected level of maturity until a measure of physiological stability is obtained.

The infant who is hospitalised is likely to experience emotional distress in several different areas. There is exposure to a strange environment and a variety of people who will interact with the infant in different ways. Nurses may be nurturing at times and at other times inflicting pain as a result of necessary interventions. With babies and infants, if the parents are not present at the time of handling by strangers, the infant experiences abandonment and distress. The infant who has not left hospital is unable to establish the predictable daily routines that help the infant to organise her day-to-day life experiences. Each time the infant is readmitted, this predictability of routine is ruptured. Of course, there are some infants in chaotic environments where hospitalisation provides order not experienced at other times. This type of variation in the familial backgrounds of infants emphasises the difficulty of determining the effects of hospitalisation alone.

EFFECTS ON PARENTS AND SIBLINGS

A sense of control in the care of the infant seems to be crucial for the development of the infant–parent relationship. Parents of a sick infant are trying to develop a relationship with their infant in an artificial situation, sharing the care of their baby with strangers. It has been found that where the infant has been at home in the care of the parents for at least two weeks in the first three months, mothers were more likely to visit their hospitalised infants every day in contrast to those who had not as yet taken their infants home (Lampe, Trause & Kennell, 1977). Lampe and colleagues suggested that total care of the infant at home strengthened the relationship and the mother's commitment to her infant.

If there are other children, the parents have the conflict of balancing time with the sick infant or siblings who are with grandparents or some alternative care. There is also the parent's perception of the infant as a consequence of hospitalisation. Will the infant be perceived as fragile and thus over protected in terms of exploration or in relationship with siblings and peers?

EXAMPLE: VIVIAN, ARI AND ESTHER

Vivian and Ari were the proud parents of Jacob, four, and Joshua, two, when Esther was delivered at 30 weeks gestational age. The family was thrilled to have a beautiful daughter and sister. Neither Vivian nor Ari had family in the city where Esther was born. When they visited the hospital they had to use the occasional care at the hospital, visit on one of the days Jacob was at preschool and take Joshua with them, or go independently and the other parent staying home with the boys. Occasionally a neighbour would help out but they could not leave the boys with a neighbour for too long. Vivian, in particular, was torn, longing to spend more time at the hospital with their daughter. Also, it was easier to express the breastmilk there, it was calmer. She felt she was always on the go, rushing from home or preschool to the hospital and back, desperately trying to be there for each of her children. She felt she and Ari were like ships in the night and that they hadn't had a proper conversation in days. Vivian thought that things might be better when Esther came home but was terrified of how she would care for her. Vivian felt she only knew about boys, and robust healthy ones at that.

The relationship between the parents is placed under enormous strain with the birth of an ill baby. The parents are hurting in numerous ways and may not be able to support each other. Unless there are supports for the parents, the relationship deteriorates with the risk of separation—an additional stress on their relationship with their infant (Mayes, Gabriel & Oberfield, 2002).

With the birth of twins or triplets it is not unusual for one infant to be sicker than the other(s) and therefore to require longer hospitalisation. In this context, the infants develop their attachment to their parents at different rates. The relationship with the infant at home develops earlier.

Developmental delay

Developmental delay is when an infant does not meet developmental milestones at an expected age, even with a wide variability of the normal range. Delay may occur in four main areas: motor, fine and gross; language and communication; adaptive/personal and social; and cognitive. Infants who are born with specific syndromes and diagnosed conditions may be delayed in any or all areas of development to varying degrees.

Factors that cause developmental delay

In the majority of developmental delays or disabilities, specific genetic defects have not been identified but there is increasing acceptance that genetic factors are involved in many cases of delay. Three categories of risk have been identified (Tjossem, 1976):
- established risks are medical disorders, such as Down's Syndrome, with known association with developmental disorder
- environmental risks encompass limited social and experiential opportunities, and poor quality family interactions (see Chapter 3 for discussion of these risk factors)
- biological risks include potentially noxious ante-natal and post-natal events, for example, infection, peri-natal asphyxia and sensory impairments.

Infants may be exposed to more than one risk factor, with a subsequent increase in risk of development delay.

AUTISTIC SPECTRUM DISORDERS

In 1943, Leo Kanner first described the triad of features that he named autism: extreme social isolation, severe language abnormalities, and unusual responses to the environment. He believed that it represented some kind of inbuilt deficit. Today autism is defined as a biologically determined disorder (Gillberg & Coleman, 1992), a clinical expression of an underlying abnormality of brain function that produces disordered development.

Effects on infant and parent mental health

As noted previously, there is little evidence available on the effects of disability or delay in an infant on infant mental health. It is clear, however, that there is a process of grief that parents go through and there are possible effects on the establishment of the attachment relationship. Bonding will be affected with infants who are difficult to hold or do not respond with eye contact, smiles or other signs of developing attachment, however, it is not necessarily the condition itself that affects parents' mental health. In a study of maternal depression in mothers of premature infants at risk of cerebral palsy, development of depression was found to be linked to psychosocial stress, rather than to the infant's disability (Lambrenos, Weindling, Calam & Cox, 1996), demonstrating the significance of social and family support for families with a disabled child.

ASSESSMENT, FORMULATION AND INTERVENTION

With a premature birth or a medical problem identified at birth, the baby becomes the focus of medical attention in an alien situation and the mother is often left in the labour ward as the partner accompanies the baby to the nursery. This means that the parents are very vulnerable from the beginning. Ideally, the hospital addresses that vulnerability by providing emotional and social support for the parents from the time of admission to the hospital and easy access to their baby. In tertiary hospitals, where patients are often from 'out of area', a particular effort is often made to identify families isolated from their normal supports. However, hospitals vary in their recognition of the need for parents to be emotionally supported and given every opportunity to be involved in the care of their baby.

Parents of premature or ill infants continue to require support from the time of the birth or diagnosis through the early years of their infant's life. Initially, there is the trauma of the interrupted pregnancy or the early development of intimacy between the mother and infant, the anxiety of whether or not the infant will survive, and sometimes there is also anxiety about the mother's well-being. Once the premature or ill infant is stabilised, parents need to grieve the loss of the pregnancy they did not have and the ideal birth experience with the perfect baby. However, parents vary enormously in their response to the birth of their baby and the timing of their need to grieve.

For many parents, in the early weeks of their baby's life, these emotions are put on hold, perhaps surfacing as the baby grows healthily, or in some cases not until months later, during preparation for another baby.

Lengthy hospitalisation means that families have become known to nursing staff, impressions are formed and assessments made. There are expectations about visitations and behaviours; for example, visiting often enough not to be labelled as neglectful parents, but not too often to become labelled as anxious, intrusive parents. Fortunately, in recent years in many hospitals with the introduction of a family-centred approach, nursing staff are being supported and thus can acknowledge their own emotional stress and can identify signs of anxiety in the parents and be more empathic.

Risk and protective factors

It is well known that premature and very sick infants are at risk for developmental problems (Bennett, 1988). Most studies initially focused on neurological and cognitive outcomes, although some studies have also included behavioural outcomes (see Minde, 2000, for studies). More recently, studies have included emotional development and mother–infant relationship in outcomes (Veddovi, Gibson, Kenny, Bowen & Starte, 2004; Wolke, 1998). Other factors that may have an impact on the outcome for a premature infant include:
- the amount of separation of infant and parent while in the hospital
- the opportunity the parents have had for talking through the pregnancy, birth and hospitalisation experience
- the neurological impairment of the infant
- the parents' perceptions of this baby—the pregnancy and birth
- the couple's relationship
- family support
- knowledge of infant development, in particular, development of premature infants
- the parents' capacity to read their baby's cues.

Biological risk factors

The dramatic increase in survival of low-birthweight infants, especially the ELBW, has been accompanied by a higher incidence of neuropsychiatric disorders in this population (see Minde, 2000, for studies). Lorenz et al. (1998) have suggested from their recent study in a population of ELBW infants, that each 1 per cent increment in survival increased the population of children with disabilities by 2 per cent.

Minde (2000) makes the point that although there has not been a similar increment in developmental disorders in premature infants with a birthweight of more than 1000 grams, VLBW children on average still show a 5–7 point lower IQ than same age controls and 25 per cent exhibit significant abnormalities of cognition and/or behaviour. This is probably a conservative figure for other studies have found up to 40 per cent with behaviour difficulties (see Minde 2000, for details of studies).

Behavioural risk factors

It has been observed since 1964 (Drillien) that VLBW infants are at risk for a range of behavioural difficulties including major and minor psychiatric disorders. Even earlier, Benton (1940) described children born prematurely as restless, easily tired and nervous, which resulted in distractibility and poor concentration.

However, most studies of the 1970s and 1980s only looked at physical and cognitive development and did not look at behavioural characteristics.

Minde's study (Minde, Perrotta & Hellmann, 1988) looking at outcomes of a premature birth and the experience of NICU, found at four years that all the children showed normal intelligence and good physical health. However, 43 per cent of the children scored within the abnormal range on a behaviour questionnaire completed by the parents, which indicated a likelihood of a behaviour disorder. This was four times higher than found in a nonclinical group. Teachers rating a preschool behaviour questionnaire found 24 per cent of premature children scored in the abnormal range. After analysing the problems indicated by parents and teachers, Minde conceptualised the symptoms to represent a general immaturity, possible hyperactivity, or an overall poor behavioural organisation. However, only 10.9 per cent received a psychiatric diagnosis.

The same population was assessed on the Ainsworth Strange Situation Procedure (SSP) at 12 months (see Chapter 2 for a description of the SSP) and differences between secure and insecure attachment did not predict high or low scores on the behaviour questionnaire at age four. However, 75 per cent of children who were given a 'D' (disorganised) classification at 12 months were given a psychiatric diagnosis three years later. Minde et al. (1988) suggest that the disorganised attachment classification may predict premature children's emotional disturbance. For the teacher's ratings, it was the mother–child relationship and family functioning that were the best predictors of behavioural difficulties. This confirms what other authors report; that for premature infants, as for all infants, the best predictor for emotional outcome is the infant–mother relationship and family variables.

Heidelise Als has focused on the NICU environment and its effects on infants who have suddenly been displaced from the 'econiche' of the maternal womb, which functions to nurture neurodevelopmental progress to an 'unecological' environment. Als refers to the severing of continuous organism–environment interaction and other developmental principles, which explains many of the neurodevelopmental problems these infants experience, and the difficulties for parents (Als & Gilkerson, 1997). For example, the interference with the development of cortical neurones, which occurs at a phenomenal rate in the middle and later part of the pregnancy, would affect infant attention and self-regulation, making the infant more difficult to 'read' by the parent.

Relationship between the premature infant and caregiver

Many researchers of prematurity have looked at the relationship between the infant and her caregiver and the effect of prematurity on that relationship. The interaction between parent and infant, and caregiver responsivity, is a key component of the child's final intellectual and behavioural outcome.

It has been noted, for instance, that the mothers of premature infants show continuing anxiety and lack confidence in their caregiving, at least in their infant's first year (Mayes et al., 2002). It is hypothesised that premature infants, who are often erratic in their behaviour and are less attentive, make it difficult for the parents to read their infant's needs and respond appropriately to facilitate the infant achieving regulation. Parents who have risk factors of their own, for example, drug addiction or no social supports, will have more difficulty focusing on the often difficult to interpret needs of their infant. Also, the trauma of a premature birth may often awaken earlier traumatic experiences of the parent, which will interfere with the parent's capacity to be sensitively attuned to the premature infant's needs.

Montrasio (1997) discusses the inherent and possible difficulties of a premature birth or illness in infancy and the possible consequences on the relationship. Montrasio states 'every infant, and a premature child more than other children, can be competent only to the extent that the caregiving context is responsive to the reflexive self-functioning in the child' (p. 12).

Minde (2000) refers to 'process studies' (p. 182), which acknowledge that many events and interactions interweave to determine outcomes for premature infants. This is a very important point to note. The recent work by Brisch et al. (2003) indicates that for the high-risk, VLBW infants the quality of attachment could be influenced by cerebral risk factors and neurodevelopment. Without intervention, the mother's responsiveness to her infant with serious neurological disability was not sufficiently protective to ensure a secure attachment.

On the other hand, where the attachment classification of the infant at 14 months was identified as disorganised, this was independent of the premature infant's neurological profile, indicating that this pattern of attachment was more likely to be as a consequence of infant–mother interaction than of neurological impairment.

Another recent study (Keren, Feldman, Eidelman, Sirota & Lester, 2003) examined the relationship between mothers' representations of their infants, pregnancy and premature birth and mother–infant interactions. The authors found that mothers with positive maternal representations of their premature infants, the pregnancy, birth process and experience in the NICU, a factor labelled 'Readiness for Motherhood' (as obtained from a semi-structured interview), had more optimal interactions with their babies in the NICU than mothers with negative representations. Better maternal adaptation to the infant's signals and maternal positive touch were negatively related to maternal depression. The maternal negative representations factor of 'Maternal Rejection' predicted the interaction behaviour, 'Infant Withdrawal'. Maternal rejection included items such as unplanned pregnancy and negative first reaction to pregnancy, revealing that maternal negative attitudes towards the infant started well before the infant was born and were later linked to negative perceptions of the born baby.

Keren et al. (2003) found that the infant's medical condition did not affect the mother's level of anxiety or depression, but was an important factor in the parent's representations. Mothers of high-risk infants scored less on readiness for motherhood, touched their infants less often and were less adaptive to their infants than the mothers of low-risk infants. The infant's medical condition did not affect the negative attitudes as depicted in the maternal rejection factor that were linked more to prenatal representations.

These findings stress the importance of obtaining the parents' narrative about their baby to determine those at risk of having difficulties in their interactions with their infant and depression. It also confirms that the sickest infants were vulnerable to less optimal interactions with their parents.

Parental trauma

There are individual differences in the experience of trauma for each parent of any premature infant. A premature birth can hold different significance depending on factors in the parents' lives and experience, and their effect on the birth experience.

Some of the common characteristics of the experiences of parents of premature infants have been described by researchers interested in the psychological impact of this abrupt transition to parenthood. Tracey (2000) has identified the following features:

- an initial lack of affect when describing the experience of the birth—a lack of a sense of the internal meaning of events
- later return of emotion as the infant is gradually handed over to the care of the parents
- terror of death; always for the infant and sometimes for the mother
- shock
- marked differences in feelings and attitudes towards parenting compared with parents of full-term infants
- increased period of early preoccupation with the infant after return home from hospital
- ambivalence towards staff who both protect and sustain the life of the infant, but also come between the mother and infant.

Tracey (2000), in a study of the emotions of parents of premature infants, found that the rupturing of normal birth processes also had a significant effect on the emotional connection within the family unit. Tracey conducted research on 12 couples over 12 weeks, identifying emotional processes affected by the premature birth of an infant. The experience of trauma was found to be significant to all parents, and to have a range of effects. According to Tracey, trauma affects a range of emotional processes and therefore has an effect on the way that parents of premature infants behave, think and gradually come to terms with what has happened.

Hospital ecology

For many parents of a premature or very sick infant, the first real meeting with the baby is in the NICU. The baby is in a Perspex box, attached to machines that emit intermittent electronic sounds. There is no privacy. Often, parents are shocked at the size and colour of their baby, expressing their observations in tones of disbelief: 'she looks like a hairy monkey' or 'he looks like a skinned rabbit'. They cannot touch their baby, they can only sit and look.

Instead of being able to get to know each other in the quietness and intimacy of their own home, the new family has to do so in the rarefied environment of the NICU. The family has to accommodate nursing and medical staff and negotiate opportunities to hold, feed and bathe their baby. Ordinarily, in the first days and weeks of the infant's life there are hundreds of acts of intimacy between new parents and their baby, which are the building blocks of the relationship. For the parents of the premature and very sick infant there is limited contact and the parents struggle with their identity as mother and father.

At the point of discharge, reality dawns. They did have a baby and suddenly they are totally responsible for her welfare.

Availability of social supports

Lack of social supports when parents take their premature or sick infant home is a definite risk to the relationship between parents and infants. The parents are traumatised, often highly anxious, and fearful of their infant getting sick, getting an infection, or dying. They sleep lightly or fitfully and are likely to be sleep deprived. Family or other support whom the parents can trust to care for their baby enable the parents to have essential respite.

Where there is no family support, community supports may help to relieve the stress on parents.

Infant regulation

A feature of prematurity is a delay in the process of the infant obtaining self-regulation. As with sick infants and infants with neurological problems, often their early signals for tiredness, hunger or readiness for communication are subtle and easily missed and the infant moves quickly to intense distress. These signals are more difficult for parents to read, creating more anxiety in the parents and professionals.

Experience of pregnancy and past obstetric history

The experience of adverse pregnancy and past obstetric history is potentially a risk factor for the ongoing mental health of most parents who have had a premature or sick infant. Often, with women who have a premature birth, there have been past terminations or miscarriages of previous pregnancies. A number are associated with fertility assistance. Sometimes, the disruption or loss of the previous pregnancy has been so traumatic, associated with serious illness in the mother, that the mother's capacity for connecting with her live infant is delayed or seriously disrupted. In other situations, the trauma is put aside and resurfaces when the mother is pregnant with another baby.

Some abnormalities are identified in utero; for example, a history of polyhydramnios in the pregnancy indicates the likelihood of tracheo-oesophageal fistula in the newborn. Identification of a problem in utero cements an anxiety often experienced by pregnant women, that of having a disabled child. This knowledge, with its uncertainty of outcome, may interfere with the work of emotionally preparing for the baby. In addition, the mother is often hospitalised for several weeks prior to the birth of the baby, interfering with the relationship between the couple and the physical preparation for the baby.

Assessment and formulation principles

A careful history and clinical interview needs to be taken to establish factors that interfere with the parents' capacity to care for their infant, including:
- the parents' prior opportunity to debrief the experience
- the parents' representations of this infant
- family and social supports
- whether this was a planned and wanted baby
- what community supports are available
- economic pressures on the family
- knowledge the parents have about premature development or their baby's illness.

Infant developmental assessment

A developmental assessment, for example, using the Neonatal Behavioural Assessment Scale (Brazelton & Nugent, 1995), shared with the parents at the time of taking their baby home gives important information to the clinician and the family. The assessment allows the parents to observe their baby's unique characteristics, response to handling, and strengths, and where the baby needs extra support. The clinician obtains a clear picture of the baby's tolerance of handling, signs of stress and availability, and how much support the infant requires to return to a calm state after stimulation. The information gained from the assessment forms the basis of the intervention with the family to address the developmental needs of the baby.

Once a careful history has been taken and an assessment of the infant has been obtained, an agreement is made between the clinician and the family as to ongoing involvement by the clinician or other agencies.

At the very least, these parents usually need to have the opportunity to debrief the experience of the previous weeks and sometimes months. They also frequently require some information as to the developmental needs of their particular infant. For example:
- how their premature infant has two birthdays, the day on which she was born and the day on which the baby was due to be born
- that for developmental purposes, for at least the first three years, it is the day on which she was due to be born that is significant
- the importance of sleep and a rhythm of light sleep, deep sleep, quiet alertness and active awake time to their infant's development
- that premature babies and babies who are ill or have developmental delay often require assistance to get to sleep, assistance in the form of wrapping and/or holding until the baby's body is relaxed before placing her in a bassinette or carrying her in a sling (to allow the infant to feel human closeness and relax to sleep, as infants prefer to sleep in the company of others)
- that many premature, ill, or infants with developmental delay are inclined to be extended in their bodies and thus benefit from being carried in a sling to enable them to maintain a curled posture, which assists them in getting to sleep
- that their particular baby has been denied the normal closeness experienced by healthy full-term infants and will require extra holding and body-to-body contact in the first few months of their time together and that infants cannot be spoilt when their needs are met in this way
- that the more extreme forms of behavioural techniques to get infants to sleep through the night are completely inappropriate for their baby, given the baby's history to date. A more appropriate approach would be to find respite for the parents to enable them to get uninterrupted sleep.

Most families with a premature or sick infant will have ongoing appointments with medical services, either at specialists' rooms or at the hospital, and with a follow-up clinic with allied health services. Very often these parents require someone who can monitor their baby's progress and their well-being in a holistic way, with whom they can share their ongoing concerns and often their stages of grieving as they adjust to the baby they have, rather than the baby of their dreams.

Often the clinician will recommend referral to additional services as the need arises.

Intervention principles

The developmental challenges are the same for premature, ill or developmentally delayed infants as they are for full-term healthy infants, but the parents have to be more sensitively available. This often requires professional help, for the social myth is that the baby will be 'spoilt' if her particular needs are addressed. Intervention offered at key points of change is particularly important; for example, at discharge, three months, six months, 12–18 months and three years (Brazelton, 1993).

Intervention based on the assessment of the infant and offered in the context of the parents' concerns will be incorporated into the parents' handling of the infant (Dolby, Warren, Meade & Heath, 1987).

The example of Rosemary, John and Alexandria, below, illustrates that issues the parent has will become apparent as the infant's behaviour challenges the parent's vulnerabilities. Sensitive listening to the parent and helping the mother to distinguish between her 'ghosts from the past' and the infant's behaviour will allow more responsive attention to her infant.

EXAMPLE: ROSEMARY, JOHN AND ALEXANDRIA

Alexandria was born at 28 weeks gestational age by caesarean section, weighing 825 grams, parity 2 and gravida 1. At the time of Alexandria's birth she was admitted to the Neonatal Intensive Care Unit (NICU) because of respiratory distress and very low birthweight. Apgars were four and nine. Pathological disease processes documented in the NICU unit were:

- *hyaline membrane disease*
- *apnoea*
- *chronic lung disease*
- *necrotising enterocolitis*
- *no periventricular haemorrhage.*

Alexandria required mechanical ventilation for 36 days, multiple peripheral arterial lines, phototherapy as the bilirubin level rose to 117 (mc Mol/L) and blood transfusion and TPN for 10 days.

Rosemary and John, both professionals, were first-time parents with no family in the city they live in. They visited the NICU regularly, Rosemary often twice a day to express breastmilk and bathe her baby. Staff noted that Alexandria was slow to put on weight and that the parents were very anxious.

As the time approached for Alexandria's discharge from hospital, Rosemary and John expressed a desire to receive as much information as possible about how to care for her at home. They had heard a talk given on prematurity at the parents' group in the nursery by a staff member from a home-visiting program attached to the hospital. The nursery staff made a referral to the program, noting that

Alexandria was 'hard to settle' and 'wound up'. The referral also noted the parents' expressed wish for more information about the development of premature infants. It was arranged that someone from the program would see both parents the next day after they had a night with their daughter in the room with them. At the time Rosemary and John were having their first night with Alexandria, she was two and a half weeks post due date, having been in hospital for over 100 days.

The day after the referral to the home-visiting program, the nurse from the program made contact with Rosemary and arranged to call at the end of the day: they had roomed in for the first time the previous night. Rosemary presented as a well-dressed, good-looking articulate woman in her thirties. As the brief was that she wanted information about premature development, during the first contact the nurse talked about the developmental issues for Alexandria, that is, achieving a calm base of deep sleep (16–18 hours in 24) and brief periods of quiet alertness. She explained that their reciprocal role as parents was to be a stimulus buffer or filter to protect Alexandria from being bombarded. On asking how things had been since Rosemary had roomed in, Rosemary explained that Alexandria had been restless that morning, not settling into a deep sleep.

The nurse spoke of Alexandria's need to achieve a curled posture to be still and demonstrated wrapping to keep her flexed, whereupon Alexandria went into a quiet sleep. It was stressed that Alexandria had two birthdays, and how, for all developmental purposes, she was a couple of weeks past her due date, that is, two weeks corrected for prematurity.

Rosemary responded with great interest, and seemed to absorb all that was said. Although the nurse recognised Rosemary's anxiety, it seemed manageable. The next day the nurse called again to be told Alexandria was back in the nursery. Rosemary and her husband were sitting in the lounge room and Rosemary said that Alexandria had a cold, and so they were not going to take her home—they had waited so long another few days wouldn't matter. The nurse was sympathetic and they talked for a few moments.

Rosemary said she was booked to room in again the following Monday. The nurse suggested she would probably only stay one night. Rosemary gasped and the nurse suddenly understood how terrified she was of taking the baby home. Quietly it was suggested that it was scary and Rosemary agreed and burst into tears. Empathy for Rosemary's anxiety was expressed, possible supports were discussed and arrangements made to meet the next week when she returned, and an assurance was given that they would be visited at home.

The next week the nurse again met with Rosemary and John while they were still rooming in with Alexandria, and their concern was Alexandria's irritability. Rosemary had found the wrap useful the week before and now discovered she had to hold Alexandria for some minutes after she was wrapped, before her body relaxed and the 'noises ceased'. It was only then Rosemary could put Alexandria in the bassinette and know she would remain calm.

Rosemary's question was what to do if Alexandria didn't settle? They were assured that she would if Rosemary and John stayed with what they had decided to do. Once they knew she was well fed, had a clean nappy, then they were to wrap and hold her. It was explained that it was important for Alexandria to know there was someone there for her, who was going to hold and contain her in her discomfort.

Alexandria was discharged the next day after 15 weeks in hospital, at almost four months of age, one month corrected age. Intervention was to continue at home.

During the first visit at home to Rosemary, John and Alexandria, Rosemary described her experience of the pregnancy and birth. Rosemary shared the details of her previous miscarriage and the difficult pregnancy. The previous year Rosemary had had a miscarriage at eight weeks. She found this distressing. Rosemary felt the doctor was not caring and was critical when she became pregnant again in two months. It was then that the nurse understood Rosemary's extreme anxiety and doubt about her ability to successfully nurture her baby.

During the first pregnancy she had a lot of energy. During the second pregnancy she was not happy, not sad, never 'super duper' and put this down to hormones. Things went quite well until six months. Her diet changed during the pregnancy—she got gastric reflux, indigestion—the beginnings of a hiatus hernia. Rosemary visited a doctor while on holiday who thought it might be gallstones. Her local GP suggested she change her diet. The baby had moved, pushing up under her ribs. In the seventh month she began to feel well. However, she went to her scheduled appointment with the obstetrician and her blood pressure was high. She was put into hospital overnight because of hypertension and then transferred to a teaching hospital with a Level 3 NICU.

The next morning Alexandria was delivered at 6.15 a.m. by caesarean section. Rosemary's blood pressure was down within a week and two weeks later it was back to normal. Rosemary reflected that it hadn't been a pleasant pregnancy and she was relieved when that period was over.

Rosemary went on to say that before the family left the hospital, the staff had expressed concern about Alexandria's weight gain and wanted Rosemary and Alexandria to stay in hospital to sort out feeds. Rosemary decided she wanted to get home and so went home with a supply line. On this first visit, Rosemary felt depressed at home—missed the company of the hospital. She felt more exhausted especially when Alexandria woke for protracted periods in the early hours.

Both Rosemary and John, but especially John, found they could settle Alexandria if they wrapped her firmly and held her until her body stilled and she was quiet, then put her into her bassinette. They had attended a Family Support Cottage during the week and confidently shared their knowledge of 'premies', that is, how premature infants have difficulty settling and need to be wrapped and held and how it was inappropriate to put a premature baby in the pram and 'let her cry'. Another visit was organised for the following week.

As no developmental assessment had been done with Alexandria prior to discharge it was decided that an assessment would be carried out at the next visit when Alexandria was five weeks corrected age. The behavioural assessment was the Neonatal Behavioural Assessment Scale (NBAS). The assessment revealed Alexandria's difficulty in regulating her attention, shown by her inclination to hyperalertness, her increased muscle tone and jerky movements, and her poor state control indicated by her persistent fussy state. Alexandria's strengths were that she was responsive when cuddled and held curled, relaxing and looking into the face of the person holding her and she quietened when spoken to. It was apparent that Alexandria was going to need assistance in gaining regulation of her states, and also wrapping and being curled in, to help her flex and reduce the increased muscle tone.

The parents observed the assessment and noted Alexandria's responses when wrapped and held firmly and also how she quietened and paid attention when spoken to. The parents were growing in confidence in being able to contain and read Alexandria.

Rosemary and John reported that they heard Alexandria's cry as a plea to be held. In the holding Alexandria gained control of her body and was able to be still and settle. And Rosemary gained confidence in knowing she could quieten her baby and help her get to sleep. Alexandria gained weight, and began to have a brief awake time around the feed.

Contact with the family was maintained by phone with visits at key points of developmental change—two to three, four, nine and 12 months corrected age.

Over the early weeks, Alexandria's periods of quiet alertness and settled sleep increased. At four months the increased muscle tone remained, so the physiotherapist on the team suggested some handling techniques to further assist flexion. Alexandria struggled with getting to sleep, and at this age Rosemary had expectations Alexandria could do it alone. The issue of giving Alexandria the help she needed to get to sleep herself was discussed and a strategy implemented that reassured Alexandria that her parents were there as she needed them. This enabled Alexandria to get to sleep with minimal fuss and sleep for longer periods at night.

At each developmental challenge, when Alexandria demanded Rosemary's assistance and attention, Rosemary also felt challenged. For example, when Alexandria was four months and couldn't sit and play independently, and when she was nine months and crawled away from her mother to explore, get stuck and *demand help. In discussing Alexandria's behaviour—her assumption that her mother was there for her—Rosemary expressed that she found it difficult that 'the control is being taken by Alexandria'. Further discussion revealed that Rosemary had struggled hard for control of her own life as she was growing up in a family with a very dominating mother. Talking it through enabled Rosemary to separate her mother's desire to control from Alexandria's striving towards autonomy within the scaffolding of her mother's assistance and focus. The 'ghosts' were put to rest and Rosemary could more unequivocally attend to Alexandria's needs.*

At 12 months corrected age:
- *Alexandria was developmentally appropriate for her corrected age on both Mental and Motor Bayley Developmental Scales*
- *Alexandria was confident, had good concentration, was able to stay focused on a toy or task, and had the ability to play on her own. She enjoyed the interaction with the examiner.*

SUMMARY

Newborn behaviour is oriented towards the development of regulation in a number of systems or states. When these systems are affected by prematurity, illness or other disorders the infant's move towards self-regulation is significantly delayed or disturbed. Infants cannot be expected to begin to respond in developmentally appropriate ways until a level of physiological stability is attained. During the time of delayed connections between infant and parent, clinicians can work to foster the development of this bond by sharing the care of the infant with the parents, and actively promoting the parents' ability to understand and recognise their infant's cues and signals. By keeping the importance of the infant–parent relationship in mind, difficulties that parents may face in relating and responding to their infant can be minimised. Where a child has a chronic illness or an ongoing condition that delays development, long-term support of parents will be required. Each developmental change will bring new challenges to these parents and their infants that will require support and guidance. Opportunities for parents to debrief, grieve and reflect on past experiences are also important in fostering the infant–parent bond.

CHAPTER 7

Sleeping

KEY CONCEPTS

- Sleep–wake rhythms
- The effect of self-regulation
- The effect of the infant–parent relationship

FACTORS IN ASSESSMENT AND FORMULATION

- Developmental stage and parental expectations
- Regulatory disorders
- Parental internal working model and projections
- The caregiving environment

The development of infant sleeping patterns is a complex process with great variability between different infants. Infant sleeping patterns are influenced by biopsychosocial factors including developmental changes, self-regulation characteristics, parenting patterns and actions, and the caregiving environment. Sleep problems in infancy are a common reason for seeking clinical help. The prevalence of poor sleep habits in children under two years is approximately 15 per cent (Minde, 1997). Anders, Goodlin-Jones and Sadeh (2000) do not classify sleep problems under 12 months, as the patterns are changing rapidly.

Many sleep problems can be solved by providing information on the infant's developmental needs and requirements. But at other times, problems with infant self-regulation, disruptions or disturbances to the attachment relationship or factors in the caregiving environment may be the cause.

Infants learn to go to sleep within the context of a 'good enough' infant–parent relationship. Because of the complexity of the relationship between infant, parent and sleep, a careful understanding of the sleep problem and the context in which it is occurring needs to be obtained. The infant's sleep disturbance may reflect, for example, anxiety in the parent, difficulties in the parents' relationship, parenting lifestyle, past experiences of the parent that are not resolved, the developmental stage of the infant or a misunderstanding of the infant's ability in relation to a sleep pattern. Assessment should start with a careful history to determine possible links between the sleep problem and the past and current history of the infant, the parents and their lives together. Further assessment may include observing and testing the infant for self-regulatory problems, examination of the caregiving environment, or exploration of interactional issues between the parent and infant, such as internal representations of parenting and possible projections onto the infant. Intervention may include guiding and supporting parental responsiveness with their newborn, therapy for infant regulatory problems, or counselling for parenting issues that are unconsciously affecting the infant's sleep behaviour.

THE BASIS OF SLEEP

> The development of sleep-wake organization is intimately involved in the emerging attachment relationship and the process of self-regulation (Anders, Goodlin-Jones & Sadeh, 2000, p. 326).

In the first week or two after birth, most babies fall asleep on the breast or bottle and sleep for periods of two to four hours. It is thought that this is recovery from the birth experience. By four weeks, most babies are more alert and responsive and the early rhythm of sleep, a brief awake period including a feed, followed by sleep again, changes.

The baby's goal is to establish a rhythm of light and deep sleep, quiet awake and active awake periods. Most babies (70–80 per cent) achieve this rhythm, with longer sleep periods overnight, by four to six months (Minde, 1997). It is the 20–30 per cent who do not achieve this rhythm who present as a 'sleep problem'.

For a variety of reasons it is unrealistic to expect an infant to achieve the rhythm before three to four months. The reasons include:
- the development of the brain—the average baby of three to four months develops a regulatory capacity, which means he can inhibit arousal and drop quickly into deep sleep
- the size of the stomach
- the physiology of breastmilk production.

Some parents have concerns if their baby finds it difficult to get to sleep, is not sleeping through the night or is not achieving a predictable rhythm by four to six months, and seek assistance. Others do not see these situations as a problem and will continue to respond to the infant's needs and trust that the infant will establish his own rhythm in time.

The biopsychosocial model of sleep acknowledges that a baby has an inbuilt potential to establish sleep–wake organisation and to regulate sleep patterns, but it is not possible for the baby to do it alone. The baby requires an available parent to facilitate his emerging capacity for self-regulation (see Chapter 1). Self-regulation is fostered by the parent's ability to meet the baby's need for nurturing and social interaction, that is, the parent's ability to read and respond to the baby's cues for food, sleep and quiet conversation when awake. Often this requires providing whatever help the baby needs to achieve sleep. Some babies, who find it difficult to still their bodies for sleep, require much more holding and containment than others. Containment means a firm embrace or wrapping of the baby, which reduces movements of the arms and legs, and back arching. Being available to a baby's needs requires that the parent is capable of emotional and physical availability, which in turn is influenced by personal and social factors, in particular, emotional, social and physical support available to the parent.

Normal development of sleep–wake rhythms

In the first few months of life, a newborn establishes internal body rhythms of sleep and wakefulness. These rhythms are known as the diurnal and ultradian clocks. When a baby is born neither the diurnal nor the ultradian clock is organised or 'set'. With time and the availability of a responsive carer, the patterns emerge.

The diurnal clock

The diurnal clock drives the day waking/night sleeping cycle, sometimes referred to as the circadian rhythm. There is enormous variation in the amount of sleep occurring in 24 hours for newborns, but, in general, most infants sleep approximately 18 hours out of 24, in blocks of three to four hours, with short awake periods in between. The newborn does not distinguish day from night. The pattern of sleeping longer at night emerges gradually as the infant experiences more activity, sound and interaction with carers during the day, and less at night.

> *At eight weeks, Isabelle began to sleep from after her 10 p.m. feed through until 2 a.m. Then she would feed again and go back to sleep quickly, until 6 a.m. After a few more weeks, I could see that she was somehow losing interest in the 2 a.m. feed so I tried dropping it and settled her with patting instead of feeding. I was thrilled to see that she quickly adapted to this and began to sleep from 10 p.m. until about 4 or 5 a.m.* (Catherine, 33.)

As described by Catherine, above, a gradual process of consolidation of sleeping periods at night occurs in the first six months. By six months of age, night sleep extends to up to twelve hours, consisting of a number of coalescing sleeps, with brief wakings, sometimes for at least one feed. Wakeful periods also begin to combine during the day to produce longer periods of daytime wakefulness separated by one to three shorter sleeps of one to three hours.

By one year of age, diurnal organisation is well established. There are usually one to two long periods of sleep at night and two shorter naps during the day. This pattern gradually gives way to two periods of sleep in 24 hours during the second year—an afternoon nap and an overnight sleep. This pattern remains throughout life, however, the afternoon nap is often forgone.

The ultradian clock

The ultradian clock refers to short sleep cycles that occur within a period of sleep. These intra-sleep cycles are characterised by alternations between rapid eye movement and non rapid eye movement (REM and NREM) sleep.

> **Rapid Eye Movement (REM) sleep**
> REM sleep is light—the body may move, breathing is irregular and shallow, and the infant is more easily disturbed by the outside world. During REM sleep brain growth and differentiation of nervous pathways occur.
>
> **Non Rapid Eye Movement (NREM) sleep**
> NREM sleep is quiet—eyes are firmly closed, breathing is deep and regular, and the infant is less easily affected by the outside world. The function of NREM sleep is to rest and organise the infant's immature and easily overwhelmed nervous system.

The newborn ultradian cycle length is 45–60 minutes, 50 per cent of which is REM sleep. Newborns start a sleep cycle with 20 minutes onset of REM sleep, often after feeding and while being held. In order to sleep longer than this initial 20 minutes, the newborn must make a transition to deep NREM sleep. The newborn is easily disturbed or awakened during this transitional phase but may drop into deep NREM sleep spontaneously or if assisted to settle, for example, by holding, 'wearing' in sling, or by rocking.

By three to four months the ultradian sleep cycle is 'set' at 60 minutes. The slow drifts of light sleep are replaced by quick drops into 20-minute periods of NREM (quiet) sleep. As the infant matures, the proportionate amount of REM sleep occurring in each cycle decreases. A phase of REM sleep continues to recur every 50–60 minutes, however, the early cycles in the night have proportionately more NREM or 'quiet' sleep, and later cycles have more REM or 'light' sleep.

By four months the baby can inhibit arousal stimuli and if woken can return to sleep alone or with minimal assistance. Babies at four months usually sleep until midnight and wake every two hours after this, however. Parents are not always aware of this as the baby may not call out, however, they usually continue to have at least one feed overnight. The sleep cycle remains at 60 minutes until adolescence when the cycle lengthens to 90 minutes and remains at this length into adulthood.

Effect of sleep–wake rhythms

Although the sleep–wake rhythm is established by three to four months, it cannot be assumed that infants move between light and deep sleep without waking. Infants still wake up as part of these emerging patterns. This may be due to internal factors (for example, hunger or feeling cold) or external factors in the environment that are not conducive to sleep (for example, a loud noise). An infant who has always had help in getting to sleep and has not as yet learnt to do it alone will find it difficult to get himself back to sleep after waking. Moving smoothly in and out of deep sleep without waking is an aspect of self-regulation.

Effect of self-regulation on sleep

Infants have different capacities in learning to self-regulate (see Chapter 1). Some of this variation may reflect irregularities in maturational and constitutional factors of the infant, or the variation may be due to challenges in the interactional or family environment. Some infants have been identified as 'sensitive high needs' babies, who startle easily, are sensitive to loud noises and light, and who in general are difficult to settle and care for. Where parents are able to be sensitively responsive, recognising their infant's inability to successfully process stimuli, provide the necessary reduction or filtering of the stimulation, and contain the infant, the infant learns to regulate the sensory input and thus gain regulation.

The contemporary construct of regulatory disorders suggests that in some infants and toddlers, self-regulation may be disturbed and may underlie a number of presenting difficulties including sleep problems.

As the capacity for self-regulation develops, the infant is able to move between deep and light sleep states without waking, or, if waking, is able to get back to sleep without assistance. An infant who startles easily, and who may have an immature neurological system, has more difficulty regulating himself and requires assistance to return to sleep. A large part of a successful block of sleep is due to self-regulation, but the possible causes of why an infant is unable to self-regulate are difficult to determine.

Infant–parent interaction

The interactive nature of the rhythm between mother and infant influences the process of sleeping. Characteristics of the infant, the mother, and the father or partner (to a lesser extent), influence interactions between the mother and infant, and affect sleep processes. Constitutional factors as well as life experiences such as the birth process can affect the capacity of the infant for regulation of the autonomic, physiological, motor and state systems.

Infants with poorer regulation require more sensitive handling from their parents to establish a sleep routine. These high-need infants may include those who have experienced a difficult birth, require frequent hospitalisations or are born premature. These infants are likely to require more sensitively attuned nurturing than babies born full term without problems. The parents' capacity to be available to their infant's needs influences the interaction with the infant. Parental availability can be affected by:
- the birth process
- the parents' knowledge of and sensitivity to their infant's needs
- the parents' physical and mental health
- family and other supports
- past losses experienced by parents, the mother in particular.

A healthy full-term infant is less dependent on a sensitive environment to achieve an appropriate pattern of sleep–wake cycles.

The attachment relationship

The development of a secure attachment relationship is the optimal outcome of the infant–parent interaction over the first year. As discussed in Chapters 1 and 2, attachment involves the development of the affective or emotional bond between the infant and his mother and other significant carers in the first year. It is the culmination of all development in the first year and the basis of later relationships. It is known that infants have a hierarchy of attachment relations with the primary carers, with usually mother and father being the preferred attachment figures and optimally providing a secure base for the infant. (Patterns of attachment are discussed in Chapter 2.)

The many transitions between sleep and waking provide the opportunity for regulating experiences for the infant that address biological needs such as hunger, temperature and discomfort, and social or affective needs such as security, comfort, separation and reunion (Anders et al., 2000). Anders and colleagues argue that the repeated separations between infant and parent that characterise transitions from waking to sleep states are a simulation of the Strange Situation Procedure (SSP) developed by Mary Ainsworth (Ainsworth, Blehar, Waters & Wall, 1978) to assess the pattern of attachment between infants and their caregivers. (For a description of the SSP, see Chapter 2.)

The attachment system is activated when the infant experiences fear and anxiety, and is deactivated when the infant is consoled, comforted and feels safe in the presence of his parent or caregiver. An infant who is securely attached who awakes at night and is frightened will anticipate the parent responding to his cries and with comfort will settle back to sleep. On the other hand, insecure infants may react in different ways. If insecure/ambivalent, the infant will cry, but not be comforted by the parent and the anxiety and crying will escalate until the parent succumbs to what the infant wants, or becomes angry and, for example, feeds the infant or takes the infant into the parents' bed, begrudgingly. A child with an insecurely avoidant pattern would not anticipate the parent responding and so would learn, often prematurely, to get himself back to sleep. The consequences of this for the infant are an early emotional self-reliance, with a reduction of emotional expression, in particular, negative emotions.

The context of interaction

The context of interaction refers to the relationships in which the infant–parent relationship is embedded, including the presence or otherwise of a partner, grandparents and other children. Past relationships of the parents will also influence how the parents respond to the demands of their infant.

The environment

The infant's environment, both immediate and distant, is very dependent on parental availability and circumstances. The optimal context for the infant is to be within the parents' sensory environment (Mosko, McKenna, Dickel & Hunt, 1993). Mahler, Pine and Bergman (1975) endorse close proximity with the mother and refer to the 12 months of pregnancy—nine months in the womb and three months out, meaning that the close connection when the baby is in utero needs to be continued after the baby is born, with the baby separating gradually.

WHERE THE INFANT SLEEPS

Parents make different choices regarding where their infant will sleep, influenced by cultural norms, available space, and advice from health professionals and others. Babies prefer to sleep within the sensory environment of their parent in the first few weeks of life (Mosko et al., 1993). This means the young infant is within sensory stimulation reach, and parental sensory cues are available—touch, movement, breathing sounds, smells, temperature exchanges and partner-induced arousals. According to Stein, Colaruso, McKenna and Powers (2001), being within sensory stimulation reach allows the baby to stir and go back to sleep, being aware that he is in the presence of the other.

An example of sleeping within the sensory environment (co-sleeping) is to place the baby in a bassinette or cot next to the mother, or to extend the parent's bed with a piece of boarding and mattress. However, for some, the noises of the baby may interfere with sleep and it may be necessary to place the baby further away. What is important is that the primary caregiver is responsive to changes in the infant's state of arousal.

Sleeping with the baby (one form of co-sleeping) also brings the baby within the sensory environment of the parent. In many countries and cultures, this is the accepted practice. However, in Australia, this sleeping pattern is surrounded by controversy and guilt in parents, as there is a risk of rolling onto the baby while asleep or the baby smothering under bedding. It is not advisable to have a baby in the parents' bed if parents have been drinking alcohol, taking drugs or smoking. Also, the baby needs to sleep on a firm mattress with his head above the bedclothes at all times, and not where he could be dropped between the wall and the bed. Sleeping with the baby in the parents' bed is also not advisable if the infant is being 'used' to meet parental needs such as loneliness or conflict between the parents.

Integration of the basis of sleep

Most infants by four to six months have a sleep–wake pattern that is compatible with parental expectations. By this time parents begin to want more independence for themselves and their baby. The baby is able to drop off to sleep on his own because he can more effectively inhibit arousal stimuli as a result of his developing brain. The baby has a variety of communications and the parent is able to distinguish between the baby working on getting to sleep or requiring help, and responds. Also, as stated, the baby sleeps for longer periods at night, often interspersed with one to two feeds, and has two periods of one to two hours of sleep during the day.

SLEEP PROBLEMS

Sleep problems present in a number of ways. There are babies who find it difficult to settle to sleep, those who settle but wake and cannot get back to sleep alone and always require intervention, and there are babies who wake for long periods. When parents present with a sleep problem with their baby in the first few weeks of life it is often because the reality of the 24-hour-a-day demands of a baby does not relate to the parents' expectations. In these early weeks and months new parents need information to understand their infant's capacities in relation to sleep, and require support to help them make the adjustment to being parents.

After three to four months, parents' expectations change and they begin to expect fewer interruptions at night. From four to six months on, unsettled infants may be described in different ways.

Transient and transitional disturbances

Transient disturbances can occur because of physiological distress in the infant—'teething', rise in temperature, other transient medical conditions, developmental challenges, environmental changes such as weather changes, or changes in the sleeping arrangements of the household such as the infant being moved into his own room.

Adjustment disorders

An adjustment disorder is where there is a temporary reaction in the infant lasting days or weeks but no longer than four months, and a clearly identifiable environmental event such as the mother returning to work or the family moving house. Well-established sleep patterns can be disturbed as a consequence of change in a baby's or toddler's environment. Changes that are frequently reported to disturb sleep include the birth of a sibling, a parent being absent, a grandparent coming to stay, mother returning to work, the infant starting child care or being looked after by somebody else, or the infant and parent(s) being separated with a hospitalisation of the infant or a parent.

Nightmares and night terrors

While night terrors and nightmares usually occur in children between five and twelve years, they may begin during the toddler and preschool period. They are referred to as parasomnias, that is, disorders of arousal where motor and autonomic activation intrude on ongoing sleep. Night terrors occur in NREM (quiet) sleep, in males more than females and there is often a positive family history (Anders et al., 2000; Minde, 1997). It is difficult to know the difference between a bad dream or nightmare with a toddler as the symptoms of intense crying, poor responsiveness and inability to report the content of the dream can occur in either situation. Clinically, these children have no difficulty going to bed but wake crying one to three hours later and seem inconsolable. Very often, after one or other parent sits quietly consoling and holding the child, the crying ceases and the child returns to sleep. The next day the child has no memory of the night disturbance.

In contrast, nightmares are arousal from REM sleep, occur in the latter part of night sleep and are associated with dream accounts involving fears or anxiety. If the child has speech, nightmares can be recalled the next day. Once again, parent involvement at the time of the nightmare with lots of reassurance that the child is safe and protected, and a reduction in stress during the day, is the most effective treatment (Anders et al., 2000).

Maturational challenges to self-regulation

Situations where maturation affects self-regulation with possible effects on sleep include an infant frustrated by a desire to walk who may want to practise walking in bed, pull himself up to standing in the cot and then be unable to get back down. At this point the infant is wide awake and cries out for help to resettle.

Regulatory disorders

Sleeping problems related to getting to sleep or, when woken, getting back to sleep, are often related to difficulties with self-regulation, self-calming and the ability to manage transitions. These usually improve with maturation given a relatively consistent, sensitive and responsive environment. For some babies there can be both a distinct behavioural pattern, and a sensory, sensory–motor or organisational processing difficulty that affects daily adaptation and relationships (Greenspan & Wieder, 1993). An organisational processing difficulty implies that there are regulation difficulties in several systems, atypical patterns of sensory reactivity as well as difficulties with motor organisation and state regulation. Babies with considerable maturational or constitutional variations that contribute to specific behaviour may have a regulatory disorder (Greenspan, 1989). For example, premature infants, in the early weeks after discharge from hospital, which is around the time of the date when they were due to be born, often have difficulty keeping their bodies still, especially when tired. They also struggle with modulating auditory and visual stimulation and moving smoothly between states. This is usually a temporary situation and, tempered with sensitive, responsive care, continuing regulation difficulties can be avoided or minimised.

Behavioural patterns

Difficulties with either processing sensation (inflow) or motor planning (outflow)—that is, difficulties with being able to take in or respond back to the world—compromise the infant's ability to negotiate with and adjust to his caregivers and environment (Greenspan & Wieder, 1993). Initially, the parents present with concerns about their baby's feeding or sleeping, or express their frustration with their baby's irritability. Parents may talk of their baby being very sensitive to sound, touch or light. As toddlers, the problems may present as behaviour control difficulties, or fearfulness and anxiety. In the third year, parents may be concerned about speech or language problems, or they may speak of their child not being able to play alone or with others, or report that their child gets upset easily or has difficulty adjusting to change. Babies exhibiting these behaviours make daily caregiving and development of relationships difficult for their caregivers. These babies require very sensitive handling and more containment and holding and, in our society, parents are often accused of 'spoiling' them when they provide this level of support.

Very often a baby born prematurely, because of his organisational processing difficulty, will require much more assistance from his caregivers to achieve a rhythm of sleep and wake periods, as discussed in Chapter 6. To achieve sleep, he may require wrapping, holding firmly until the body stills, maybe gently rocking, and then placing in a crib in a darkened room.

Research into regulatory disorders is in its early days, with few empirical studies available to support the construct. The current understanding is primarily based on the clinical observations of experts in the field. Some empirical evidence is beginning to emerge from small studies, as well as from the work of occupational therapists investigating the related concept of sensory modulation, one aspect of the spectrum of regulatory disorders (Barton & Robins, 2000).

Relationship-based disturbances and disorders

When there is no evidence of regulatory involvement in the infant, and information on development and support has not changed the sleep problem, it is important to consider underlying factors in the infant–parent relationship. Unconscious feelings or past experiences of the parents may be influencing separation at sleep times. For example, has this mother experienced recent loss, or abandonment in her own childhood? Does separating from her child for sleep awaken embedded anxiety about abandonment?

Stern (1995) speaks of internal models, 'schema-of-being-with' another (p. 19), which are the template in the mind of oneself in interaction with a primary caregiver. These templates are laid down in the neural development of the brain in early infancy. The internal model determines how the individual interacts with others as he grows into adulthood, and remains as the preferred option of relationship unless other pathways are laid down as a consequence of different relationships through therapy, religious experiences or choice of partner. Thus, the model in the adult's head will largely determine that adult's interaction with her infant.

Intrapsychic factors in the mother

Several factors may make it difficult for the primary carer to allow the infant to work on getting to sleep by managing a little negative emotion or fussing from the baby. Possible causes may include:
- the death of a previous baby
- past terminations and associated feelings related to 'putting the baby down' to sleep
- how the parent was parented
- the parent's experience of abandonment.

Effect of the present and the past

Aspects of the parents' current situation have been associated with infant sleep problems: perinatal adversity, including caesarean section, neurotic symptoms, difficulties between parents, depressed mood and ambivalence towards their infant (Minde, 1997). Although the relationship between the mother's psychological difficulties and her infant's irregular sleep patterns is sometimes unclear, Minde found that the parents' contact with mental health clinicians preceded the sleeping problems of the infant. In fact, parents with insecure attachment to their own mothers were significantly more likely to have children with sleep problems (see Minde, 1997, for studies).

Possible effects on infant sleep

Fear of separation underlies some sleep problems. Being able to go to sleep and feel safe to stay asleep depends on feeling safe to be separate. Separation issues can become apparent at sleep onset and through night-time waking. Sleep-onset problems may include refusal to go to bed, crying and anxiety. These in turn may lead to angry bedtimes, punishment at bedtime, or tantrums, which of course increases anxiety in both infant and parent.

Night waking occurs when infants are unable to resettle to sleep on waking, call out for parents, cry on separations or are awake for long periods seeking parental comfort.

Parents and caregivers may have difficulty allowing their infant to fuss and settle himself to sleep alone (when it is developmentally appropriate to do so) out of concern that their infant may feel rejected, or may be harmed even though they have reassured the infant they are close by. Parents may be striving to overcome their own experiences of rejection as an infant by overcompensating with their own infant, or, alternatively, may be repeating their own experiences unconsciously.

ASSESSMENT, FORMULATION AND INTERVENTION PRINCIPLES

When an infant has problems with sleep, the whole family is usually affected. It is desirable to meet with both parents to determine their understanding of the problem, and how willing they both are to engage in the process of addressing the issue. The age of the infant is a determining factor in how to address the problem. As the family explains exactly what the problem is and how it would be if the problem were solved, it is possible to ascertain what form the intervention should take. In addition to observation of the infant and the interaction between the parents and the infant, there is opportunity to assess the capacity and motivation of the family to change. The content of the session could include developmental guidance, discussing alternative strategies, exploring the parents' supports, and the meaning of the sleep issue to them. Often the session will also include an understanding of their early parenting and how that affects how they are managing the regulation of sleep in their infant.

When assessment indicates that an underlying issue is pivotal in the sleep disturbance, then referral to an appropriate clinician may be required. Examples of this include underlying regulatory disorders, or parental issues, for example, depression, marital issues or 'projections' interfering with the infant's sleep patterns. However, in some situations parents may prefer to work on strategies to address the sleep issues, putting aside other issues in the short term. If this is the case, the clinician should keep the focus of the sessions on the sleep issues agreed upon.

Taking the history

The careful history should include:
- details of the pregnancy, including whether the baby was planned, and if unplanned, wanted.
- birth history and the infant's history since birth—the sleep pattern, any illnesses, separations from the parents, feeding and eating behaviour and general mood during the day. It is often useful to obtain a description of 24 hours with the infant. Parents are often asked to keep sleep schedules as a starting point to help gain an understanding of the basic sleeping and feeding patterns in their infant.
- the infant's age.
- how the infant indicates he is ready for sleep.
- how the infant's sleep behaviour is affecting the parents, and, in particular, how they are managing sleep deprivation.
- any concerns or symptoms that might indicate a medical problem, for example, a breathing disorder such as sleep apnoea, and if there are, has the infant been examined by a paediatrician?
- a brief summary of the parents' families of origin, relationship with parents, and any family stories and myths about the parents and their sleeping behaviour as infants.
- establishing exactly what the parents' concerns are and what they want to change.
- what they have done already to address the problem or try to bring about change.
- finding out what has worked. Does the infant have a favourite blanket or toy, or has any particular practice worked?
- observation of infant–parent interaction, looking particularly at how the parents respond to their infant's cues.

Developmental assessment

On some occasions, in particular with a toddler or older child, and depending on the observations and the history given by the parents, a developmental assessment may be required to detect any developmental issues affecting sleep. The Bayley Scales of Infant Development (Bayley, 1993) and the Griffiths Mental Development Scales (Griffiths, 1984) are two such assessments.

Both scales examine a range of skills and behaviours from one month to 42 months (Bayley Scales) and to eight years (Griffiths). The behaviours include eye–hand coordination, fine motor skills, verbal and language skills, simple problem solving, memory and gross motor skills.

The Bayley Scale has two scales in the assessment, the Mental and the Motor, each of which gives a standardised numerical score, the Mental Development Index (MDI) and the Psychomotor Development Index (PDI). There is also a Behavioural Rating Scale (BSR), which assesses the infant's capacity for regulating state, social engagement, emotional regulation and the quality of motor behaviours.

The Griffiths Scales have five scales—locomotor, personal–social, hearing and speech, eye and hand coordination, and performance. Once scored, a profile of the child's behaviour indicates strengths as well as areas of difficulty for the child.

Both scales give an indication of the infant's competencies and emerging skills. Areas of difficulty for the child that may contribute to sleep problems can be identified and shared with the parents. The scales give an indication of the child's current developmental status and are not found to be predictive of later development.

Assessing the caregiving environment

Factors in the caregiving environment that may influence sleep patterns include:
- stress, including the accumulative impact of maternal sleep deprivation
- availability of social supports for caregivers
- lack of attunement to infant caused by disability, drug and alcohol abuse, or lack of time
- difficulties for infant and parent with managing separation and transitions such as getting to sleep or getting back to sleep once woken.

Formulation principles

The basic formulation question is: 'Why is this infant in this family having difficulty getting to sleep or staying asleep?' The following formulation principles apply to all situations where parents are concerned about their infant's sleeping patterns:
1 Having heard what parents want to address, establish that their developmental expectations are appropriate.

2 If not, offer information about infant development and developmental needs. Ensure that any guidance or specific intervention strategies are also developmentally appropriate.
3 Return to any issue that may have been raised during the interview that might be linked to sleeping difficulties (part of the assessment). Identify risk and protective factors for this infant and parent; for example, lack of support for the caregiver may be the main contributing factor to a sleep problem.

Intervention

Most approaches to treatment described in the literature for managing sleep problems have been reported as effective, either alone or in combination. The efficacy of one treatment over another has not been established (Anders et al., 2000). In clinical settings, the skills and background of the clinician may often influence the approach used.

Developmental guidance

Supporting parents in the early weeks and months of their infant's life with education and guidance may prevent or solve some sleep onset and night-waking problems. Clinicians may be able to assist parents to enable their babies to develop their own self-regulatory capacities around going to sleep by:
- giving information about the development of the infant's sleep rhythms and sleep–wake patterns
- explaining the difference between fussing, grizzling and crying, and that it is necessary to tolerate some fussing behaviour at appropriate ages and stages so that the infant learns to manage negative emotions
- communicating the vital importance of the parent as an available and responsive 'other' for up to three months and beyond, as a continued source of external regulation when the infant requires help to regain a calm state of quiet awakeness or deep sleep
- sharing observations of the infant's constitutional presentation that may affect self-regulatory capacity
- explaining the significance of developmental age, attachment and emotional regulation on sleep.

DEVELOPMENTAL GUIDANCE IN THE FIRST YEAR

Newborn

Wrapping, snuggling in mother's arms, 'wearing' in a sling or patting may assist transition from REM to NREM sleep. A degree of maturity is needed before an infant can develop self-comforting means (such as sucking hands) to assist frequent transitions between REM and NREM sleep.

One month

The infant continues to need assistance to move between different sleep states. Wrapping, rocking, and allowing sucking hands, thumb or dummy for comfort will help settle the infant to sleep. Wearing in a sling is particularly successful in aiding transitions.

Three to four months

Help to resettle overnight may not be needed as capacity for self-comforting increases. Infants can hold hands together and suck fingers for comfort. Peripheral movements have decreased so often less wrapping is needed. For full-term healthy babies, four months is the optimal time to begin to encourage self-settling. This may mean being able to tolerate a small amount of grizzling at appropriate times for the infant to develop self-comforting methods.

Older infants—from six months

Many infants are able to self-settle to sleep from six months. If not, and assistance is sought, assessment involves establishing whether the infant has had an established satisfactory sleep rhythm and there has been a change, or whether a rhythm has never been established. Assessment also focuses on when the change in sleep pattern occurred, what event or change in circumstance coincided with the change in behaviour, and how the parents responded. Very often parents are not aware of how their behaviour might cause anxiety in the infant or how the anxiety might find expression in the infant.

Intervention aims to help the parents understand the emotional effect of the event or change on their infant. The age of the infant influences what advice is given to parents on responding to their child. The parents may need to return to a settling pattern that was appropriate when the infant was younger, for example, being more available at bedtime or when the infant wakes through the night, until the infant is reassured and feels safe to sleep again.

For the older infant, changes or events that may be contributing to sleep disturbances should be discussed, with sensitive reassurance that the child is safe and loved no matter what has occurred. If the child can talk, allowing him to express his concerns can be helpful. Providing opportunity to play out family interactions without judgement can also help children adjust to changes in family constellations. This play can occur at home, in day care or preschool. Parents and staff may need guidance and support to understand the importance of the play to the child and allow its occurrence.

When developmental guidance does not solve the presenting sleep problem, then other interventions may be required.

Behavioural approaches

Behavioural approaches, with the goal that infants will sleep in their own beds, with minimal interaction from parents, are sometimes recommended for sleep onset and night-waking problems. In some situations, behavioural approaches are effective. However, it is important to assess the context in which behavioural approaches are used, especially infant age, as well as developmental capabilities and the effect of developmental changes, such as the onset of separation anxiety. If behavioural approaches do not appear to be having an effect, it is important to consider other possible contributing factors.

EXAMPLE: ELSA AND MIKE

Elsa was in her mid-twenties when she married. She quickly became pregnant as she and her husband Andrew had hoped, and gave birth to a son, Mike. The early weeks and months were enjoyable, albeit tiring, and Elsa was happy with her new role. However, when Mike was two months old, Elsa was devastated by an announcement from her husband that he was leaving—he felt completely overwhelmed by his new role and the dramatic changes that had occurred in their lives. He said he was unable to cope with fatherhood, and although he would continue to provide financial support he did not intend to have an active fathering role. Despite many attempts by Elsa to find other solutions and seek help to deal with what she felt were transitional issues, Andrew left and moved interstate.

Elsa began to visit her Early Childhood Centre for regular support and told the staff of her situation. Over the ensuing months, the early childhood nurse [this book uses the term 'early childhood nurse', however, different titles are used in different states, such as 'child and family health nurse'] *became more and more concerned at the appearance of both mother and infant. Elsa reported she had begun to bring Mike into her bed when Andrew moved out, and was still breastfeeding frequently overnight when Mike was 12 months old. Mike was often whingey when seen in the clinic, and very infrequently left his mother's lap. This pattern continued into the second year when Elsa began to express concern that Mike was still waking to breastfeed extremely frequently. She was now ready to have him sleep in his own bed but found that his excessive crying when this was attempted was making this impossible.*

The nurse suggested she and Elsa meet for a longer session and discuss how Elsa might go about helping Mike sleep in his own bed. When they met, Elsa was encouraged to talk about the situation and she revealed how devastated she felt at Andrew's departure. She was very angry with Andrew for she felt that it was a shared dream to have a child. She loved Mike dearly but felt so bad that he didn't have a father to share his life. She felt she had to make up for the absence of Andrew by being constantly available to Mike: that if Mike cried then she had to give him what he wanted. Elsa wept. She said she knew she was creating an impossible situation but didn't know how she could change things.

It was agreed that the first thing they would address was Mike sleeping in his own cot. The nurse talked about Mike's tears when this had occurred before and suggested that the tears indicated Mike's objection to this move; that he was entitled to express his anger, but that Elsa was entitled to have her bed back. Elsa said she thought he was crying because he felt abandoned. It was suggested that perhaps Mike's tears reminded Elsa of her abandonment. Once again Elsa wept. After some time she said she would put Mike into the cot but keep the cot in her room for the time being so he would know she was nearby.

A week later when Elsa and Mike returned to the centre they both looked happier and Elsa proudly reported that it had worked. The first night Mike had objected to being placed in the cot but she had persisted, remained calm, gave him lots of cuddles but kept telling him that it was his own special bed and that was where he was going to sleep from now on. Eventually he went to sleep. He woke twice in the night and she fed him and placed him back into the cot, which he seemed to accept. Each night it got easier so by the week's end he was going to sleep within a few minutes. Elsa was happy to keep feeding once or twice a night as she valued the intimacy of that time with Mike, but she felt she had gained her autonomy again in reclaiming her bed.

In this case, the nurse focused on the issue Elsa wanted help with. When Elsa could separate her own sense of abandonment from Mike learning to sleep separately with her available, she was able to introduce the behavioural strategies. The strategies enabled Mike to separate for sleep, knowing that his mother was available as he needed. With Mike sleeping each night in his own cot, Elsa was aware that she still had issues about Andrew's departure. The nurse suggested that Elsa might want to talk through the issues of the break up of the marriage with someone and gave her the name of a family therapist.

Psychotherapeutic approaches

Psychotherapies have been repeatedly shown to improve sleep disturbances in the infant by changing parents' internal representations of relationships and consequently relational interactions between the infant and parent. Internal working models are laid down in early infancy, and are the template for later relationships, including how the parent interacts with her baby. This pattern of interaction in turn affects the baby's behaviour and the baby's emerging representations. Changing how the mother perceives herself, or her perceptions of her baby, and/or her perception of herself with her baby, will change her handling and interaction with her baby, which will in time change the baby's behaviour. (See Stern, 1995, for further discussion of the consequences of changing maternal representations.)

EXAMPLE: ANNA AND HELENA

Anna, 34, mother of Zachary, three, and Helena, four months, presented at an early childhood clinic very concerned that Helena was not sleeping at all in the day time and was waking every two hours overnight. Anna had visited the clinic previously, and in the first few months reported that her baby slept all the time but now seems to have 'woken up' and is impossible to get to sleep again. Anna reports that she has tried letting her cry, co-sleeping and feeding all night. She says that now none of these methods are working and she is exhausted.

History taking revealed that after Anna's first child Zachary was born, she went back to work when he was a few months old. Even in Zachary's early months, Anna found herself preoccupied with getting Zachary into a routine so she could go back to work. She explained that she has very few memories of Zachary as a baby, and that the period is like a blur to her. Anna said that her career was very important to her as her mother had been a 'stay at home mother' and Anna had always said she would do more with her life. Anna was less sure of returning to work quickly with Helena.

During the interview with Anna, Helena was positioned in a pram next to her mother and Zachary was held on her lap for the entire time. Helena fussed a number of times and Anna responded by rocking the pram slightly, but she did not pick her up. She appeared more responsive to her toddler than to the baby.

In Anna's case, it was not necessary to pursue sleep charts and records, as the difference in her responsiveness to her toddler and her infant were quite apparent. Bringing this disparity to her attention was the beginning of a revelation to Anna of how her unconscious feelings had been affecting her infant.

Through talks with a qualified counsellor of how little time and attention she was giving to Helena during the day, it became apparent to Anna that this was based on feelings of guilt at how little time she had had for Zachary as a newborn due to her preoccupation with her career and resentment towards her mother. These feelings of guilt only resurfaced after the arrival of Helena.

Anna had decided when pregnant with the second child that she would take extended maternity leave. Anna now had the time to give her, but instead focused on Zachary as an attempt to repair her perceived neglect of him as a newborn.

As Anna gained an understanding of how her unconscious feelings were affecting her behaviour with Helena, she was able to give more time and attention to her in the day. Anna reported a feeling of increasing sense of control, and that Helena's crying no longer disturbed her as she felt able to comfort and respond to her. The wakeful nights ceased soon after Anna developed the insight into the relational aspects of the sleep disturbance between her and Helena, and made changes in her own interactions based on these insights.

Regulation-based approaches

The routine appropriate care of babies and toddlers involves continuous sensory, motor and affective experiences. Infants require that the caregiving be sensitively administered, taking into account the individual characteristics of the infant. For infants with poor regulatory capacity this is even more important. These infants find poor reading of their cues and inappropriate responsiveness, irregularity in their daily routine and changes to their routine difficult to process and organise. As time goes on it is hard to know how much of the presenting behavioural characteristic or difficulty is due to constitutional and early maturational patterns, and how much is due to the interaction of the caregiving practices experienced by the infant with early constitutional factors.

These infants require input to help them overcome their own constitutional or maturational difficulties with self-regulation. The focus on gaining better self-regulation must occur within the infant–parent relationship and family patterns. These parents struggle with negative labelling of the behaviour, which is due to maturational difficulties. The parents require empathic understanding as they are often criticised for the lack of routine or irritability of their babies. They are often told that they will spoil their baby if they do the necessary sensitive responding and containing that the infant may require.

EXAMPLE: ROSEMARY, TOM AND PETER

Peter's mother, Rosemary, phoned for an appointment at an infant–parent unit because Peter, now eight months, was not sleeping much during the day, was demanding and irritable, and was waking several times during the night.

Rosemary and Tom (Peter's father) brought Peter to the first interview. During the interview, Rosemary outlined the problem by giving details of a typical day. Peter had three regular meals and two snacks. He went to bed easily at night following a bath, food, a play, then a breastfeed. Peter had a dummy when put to bed. During the day he was difficult to get to sleep, and was rocked by his Dad. Peter liked to be upright so Rosemary carried him around in her arms for much of the day and he had one to two hours in a walker each day. Peter was referred to as a 'sicky' baby. He had not had much time on his tummy and hadn't had 'rough and tumble' play.

Peter woke two to three times each night. On waking he had a breastfeed and was often placed in his parents' bed.

When observed on the floor, Peter was able to sit but could not move from sitting to lying on his tummy or from his tummy to his back. Peter whinged to have his position changed.

The challenges to Peter at this time were to the motor system and state regulation. Peter showed frustration with his motor skills and had not mastered getting himself to sleep, staying asleep and having enough sleep.

The following recommendations were made to the family at this time:
1 *To help develop Peter's motor skills:*
   - *Encourage more physical play time on his tummy. Introduce tummy play gradually, a few minutes at a time and change position when he showed discomfort.*
   - *Assist Peter to roll over and move from sitting to tummy and from tummy back to sitting.*

- *When Peter was trying to pull to stand encourage him to do so through kneeling, one leg at a time.*
- *Avoid using the walker.*
2. To help Peter gain regulation with his sleep:
    - *Tune into Peter's efforts to get himself to sleep. When Peter showed signs of tiredness, to go through the usual ritual of bedtime and place him in his cot with his dummy, soft toy or cuddly and say good night, not to rock or hold, and to leave the room. The parents were encouraged to observe what Peter did to get himself to sleep. If he did not manage to do so, and became distressed, they were to go in, comfort and resettle and do this as often as necessary, giving Peter the assistance he required to get himself to sleep.*
    - *Reduce the night feeds to what Rosemary felt Peter required nutritionally. Rosemary expressed that she felt comfortable with feeding once per night.*

    The parents were encouraged to phone in two weeks.

Outcome

Rosemary phoned in and stated that Peter was now enjoying playing on his tummy and was rolling around on the floor. He still liked to be on his feet but they had put the walker away, and Peter was able to get up on hands and knees and rock. In terms of getting to sleep, Peter was placed in the cot and was going to sleep within five minutes if Rosemary stayed in the room with him. He was also having more sleep. Within two months Peter was crawling. He walked at 12 months. At 14 months sleeping was a pleasure. Also at 14 months Peter was talking quite a lot, doing more verbally. However, Rosemary felt he was frustrated, for although he slept well during the day (two hours in the morning and an hour and a half in the afternoon), he could not occupy himself during the day. He constantly wanted someone to play or engage with him.

A developmental assessment was suggested and at 15 months Peter was assessed using the Bayley Scales of Infant Development. Although Peter performed on both Mental and Motor scales more than a standard deviation above the mean, there was considerable difference between the scores on the two scales, which could indicate a source of Peter's frustration. Peter showed that he was visually and verbally very competent and efficient. The area of least competence for Peter was that of hand dexterity, which possibly indicated why Peter found it difficult to sit and amuse himself by playing with objects with his hands, such as blocks. The summary of the Bayley assessment was that Peter was an infant who was developmentally advanced but showed an inability to manage the frustration he felt at not being able to work competently with his hands. He required assistance from his environment to enable him to amuse himself with satisfying hand play. After the assessment the parents were encouraged to build up Peter's enjoyment of sitting and playing by actively structuring the activity so Peter experienced success, and to talk him through games involving hand skills.

SUMMARY

The most important consideration in assessment of sleep difficulties is to be aware of the range of possible biopsychosocial factors that may contribute to sleep disturbances in infants. Realistic expectations are essential in the assessment process, so that clinicians and parents share an understanding of the developmental capabilities of the infant and are mindful of and responsive to developmental challenges. The effect of constitutional factors and the relationship between these and the caregiving environment should also be assessed.

CHAPTER 8*

Feeding

KEY CONCEPTS

- Feeding and emotional development are interconnected
- Disturbed infant–parent relationships can affect feeding negatively
- Oro-motor skills become less automatic, and more voluntary and complex with maturation
- Anatomical, neurological and medical factors can interfere with feeding

FACTORS IN ASSESSMENT AND FORMULATION

- Evaluation of the infant–parent feeding relationship
- Assessment of oro-motor skills
- Assessment of resistance and aversive reactions to feeding
- Compensatory experience for infants receiving non-oral feeds

---

Feeding should be one of the most pleasurable parts of an infant's day, intimately shared with a loving and empathic caregiver who understands the infant's cues and can help the infant learn to regulate and expand her own repertoire of feeding behaviours. The goal is independent self-feeding and the enjoyment of mealtimes with other people.

Given intact anatomical structures, and normal neurological and physiological functioning, stressful infant–parent relationships underlie many feeding difficulties. Management includes parental support and psychotherapy, to increase parents' confidence, to lessen tension in the feeding relationship and to foster the development of self-regulation for the infant. Difficulties are also caused by medical conditions, such as cerebral palsy, and these can be partially alleviated by attention to appropriate postural support and the modulation of sensory inputs associated with feeding. Temporary deprivation of oral feeding,

---

* This chapter was written by Helen Hardy.

or exposure to traumatic oral experience, because of medical conditions, can result in hypersensitivity and dysphagia. With an emotionally available caregiver, this fear can be addressed, using desensitisation and behavioural shaping techniques, but beginning to drink and eat is less easy beyond the first year of life.

The accomplishment of normal feeding development is paralleled by corresponding emotional developments, in attachment and separation, and by the motivation to reach out for the experiences that foster age-appropriate motor and cognitive development. Healthy infant–parent relationships and individualised simulation of oral feeding for non-oral feeders support these developments. In this chapter consideration will be given to the development and assessment of feeding behaviour, to aspects of the infant–parent relationship that affect infant feeding, and to the significance of oral experience for infant development.

THE DEVELOPMENT OF FEEDING SKILLS

Becoming an oral feeder is one of the dramatic adaptations necessary for survival when a baby is born. Many of the component skills are, in the beginning, substantially reflexive and innate in nature, and some appear to be the result of learning and practice that has already taken place in utero. With increasing maturity and experience, the baby expands on the repertoire of reflexes as more voluntary control is acquired. Behaviours associated with feeding become less stereotyped and more varied. Of all the physiological adaptations that the newborn infant needs to make, feeding is the first to be released from largely reflex control (Dowling, 1980). Although predominantly reflexive, sucking is not obligatory, and it will be inhibited if breathing becomes difficult.

Influences on feeding

Feeding behaviours are a reflection of the blending of a number of intricately interrelated physical, maturational and interpersonal factors. The substantially automatic responses of the newborn to root and suckle and to engage in hand-to-mouth activity begin a learning process that culminates in self-feeding. The first year of life is a particularly sensitive period for the acquisition of mature eating behaviours.

Motor, sensory, neurological and physiological functions

Coordinated sucking, breathing and swallowing, and the presence of protective reflexes, are basic to safe oral feeding. Both adaptive oral reflexes (rooting and suck-swallow) and protective (gag) are present prenatally. Also present before birth is the ability to perceive and respond to relevant sensory information (tactile, gustatory and olfactory).

Perhaps the earliest behavioural development towards eventual oral feeding is seen in the seven-and-a-half-week-old foetus who reacts to light touch in the perioral region—responding with flexion in the neck region, although it is in a direction away from the stimulus (Hooker, 1952/1969; Humphrey, 1968). At nine-and-a-half weeks mouth opening can be elicited by stimulation of the lower lip. By 10 weeks, stimulation of the lower lip and mandible produces flexion towards the stimulus, and at 11 to 11.5 weeks perioral stimulation causes rotation of the face towards the stimulus. The rooting reflex continues to mature and is complete, but slow, in the 32-week preterm infant. The foetus begins to swallow amniotic fluid at 12 to14 weeks, and rhythmic sucking is established at 34 to 36 weeks in the preterm infant (de Vries, Visser & Prechtl, 1984).

After birth, sucking is further reinforced by practice. The taste and tactile components of feeding are each independently rewarding and soothing, the tactile factor operating immediately and declining as soon as it is removed, and the effects of sweet taste persisting (Barr & Young, 1999; Blass, 1997). The experience of nutritive sucking, as opposed to non-nutritive sucking, results in a detectable cortical response (measured by EEG) that is thought to arise from responses to feeling hunger and satisfaction (Lehtonen et al., 1998). The effect is more marked in breastfed infants, as compared with bottle-fed infants, perhaps reflecting the preference for the taste/odour of the mother's breastmilk that is already established at birth (Hepper, 1996; Macfarlane, 1975; Marlier, Schaal & Soussignan, 1998). The connection between oral activity and the relief of hunger is learnt by 10 to 12 weeks (Dowling, 1980), leading to the active pursuit, and rejection, of feeding. Clinical experience suggests that the conscious appreciation of hunger and satiation is learnt. Infants receiving non-oral feeds, particularly continuous as opposed to regular intermittent (bolus) feeds, may not have enough experience of hunger to recognise this state, an effect that may persist beyond the period of non-oral feeding. When the period of non-oral feeding is less than one month, subsequent oral feeding is less likely to be adversely affected (Kennedy & Lipsitt, 1993).

Both the rooting and sucking reflexes become integrated at four to six months of age, as mature sucking is emerging. This coincides with oropharyngeal anatomical changes, and digestive maturation, allowing for the introduction of some semi-solid foods. Compared with adult anatomy, the relative proportions of the oral cavity and the tongue are significantly different in the newborn, with the tongue occupying the entire oral cavity, and tongue movement dominated by extension and retraction. By six months of age, with increasing motor control and variation in tongue movement, some biting, chewing and bolus formation prior to swallowing are used when feeding.

Feeding in a more upright position and from a cup is also possible. (See Morris & Klein, 2000, for details of the sequence of developmental milestones towards independent eating and drinking.)

Infant–parent relationship

For most babies, feeding is a pleasurable and rewarding experience that enriches the infant–parent relationship. Hunger is replaced by satisfaction, and the process is accompanied by multisensory associations. These include taste, tactile, olfactory, visual and auditory stimuli, particularly linked to the parent and to the feeding situation. The experience is particularly intense for the breastfed baby, with more direct exposure to relevant odours and taste, more opportunities for mutual touching and regulation, and reinforcement of maternal feelings. Successful feeding is dependent on the nurturing capacities of the parent and on the continuing process of learning about the baby's individuality, while the baby is repeatedly experiencing the integrating cycle of hunger, followed by its resolution with feeding. It is the first collaborative activity, necessary for survival and well-being, that the baby takes part in. As such, the feeding relationship may contribute much to the templates for future social interaction that are laid down during the baby's earliest interpersonal encounters.

In addition, feeding difficulties might predispose to later eating disorders. Marchi & Cohen (1990) demonstrated significant stability in the prevalence of problem feeding behaviours over time. Maladaptive eating patterns first reported by parents when their children were one to 10 years of age tended to persist. Families were subsequently interviewed, when their children were nine to 18 years, and again at 11 to 21 years. Early eating-related family discord, problems in the self-control of eating behaviour and digestive problems were shown to be associated with subsequent eating disorders.

When feeding goes well, the baby's cues of wanting to be fed, and of being ready to end a feed, are respected so that the baby learns to regulate her own food intake (Winnicott, 1964). Parents achieve appropriate understanding of their baby's signals through identification with the baby, knowledge 'from a deeper level and not necessarily that part of the mind which has words for everything' (Winnicott, 1967/1996, p. 41). More relevant than being instructed in what to do is the parent's experience of adapting to the baby, and most feeding difficulties, in the absence of a significant medical cause, arise from the challenge of negotiating this adaptation (Winnicott, 1967/1996). This process is facilitated by a supportive social network.

As a baby matures and achieves increasing autonomy, the sensitive parent allows for growing competence, and provides opportunities for new feeding skills to be exercised. This includes weaning from breast or bottle, once cup feeding is fully achieved, and broadening the social context of feeding when it becomes a family mealtime. 'Weaning is the first experience of permanent loss'

(Salzberger-Wittenberger, Henry & Osborne, 1983), and how successfully the transition is negotiated may influence the infant's capacity to tolerate subsequent losses in life. The transition to self-feeding allows the infant more opportunities for autonomy, and for the exploration of a wider range of food tastes and textures.

Significance of oral experience for development

Developmentally, hand-to-mouth activity gives the infant strategies for self-soothing and practising self-regulation, and opportunities for the tactile exploration of objects by mouthing them (Field, 1999). Dowling (1977) studied the development of a small group of infants with oesophageal atresia (OA)—a condition, apparent at birth, in which the oesophagus is incomplete, and there is no connection between the mouth and stomach. This precludes oral feeding until the condition is corrected surgically. In reviewing the outcomes for the infants who had been deprived of varying amounts of normal oral experience, Dowling (1980) suggests that the experience of purposefully taking in, or rejecting food orally has an organising influence on behaviour. It provides motivation for gross motor activity and for engaging with the world, and this in turn enhances global developmental progress.

FEEDING PROBLEMS

Feeding problems occur in a variety of physical disorders, and can be either temporary or permanent. They may also be a consequence of immaturity, or of prolonged deprivation of oral feeding, when medical conditions preclude breast or bottle feeding. In the absence of disease, non-organic failure to thrive is associated with dysfunctional or stressful infant–parent interaction that impacts on feeding.

Physical disorders

Feeding difficulties are frequently associated with neurological, respiratory, cardiac and gastrointestinal conditions, and with anatomical anomalies of the gastrointestinal tract. Neurological conditions affecting arousal, muscle tone and primitive reflex expression can adversely affect the motor control necessary for appropriate oro-motor function, and for swallowing that does not place the infant at risk of aspiration. Respiratory and cardiac conditions can limit an infant's endurance for adequate oral feeding, and fatigue can compromise an infant's ability to coordinate sucking, swallowing and breathing effectively. Conditions such as gastro-oesophageal reflux (GOR) and oesophagitis can make feeding both uncomfortable and, if aspiration occurs, risky. Structural defects that interfere with feeding include choanal atresia, which reduces or precludes nasal breathing, cleft lip and/or palate, which makes sucking inefficient, and OA. After surgical correction of OA, GOR, strictures and dysmotility of the oesophagus may persist, creating obstacles to the introduction of oral feeds. Micrognathia, macroglossia and tracheomalacia, affecting the competency of the airway, also have a negative effect on the adequate coordination of sucking, breathing and swallowing. Other conditions, such as developmental delay, are also associated with poor feeding skills.

Failure to thrive (FTT)

FTT describes infants whose rate of physical growth is declining, or is already below the 5th centile (Casey, 1999). Although there are various further refinements in the definition of FTT, the cause is malnutrition. Non-organic FTT (NOFT) refers to infants for whom there is no identified medical explanation for poor weight gain. Population-based studies of the incidence of FTT, when preterm and small for gestational age babies are excluded, indicate a prevalence of 3 to 4 per cent (Wolke, 1996). The terms FTT and feeding disorder are sometimes used interchangeably, but feeding difficulties occur independently of FTT, and they are not necessarily a feature of FTT (Chatoor et al., 1997; Ramsey, Gisel, McCusker, Bellavance & Platt, 2002). 'Hospitalism' is a term used to describe the extreme of FTT, accompanied by severe emotional neglect due to maternal deprivation (Spitz, 1945). Maternal deprivation is synonymous with the absence of consistent caregivers and the lack of physical contact and stimulation necessary for normal development. This is not a typical feature of FFT (Wolke, 1996).

The term 'conservation-withdrawal reaction' is applied to infants failing to thrive because their nutritional needs have not been recognised or met, who have passed beyond the stage of crying, and passively tolerate inadequate feeding (Menahem, 1994). Such infants have adapted to the futility of protesting, and to the need to conserve energy. With less frequent feeding the hunger–satiety cycle becomes reprogrammed and hunger is experienced less intensely (Wolke, 1996). This is seen as a survival strategy.

Even mild FTT, especially during the first six months of life, is associated with delayed cognitive development, which is likely to arise from poorer brain development resulting from malnutrition (Corbett, Drewett & Wright, 1996; Wolke, 1996). Compared with thriving infants, babies with NOFT are frequently:
- more fussy
- more demanding

- more unsociable
- more inconsolable
- less happy

and they have:
- below average development
- immature or abnormal oral-motor skills, making them more difficult to feed
- more negative affect associated with feeding (Oates, 1996).

Initially, it may not be clear whether these infant behaviours are secondary to FTT or are primary characteristics of a baby whose temperament and ability to respond to care are mismatched with a discordant parenting style. Studying interactional feeding behaviours, Drotar, Eckerle, Satola, Pallotta and Wyatt (1990) compared NOFT babies, after discharge from hospital, with healthy babies. The mothers whose babies had been underfed demonstrated less positive and appropriate behaviours, and were more likely to arbitrarily terminate feeds. Such mothers may be less inclined to touch their babies during feeding and play (Polan & Ward, 1998). Parental psychopathology is a frequently reported association of FTT (for example, Chatoor et al., 1997). This suggests a possible causal link between psychopathology and FTT (Duniz et al., 1996). A distinction also needs to be made between mothers who are capable but overwhelmed by external factors such as poverty, social isolation or stressful life events, and those with limited emotional resources (Derivan, 1982; Oates, 1996). Atypical feeding behaviour can also be the overt symptom of intra-psychic conflicts within the family (Stern, 1985).

Infants with either organic or non-organic FTT may be at increased risk of insecure attachment (for example, Ward, Lee & Lipper, 2000), however, Chatoor, Loeffler, McGee and Menvielle (1998) also demonstrated high rates of secure attachment among toddlers with infantile anorexia. While disturbed feeding relationships are more likely to be a feature of NOFT (Lucarelli, Ambruzzi, Cimino, D'Olimpio & Finistrella, 2003), feeding problems and FTT can also be present in securely attached infants (Chatoor, Ganiban, Colin, Plummer & Harmon, 1998). NOFT and hospitalism are sometimes classified as psychosomatic disorders of attachment (Brisch, 2002). In contrast to DSM-III, DSM-IV no longer includes FTT as a defining feature of reactive attachment disorder (Casey, 1999). NOFT has been shown to be frequently associated with oro-motor dysfunction, suggesting that a diagnosis of NOFT may sometimes in fact have an unrecognised organic basis (Ramsay et al., 2002; Reilly, Skuse, Wolke & Stevenson, 1999).

Wolke (1996) suggests that there are several subgroups in infants with NOFT, reflecting multiple pathways to malnutrition:
- undemanding, sleepy babies, possibly hypotonic and with weak suck, who are not woken for feeds

[CLINICAL SKILLS IN INFANT MENTAL HEALTH

- infants with subtle oro-motor dysfunction who do not negotiate the transition to more textured and varied food, remaining exclusively breastfed beyond six months, and therefore likely to be undernourished
- infants who refuse to feed, possibly because of oro-motor problems, although refusing food does not necessarily lead to poor weight gain
- a small group of infants on restricted diets because their overweight mothers prefer slimmer babies
- a very small group of infants, exposed to neglect and deprivation, and likely to be referred to clinical services.

ASSESSMENT, FORMULATION AND INTERVENTION

The assessment of infant feeding difficulties requires a multidisciplinary approach since there may be a number of factors contributing to a problem. If there is any question that the infant could be at risk of aspiration when swallowing, this should be investigated medically, often by means of a modified barium swallow, before beginning oral feeds. Naturalistic observations of feeding behaviour, with a primary caregiver and in the infant's home, will provide a realistic picture of the strengths and limitations of a feeding interaction. For sensitive infants, transfer to an unfamiliar setting and carer for assessment may adversely affect their feeding performance. Because feeding is a many-faceted system, interventions that target one feature of the gestalt (that is, an organisation of interrelated components, the whole being greater than the sum of the parts), are likely to effect changes in other aspects of the system.

Risk and protective factors

Characteristics of the infant and/or the parent may have an impact on the success of infant feeding. These include infant neurological integrity, parental psychopathology, infant oropharyngeal trauma, infant characteristics and infant–parent fit.

Infant neurological integrity

Neonatal encephalopathy, resulting from insufficient oxygen reaching the brain, can involve the suppression of the gag reflex. Without this protection of the airway, oral feeding is unsafe. Efficient infant feeding behaviour is a reflection of neurological integrity, and poor feeding neonatally may be an early indication of compromised neurodevelopmental potential (Mizuno & Vedi, 2005).

Severe encephalopathy results in cerebral palsy. In older infants, with cerebral palsy, abnormal muscle tone and movement patterns and the persistence of primitive reflexes frequently affect oro-motor function and limit the ability to achieve normality or independence in eating and drinking. The quality of feeding interactions for children with cerebral palsy appears to be related to the abilities of the child, and not affected by maternal factors, such as the mother's psychological status with respect to the resolution of grief associated with the child's diagnosis (Welch, Pianta, Marvin & Saft, 2000). However, Sayre, Pianta, Marvin and Saft (2001) found that the mothers experiencing emotional pain displayed more hostility, those with compliance-related concerns displayed less sensitivity, and those worried about their child's future displayed sensitivity and delight in their children.

Inefficient neonatal sucking, in otherwise healthy babies, can be transient, and does not predict later feeding difficulties (Ramsay et al., 2002). As with other developmental achievements, there are individual differences in the ease with which new skills are learnt, so some infants take a little longer than others to become efficient feeders.

Parental psychopathology

Researchers have identified a number of diagnostic categories for feeding disorders in infancy (Chatoor et al., 1997). A review of these categories illustrates the effect of parental psychopatholgy on infant feeding. Some specific disorders in the parent such as eating disorders and depression have not been shown to be predictive of FTT.

DIAGNOSTIC CATEGORIES

In *Feeding Disorder of Homeostasis*, when an infant is attempting to master the first self-regulatory skills around feeding, and learning to regulate the intake of milk, parental anxiety, depression, psychopathology and/or psychosocial stressors have been identified as interfering with the parent's ability to assist the infant in achieving these goals (Chatoor et al., 1997). During the second phase of feeding development, *Feeding Disorder of Attachment* is seen when there is lack of engagement between the infant and parent. This leads to lack of pleasure in feeding, reduced appetite and, in extreme cases, vomiting and rumination. The contributing parental psychopathology is acute or chronic depression and/or personality disorder, drug or alcohol abuse and/or high psychosocial stress. In *Infantile Anorexia* (IA) (*Feeding Disorder of Separation*), toddlers are perceived by their mothers to be difficult, arrhythmic, negative and wilful in temperament (Chatoor, Ganiban, Hirsch, Borman-Spurrell & Mrazek, 2000). These mothers, who are highly anxious about their toddler's food intake, also show greater adult attachment insecurity, as assessed on the Adult Attachment Interview (Main & Goldwyn, 1991), when compared with mothers of healthy eaters (Chatoor et al., 2000).

PARENTAL EATING DISORDER

Chatoor et al. (2000) in comparing the mothers of infantile anorexics, picky eaters and healthy eaters demonstrated no differences between the three groups of mothers in the prevalence of eating disorders, indicating a lack of association between FTT and maternal anorexia. Infants of mothers with eating disorders tend to be smaller (Stein, Murray, Cooper & Fairburn, 1996; Stein, Woolley, Cooper & Fairburn, 1994). However, this does not seem to be due to an extension of maternal psychopathology to the infant. Stein et al. (1994) observed that mothers with eating disorders, compared with controls, were more intrusive during both play and mealtimes with their 12- to 24-month-old children. Expressions of negative emotion towards the children were more frequent at mealtimes, but not during play. Compared to controls, the mothers did not appear to misjudge their children's size, and they were very sensitive to their children's shape (Stein et al., 1996).

MATERNAL DEPRESSION

Maternal depression per se does not appear to be predictive of FTT (Ramsay et al., 2002; Stein et al., 1996). Ramsay et al. (2002) noted that depressed mothers had a tendency to be overstimulating in feeding their babies, but without any negative effect on weight gain. Depression may, however, be associated with disorganised feeding relationships (Chatoor et al., 1997; Duniz et al., 1996). It may interfere with a mother's ability to read her infant's cues, and to facilitate calm and satisfying feeding. Feeding patterns may become erratic and intake variable. Weight gain may then be compromised.

Infant oropharyngeal trauma

Post-traumatic feeding disorder (PTFD) is diagnosed when food refusal follows trauma to the oropharynx or oesophagus, but it is not necessarily, or commonly, seen among groups of infants in whom it might be expected to occur, for example, infants with OA. This suggests that other factors, such as oro-motor dysfunction, hypersensitivity to food taste, temperature or texture, temperament or pre-existing anxiety, may contribute to the response (Chatoor, Ganiban, Harrison & Hirsch, 2001). PTFD can be distinguished from IA by the intensity of the toddler's resistance to feeding, although toddlers with IA who have been force-fed also exhibit intense resistance. Chatoor et al. (2001), in comparing the feeding relationships between PTFD and IA toddlers and their parents, found that feeding between PTFD toddlers and their mothers was more synchronous and less negative than for the IA group. They observed that food refusal in IA appeared to be due to lack of appetite, whereas fear of swallowing seemed to be the precipitating factor for PTFD.

Infant characteristics

Infant characteristics that may have a bearing on the feeding relationship include:
- temperament
- individuality, within the normal range, in the ease with which infants master motor skills
- the way in which sensory information is processed.

These factors create a different behavioural profile for each infant.

Within each sensory modality (such as touch, taste, vision and hearing) an infant has an individual threshold of neurological responsiveness, ranging from low (sensitisation) to high (habituation), together with a typical style of behavioural response that ranges from extreme passivity to extreme activity (Dunn, 2002). Sensitisation is characterised by hypersensitivity to stimulation, whereas habituation requires novel stimulation in order to elicit a response. An infant's behavioural response style determines how much she seeks out stimulation, or avoids it. The various combinations of sensitisation, habituation, passivity and activity influence infant feeding behaviour. This is seen in particular reactions to oral touch, odours and tastes, to being held and in being able to ignore distractions appropriately when eating and drinking.

When habituation is coupled with passivity, an infant may seem uninterested, and respond more engagingly with increased sensory novelty, such as a variety of flavours. Habituation with high activity is indicative of attempts by the infant to achieve enough stimulation to meet her required threshold for stimulation, and the need to incorporate more sensory input with everyday activities. Sensitisation combined with passivity is evident in distractibility. For more focused attention, parents may assist their infants to dampen sensory arousal by firm touch-pressure and by the provision of predictable patterns of sensory input rather than unexpected stimulation. Sensitisation combined with an active response reflects an infant's attempts to avoid overwhelming sensation. This requires the limiting of unfamiliar sensory experience, and gradual exposure to increasing amounts of input. Sensitisation, with a mixture of active and passive self-regulatory strategies, is often a feature of fussy, difficult feeding behaviour.

Atypical infant behaviour may be seen in particular conditions, such as visual or hearing deficits and prematurity, and this will also modify the feeding relationship.

Infant–parent fit

Parenting styles have been described as facilitating, reciprocal or regulating (Raphael-Leff, 1993). The facilitator adapts to the baby on the basis of identification with the baby, the reciprocator negotiates her interaction with the baby on the basis of intersubjectivity, and the regulator expects the baby to adapt on the basis of detachment. In feeding relationships, the negotiated position best provides the flexibility that is needed in both responding in an age-appropriate manner to the baby's or toddler's cues, and in providing the individualised structure around feeding that enables the baby to achieve optimal self-regulation. It also allows both the mother and baby to manage the ambivalence associated with weaning more comfortably. The capacity to mourn, and to tolerate ambivalence within a loving relationship, is facilitated by the mother's capacity to gently bear the feelings of sadness and anger, together with the baby (Lubbe, 1996; Salzberger-Wittenberg et al., 1983; Winnicott, 1964). For a mother who is less comfortable with ambivalence, and so either reluctant to wean, and less at ease with negative feelings, or too ready to let go, and more dismissive of the value of attachment, the transition of weaning will be more challenging. Winnicott (1975/1982) identifies the infant's game of playfully dropping objects, occurring between the ages of five and 18 months, as an indication of the infant's growing capacity to master loss and to be ready for weaning.

Assessment, formulation and intervention principles

In the context of oral feeding, three areas of consideration are important:
- the quality of the infant–parent relationship
- the infant's neurobehavioural responses to oral feeding
- the special needs of infants receiving non-oral feeds.

(Medical and nutritional assessments, which are not included here, must also be undertaken.)

The quality of the infant–parent relationship

Formal observation of feeding situations is covered by a scale such as the Observational Scale for Mother–Infant Interaction During Feeding (Chatoor et al., 1998). Noted are the mother's affect (inferred from posture, facial expression and attitude towards the infant), sensitivity to the infant's cues and comments about the infant, verbal and non-verbal communication with the infant (for example, the way she positions and holds the infant, speaks to and touches the baby), and the feeding techniques used. Also documented are the infant's affect (as reflected in body posture and facial expression), communicative gestures (such as smiling and looking at the mother, as opposed to gaze aversion), vocalisation and feeding behaviours. From these observations, measures of *Dyadic Reciprocity*, *Maternal Non-contingency*, *Dyadic Conflict*, *Talk and Distraction* and *Struggle for Control* can be obtained. These, in turn, identify disorders of *Homeostasis* (in infants from birth to two months of age), *Attachment* (from two to six months of age) and *Separation* (from six months to three years) (Chatoor, 1986).

Subtle differences in feeding interactions among mother–infant pairs of preterm infants, as opposed to full-term infants, at eight months of age, with age adjusted for prematurity in the preterm group, were reported by Stevenson, Roach, ver Hoeve and Leavitt (1990). Reciprocity, that is, systematic turn-taking, was established in both groups. In the full-term group, well-organised, rhythmic interactions typical of a reliable, routine practice were seen. In contrast, the mothers of the preterm group were more attentive, and reliant on vocal cues, offering food in response to infant vocalisations, and using vocalisation to comment on the infant's intake, possibly to stimulate the baby and encourage further feeding. Stevenson et al. (1990) suggest that the pattern for the preterm mothers might stem from the infant's disorganised feeding ability early on, and initial difficulties in reading the infant's cues, so that reliance on the clearest signals has become embedded in their feeding relationship. Neonatal intervention, both to help parents better understand the behaviour and development of preterm infants, and to assist families in adjusting to the demands of caring for a fragile baby, has been shown to enhance mother–infant feeding interactions (Meyer et al., 1994).

Family interventions that dealt with concerns that parents raised included counselling for issues such as maternal depression and stress, and marital tension, involvement of the parents in the care and discharge planning for their babies, and practical assistance in arranging for social support and appropriate services after discharge. Interventions aimed at addressing parents' concerns about their infant's behaviour included help with recognising signs of overstimulation, and finding ways of limiting stimulation to appropriate levels, together with demonstrations of the infant's behavioural and developmental progress, using the Neonatal Behavioral Assessment Scale (NBAS) (Brazelton, 1984). (This scale is described in Chapter 3.) With this support, more positive and fewer negative infant and maternal behaviours associated with feeding were seen. For example, the infants were less likely to grimace or gag, and the mothers were less likely to interrupt the feeding noncontingently, they stimulated sucking less frequently and showed more positive affect.

CLINICAL EVALUATION

Clinical evaluation of the mother–infant feeding relationship at six weeks, by Sewell, Tsitsikas and Bax (1982), was shown to be an effective way of identifying dyads requiring more support, to enable them to achieve more optimal parenting and infant behaviour. There were correlations between aspects of this assessment and infant behaviour neonatally, as evaluated by the NBAS, performed between 12th and 15th post-natal day. This suggests that babies at

greater risk of poorer feeding relationships later on might be identified by their neonatal behavioural profile. In the study by Sewell et al., the assessment questionnaire enquired about feeding and sleeping behaviours. The questions relating to feeding included:
- the type of feeding—breast, bottle, combination
- strength of sucking
- regurgitation—amount
- whether feeding was going well at the time of the assessment (six weeks)
- whether there had been any feeding problems—minor or serious
- frequency of feeding—and whether on demand, a flexible schedule or a rigid schedule
- amount of feed taken
- the baby's weight.

There were also observations of the family environment, and of the mother–infant interaction. The latter included:
- Does the mother appear to be in love with the baby?
- How often and appropriately does she talk to the baby while caring for her?
- Does she think the baby will be spoilt if picked up too often?
- Does she appear to enjoy physical contact with the baby?
- Does she handle the baby awkwardly?
- How attentive and responsive is she to the baby's needs?
- How confident does she feel about day-to-day care of the baby?
- How does she find motherhood—totally enjoyable, restrictive, depressing?
- Did she wish for a boy, a girl, or didn't mind?
- Does she worry about the baby's health—a lot, occasionally or not at all?
- Is this worry justified?

In the Sewell et al. (1982) study, Interactive Processes on the NBAS, that is, alertness, consolability and capacity for processing visual and auditory stimuli, correlated positively with breastfeeding and with the mother–infant interaction. The infants with optimal interactive processing were significantly more likely to be breastfed on demand, and to have confident mothers who openly enjoyed affective interaction with their babies.

Infants with optimal Motoric Processes, for example, muscle tone, motor maturity, activity level and hand-to-mouth facility, were likely to have developed rhythmic sleeping patterns over the first six weeks, to be sleeping longer between feeds, settling quickly after waking at night and crying less overall. There was a trend for these babies to be the most responsive and least demanding. Motor competence also contributes directly to successful feeding, with normal muscle tone and posture making sucking and swallowing most efficient (Wolf & Glass, 1992). This enables an infant to be comfortably held by the caregiver.

In the Sewell et al. (1982) study, the measure of Organizational Processes–State Control on the NBAS, for example, irritability, changes in states of arousal and self-quieting activity, identified three disorganised infants. The mothers of these infants were among the small number who least enjoyed physical contact with the baby, who handled their babies more awkwardly, and appeared less confident and attentive. Their babies slept for shorter periods through the day, and tended to stay awake and fuss during the night.

The least positive observations of the mothers in this study are among the characteristics often seen in mothers of infants with the nutritional and emotional deprivation manifesting as NOFT, which is seen as part of the spectrum of child abuse (Derivan, 1982; Oates, 1996). These include:
- poor self-esteem
- depression and/or anger
- anxiety
- holding the baby clumsily or facing away from her
- having poor eye contact with the baby
- poorly perceiving the baby's needs, and often seeing them as demands
- attributing mature emotions and motivation to the baby
- having a negative or ambiguous perception of the mothering role.

INTERVENTION PRINCIPLES

Depending on the particular family circumstances, intervention might include:
- 'mothering' the mother as she cares for her baby (when a mother is emotionally deprived and unavailable to her baby)
- providing for psychosocial support in the community (in the absence of family, or other psychosocial support), and help in managing external stresses (such as poverty or marital disturbance)
- speaking for the baby (in order to change distorted perceptions by the caretaker of the meaning of the baby's cues)
- suggestions and modelling of more appropriate parenting skills (for example, if the mother is inexperienced, or holds unusual beliefs about child care or infant nutrition)
- acknowledging the challenge of fitting in with the baby, and accurately identifying the baby's needs (when the baby's temperament and the mother's parenting style are mismatched), and exploring with the mother what the most compatible options for managing feeding may be
- focusing on lessening the tension in the infant–parent relationship, rather than on improving weight gain, offering feeds only when hunger cues are shown, and not overriding an infant's wish to cease feeding. Applying this strategy and combining it with psychotherapy Duniz et al. (1996) have demonstrated a significant reduction in parental psychopathology, other than personality disorders, together with significant weight gain in the infants. A variety of therapeutic approaches were used. Compliance with therapy appeared to be the most important factor in success.

EXAMPLE: THOMAS

Thomas was a four-month-old baby presenting with refusal to feed. He had been born by caesarean section at 38 weeks, after an uneventful pregnancy. Birthweight was appropriate for age. From the beginning feeding was problematic, but in other respects Thomas had been well. No neurological abnormality was detected. He was breastfed for several days, but this had been discontinued due to an 'inadequate supply'. Over the next few weeks several infant formulas were tried until one was found that did not cause diarrhoea. At one month of age a formula that appeared to suit him was commenced, but his intake was poor, and there was some vomiting and back arching associated with feeds. A modified barium swallow and other medical investigations excluded a major organic cause for his refusal to feed, except for mild GOR. Medication was prescribed for this. He still failed to gain weight, until additional calories were added to the formula.

Solids were also started early, at three months. At four months, Thomas was alert and responsive, but an undemanding baby. He was frequently distressed by bottle feeding, but able to accept solids well from a spoon. Tom's mother acknowledged her anxiety and the likely adverse effect that this could have on her relationship with Thomas. In addition, social support was limited as her husband was often away from home, and she was largely housebound, preoccupied with managing Tom's feeding and caring for another preschool child. Both his mother's anxiety, and the association of earlier unpleasant experiences with feeding with unsuitable formulas, could have affected Tom's reaction to bottles. When fed by a therapist, Thomas was able to take his full feed. Tom's mother expressed relief that he had demonstrated the necessary skills for feeding. Exploring and discussing with her some factors that may have contributed to this improvement, helping him to relax and feel safe, with secure holding, eye contact and speaking reassuringly to him, seemed to have been helpful. Waiting for him to wake for feeds, instead of waking him up, and offering him his bottle when he was most hungry, and before giving solids, were also identified as strategies that had enabled him to take enough milk. Being supportively with Tom's mother while she fed him, and in her own home, maintained the improved feeding and made feeding a more rewarding experience for both Thomas and his mother. She also learnt baby massage, to further build their relationship, and to help Thomas to be more relaxed before his feeds.

Neurobehavioural responses to oral feeding

Clinical evaluation of functional feeding behaviour in very young infants (for example, Wolf & Glass, 1992, pp. 154–7) includes the assessment of:
- state—state of arousal before, during and after a feed is observed as the baby needs to be sufficiently awake and calm in order to feed
- motor control—normal muscle tone and posture, and age-appropriate

primitive reflexes allow the baby to be held and positioned comfortably, facilitating engagement with the caregiver and a head position (without excessive neck extension or neck flexion) that makes swallowing easy
- tactile responses—the presence of oral reflexes (rooting, sucking, cough and gag) necessary for the commencement of feeding, and the quality of responses to touch (ranging from absent to hyporesponsive, through normal, to hyperresponsive, to aversive) will influence the way an infant reacts to oral and perioral contact and to being held
- oral-motor behaviour—the position and movement of the tongue, jaw, lips/cheeks and palate influence the efficiency of feeding
- sucking/swallowing/breathing—coordination, rhythm, strength, suction, compression, and duration of sucking bursts affect the efficiency of feeding
- physiological control—maintenance of adequate heart rate, respiration rate, oxygen saturation and skin colour reflect appropriate endurance, without physiological stress
- medical conditions—identification of medical conditions that may have a negative effect on feeding performance, for example, respiratory disease, GOR or cardiac conditions.

INTERVENTION PRINCIPLES

Physiological stability is an essential prerequisite for commencing feeding, and needs to be constantly monitored while feeding an immature or medically fragile baby. Other interventions may include postural support for the baby, desensitisation of hypersensitive responses, and the graded introduction of oral feeding so that it remains a pleasant and positive experience. Partial non-oral feeding, such as via nasogastric tube or gastrostomy, may be necessary until full oral feeding is established. Not only is this necessary for adequate nutrition, but it also allows oral feeding skills to be learnt at a pace that is not stressful for the baby, and without parents becoming anxious that the baby is not taking enough.

EXAMPLE: JANE

Jane, born at 35 weeks, was the youngest child of a large family. Gastroschisis (a congenital defect of the abdomen, which remains open) and growth retardation had been diagnosed prenatally by ultrasound. This required several operations during the neonatal period, before partial gastric feeding could be attempted. For many weeks, most nutrition was given slowly, directly into a vein. This feeding was stopped for a few hours each day, so that Jane could have small bottle feeds of expressed breastmilk, which were given by her mother. She was always alert, but often seemed fragile and listless. She sucked a dummy well, but was generally reluctant to try a bottle. Several factors contributed to this—the fact that she was never really hungry, because of the continuous feeds; the negative associations of frequent vomiting when feeding orally; and lack of practice. Feeds were stressful for both Jane and her mother. It was noticed that when given her medication prior to feeds, from a syringe and with her dummy to facilitate swallowing, she managed this more successfully than her feed.

The medication was more viscous than the milk, so her milk was thickened to a similar consistency. This was given from a syringe, like the medication, and later from a squeeze bottle, using a teat shaped like her dummy, with varying acceptance and success from day to day. Rice cereal was also introduced, and spoon feeding proved to be more enjoyable. It provided Jane with opportunities to experience some control over what was in her mouth and some choice as to when she would swallow, and to experiment with different oral movements and hand-to-mouth play. Jane's mother received regular support during feeding sessions, and throughout the hospitalisation. This was for practical assistance, and also to make it easier for her to remain emotionally available for Jane, given her anxieties about the baby's condition, discomfort and separation from family, and the strain in balancing the needs of other children as well as spending as much time as possible at the hospital. Bolus tube feeding gradually replaced the continuous feeding, and supplemented what Jane could manage orally. This continued after discharge from hospital at five months of age, but was gradually replaced with full oral feeding. By 12 months, Jane was giving herself small pieces of food. She remained a quiet little girl, but was progressing developmentally and enjoying playtime with her siblings.

The special needs of infants receiving non-oral feeds

Scott Dowling's (1977, 1980) conclusion from the study of impoverished development in infants with OA, who had been exposed to prolonged deprivation of normal oral experience, was that the normal experiences of knowing hunger, actively taking in nourishment and achieving satiation, constitute an organising stimulus for other areas of development. Even in the absence of oral intake, some simulation of the normal experience resulted in better developmental outcomes for the infants studied by Dowling (1980). The inclusion of feeding-related routines in the care of such infants appears to be essential if they are to have an adequate sense of reaching out and incorporating experience from the outside world. In addition, aversive medical and nursing events, such as intubation, suctioning and surgical procedures, around the infant's nose, mouth, throat and oesophagus, can result in oral hypersensitivity and dysphagia (PTFD), and rejection of oral feeding once this becomes possible medically.

INTERVENTION PRINCIPLES

Intervention consists of providing the same holding and individual attention as would be given to a baby who is feeding normally, and coupling non-oral feedings with as many as possible of the social, tactile, olfactory and gustatory experiences that normally go with oral feeding. This means that non-oral feeds are offered in response to the infant's hunger cues, and that feeds are discontinued when the infant signals satiation. The younger infant is nursed engagingly by the mother for the duration of each feed, and offered a dummy. While the infant remains in hospital, it may not be possible for the mother to be present for every feed, so consistent alternative caregivers may also be needed. Expressing breastmilk for the baby is encouraged, and 'kangaroo' cuddles, even if breastfeeding may not ultimately be feasible. An older infant is sat up for feeds and included in family mealtimes, or given opportunities to see other people eating if it is necessary for the infant to stay in hospital.

Because non-nutritive and nutritive sucking are organised differently, sucking on a dummy does not necessarily mean that this skill will transfer to bottle feeding, especially if oral feeding is precluded for a long time. For full-term infants, Mizuno & Ueda (2001) found that the time taken to establish efficient oral feeding, after two months of deprivation, was similar to that taken by non-deprived newborn infants, and that non-nutritive sucking during the period of deprivation did not make a difference. For preterm infants, non-nutritive sucking, associated with tube feeding, has been shown to facilitate the acquisition of oral feeding skills and to improve weight gain (Bernbaum, Pereira, Watkins & Peckham, 1983; Field et al., 1982). If the period of non-oral feeding extends beyond a month, the transition to oral feeding may become more difficult (Kennedy & Lipsitt, 1993) and, after about six months of age, sucking feeds may not be achievable, with cup feeding a possible alternative. Oral sensory desensitisation will also be necessary if aversion is present, though this may be averted if a dummy is used consistently, enabling the gag reflex to mature appropriately and to move towards the pharynx (Senez et al., 1996).

If PTFD is diagnosed when oral feeds are introduced, the task can be analysed into small components and presented in a graded fashion, together with reassurance and positive reinforcement. For example, working for acceptance, in sequence, of non-food oral play, spoon to lip, taste of liked food on spoon to lip, spoon in mouth, spoon with taste of food in mouth etc.

An alternative approach is to withdraw all non-oral feeding, and even allow some loss of weight, so that the infant feels hungry. The infant is fed only in accordance with hunger and satiation cues, with the infant choosing what to eat and the parent, rather than hospital staff, helping the infant (Dunitz-Scheer, 2002; Dunitz-Scheer, Wilken, Walch, Schein & Scheer, 2000). This is combined with individualised psychotherapy for the parents. Another approach, advocated by Benoit, Wang and Zlotkin (2000), is to challenge the infant with systematic exposure to feeding, despite distress, while ensuring that the infant remains safe. For example, if spoon feeding causes gagging, 'feeding' continues using an empty spoon, so that the infant does not learn that gagging is a means of avoiding being fed. Although effective in achieving oral intake for some children, this type of treatment does not appear to take into account the negative emotional and interpersonal effects that might also occur when distress is ignored.

EXAMPLE: EMILY

Emily, the first child of her parents, was born by emergency caesarean section at 28 weeks, with very low birthweight, low Apgar scores and with oesophageal atresia and tracheoesophageal fistula. She had respiratory distress syndrome, and was ventilated for nearly four weeks. A gastrostomy was performed soon after birth, and final corrective surgery took place when she was three months old. She remained in hospital for another month, during which time her parents learnt to give gastrostomy feeds (which continued until she was 14 months old). From the beginning of the hospitalisation, Emily's mother was with her every day, and her father visited every evening. Encouraged by the nursery staff, they became attuned to every nuance of her behaviour, and sensitive to her cues, including those that meant she wanted a dummy, or did not. She began to take small amounts from a bottle shortly before going home, while continuing gastrostomy feeds, but was slow to gain weight. At home, Emily was offered a bottle at each feed, but only for as long as she wanted to suck. She sucked her dummy while receiving the gastrostomy feeds. Emily's mother was consistently patient and gentle in her approach, and always supported by her husband. Home visits from hospital staff continued until about six months, as the extended family were not available at that time for support. By then Emily had just started spoon feeding, taking small amounts of appropriate family food (soup). Spoon feeding became Emily's preferred way of taking food, although she also managed to bottle feed, allowing for closure of the gastrostomy. A month later, at 15 months of age, she was partly self-feeding with a spoon. At this time her gross motor development was slightly delayed, but in other respects was appropriate for her corrected age.

SUMMARY

Successful infant feeding depends on the integration of complex motor, sensory, neurological and physiological functions, and it is the infant's first experience of a mutually satisfying social interaction. It also provides repeated experiences of self-efficacy as the infant actively participates in overcoming feelings of hunger. This may have positive effects on other areas of development besides feeding.

An appreciation of both the biological and psychological processes that contribute to successful infant feeding is important for an understanding of the psychosomatic nature of many feeding difficulties.

ADDITIONAL READING

Benoit, D. (2000). Feeding disorders, failure to thrive, and obesity. In C. H. Zeanah (Ed.), *Handbook of Infant Mental Health* (2nd ed., pp. 339–352). New York: Guilford Press.

PART C

The toddler period

CHAPTER 9

Behavioural and emotional difficulties in toddlers

KEY CONCEPTS

- Emotional development in toddlers
- Influences on toddler development
- Importance of language development
- Self-regulation in toddlers
- Disruptive behaviour and aggression

FACTORS IN ASSESSMENT AND FORMULATION

- Risk and protective behaviours of toddlers
- Developmental history
- Conflicts and challenges associated with parenting

As discussed in Chapter 1, models of infant development have become more complex with the development of the field of infant research and increased knowledge of the innate capacities of infants to enter into social relationships and engage with the environment from birth. Infants are now seen as active partners in relationships and as having a 'hard-wired' capacity to develop attachment relationships. Earlier developmental models saw the infant as a passive player in the process of development as expressed in simple stage theories (such as Freud's psychosexual stages, described in Chapter 1).

Current developmental models look at the interaction of both infant and environment and include the effect the infant can have on the environment. The transactional model of development (Sameroff & Fiese, 2000) looks in a complex way at the transaction between genetic and environmental factors over time. For infants, this involves the interaction of cultural, social and parenting factors with intrinsic and biological factors. Risk and protective factors can occur in all these areas.

EARLY DEVELOPMENT

As described in Chapter 1, there are numerous accounts of early infant development, including psychoanalytic, cognitive and psychosocial models. Research has contributed an understanding of the capacities of the infant to interact with the environment and begin organising the self and learning from birth. Most accounts of early development stress the infant's move from dependency towards self-organisation and the development of identity.

Development occurs in the context of a caretaking relationship and the carer is vital in supporting the unfolding of the infant's capacities. Even though the infant is genetically and biologically programmed for development, certain environmental experiences are required at specific times, known as 'critical periods' in development.

The first year involves the development of the basics for language and the establishment of attachment relationships. The second year of life involves two major achievements: the development of language and symbolic play; and the development of mobility. Mobility allows the child to explore and develop cognitively and to develop independence from the caretaker. The toddler experiments with separation and is developing his own sense of identity and autonomy. During the third and fourth year of life the toddler is consolidating, refining and expanding these abilities to consolidate the sense of self; in particular, in relation to others, a sense of his place in the world. The developmental changes throughout infancy are summarised below.

Table 9.1 **Developmental changes throughout infancy**

Development in the first year

- Development of basic trust (Erikson, 1950), a secure enough emotional base from which to explore the world.
- Beginnings of self/other awareness.
- Advances in social behaviour and interaction.
- Cognitive development (sensorimotor period).
- The basics for language development.
- Locomotor development, to be ready physically and psychologically to take off.

Development in the second year

- Development of language and symbolic play and development of mobility, which enables secure base behaviour and exploration.
- Development of verbal self-identity with the beginning of language.
- Beginnings of regulation of affect and aggression.

Development in the third year

- Development of interpersonal style.
- Understanding others (empathy).

- Consolidation of a sense of self (verbal).
- Range of words for own emotions (internal state language) (Fonagy, Steele, Steele, Moran & Higgitt, 1991).
- Physical competence.
- Increased mobility.
- Network of relationships.
- Learning to manage interactions with others, including peers.
- Learning to tolerate longer separations from parents and beginning to predict events.
- Wilfulness, possessiveness.
- Experimenting with control and power—may become ritualistic or picky about food or clothes and unpredictably oppositional.
- Able to be fully collaborative partners in activities and in anticipation of events.

Development in the fourth year

- Dramatic integration and organisation that prepares the child for school years.
- Language elaborated, also symbolic and imaginative play.
- Increasingly aware of social expectations and responsibilities.
- Beginnings of capacity to know that others have thoughts and feelings separate from our own, linked with a capacity for empathy.

The period from 18 months to four years of age is a period of extraordinary development and learning. Not only is the toddler acquiring external skills, for example, mobility and language, he is also becoming acquainted with the world of feelings.

The toddler is discovering feelings, learning to name and share those feelings and to develop an understanding that those feelings are shared by others. With the discovering of feelings and their expression, the toddler is learning about social rules and constraints. The toddler begins to develop the capacity to regulate those emotional states, dealing with frustration and managing impulses.

By the end of this period the toddler has the necessary social, physical and language skills of a preschooler, together with the capacity to regulate emotions that enable satisfying interpersonal relationships to develop with peers and adults.

Emotional development in the toddler

During the toddler years a number of important emotional developments occur. These include:
- self-awareness and self-assertion
- emotional processing and control
- language and symbolic capacity
- development of empathy.

Self-awareness and self-assertion

'Toddlers are coping for the first time with a lifelong existential dilemma: having to negotiate a balance between relying on others and doing their own thing' (Lieberman, 1994, p. 1). Stern (1995) makes the cogent point that the essential issues of emotional development—'trust, attachment, dependence, independence, control, autonomy, mastery, individuation and self-regulation are life-course issues' (p. 70). Stern maintains that the issues are not resolved at a particular age or phase of development, but are constantly being reworked as the child develops and acquires new skills in other spheres of development and thus challenges the parent to interact in different ways.

With the ability to crawl and walk, the infant is self-evidently a separate person and will explore. Initially, the infant is content to crawl in a limited area, preferably where he can still see or hear the parent. Within this confined area it is possible to ensure that the infant 'doesn't get into things' and is safe.

With walking and increasing competence with mobility, the toddler's goal is exploration in the fullest sense of the word, to acquire information from the external world, to satisfy curiosity. If inside, once the toddler realises that a cupboard can be opened, then that becomes a goal; once he can see a bench or table top, the toddler will reach for what is on the edge. Outside, the toddler will explore the limits of the boundary and want to touch, perhaps taste, everything that is within reach, with ignorance or complete disregard for possible danger.

A preverbal toddler can often be diverted from proceeding in one direction or playing with a particular toy or object onto something else. In the second half of the second year diversion is less effective and there may be physical resistance. With the beginning of language, 'no' will become the response to a request or prohibition. The toddler's sense of self is being asserted and the parent is challenged to negotiate limit setting. 'Me do it' is the favourite phrase of a two year old. Asserting and satisfying oneself within an approving social context are constantly being juggled in toddlerhood. As Lieberman (1993) describes, 'Paradoxically, the toddler wants to please but also needs to risk parental anger and disappointment again and again. This is because being true to oneself becomes a compelling motive at this age. The cycle of disagreement, resolution and reconciliation, occurring with greater or lesser intensity throughout the day, is a cornerstone of the toddler's psychological growth' (p. 22).

The toddler is able to explore and discover with abandon because he has an awareness of the parent or caregiver's physical and emotional presence, referred to as secure base behaviour (Ainsworth, Blehar, Waters & Wall, 1978). Toddlers learn to trust that other adults can substitute for the primary caregivers when the need arises.

EXAMPLE

> *Maaike, an almost three-year-old, was at her seven-year-old cousin's birthday party enjoying playing with her cousins and sharing in her cousin's joy as he opened presents. Adults not familiar to Maaike arrived and she slipped her hand into the hand of her grandmother standing beside her, for the courage necessary to manage introductions to the strangers.*

Emotional processing and control

There are two predominant anxieties of toddler years—separation anxiety and fear of disapproval (Lieberman, 1993). The toddler has to learn to satisfy curiosity and explore while remaining close enough to the parent to feel safe, and balance asserting his own will with maintaining the parent's approval.

As an intensely curious being and explorer the toddler experiences a range of emotions in pursuit of goals, for example, sharing with the parent or caregiver delight in discovering a butterfly in the garden. However, a toddler can just as easily be apprehensive about a discovery.

EXAMPLE

> *Sixteen-month-old Harper noticed the leaves of a plant swaying gently in the breeze. She ran to her grandmother, pointing at the leaves and making apprehensive sounds. Her grandmother squatted to Harper's level and in a very reassuring tone assured Harper that it was nothing to be afraid of, pointing to other evidence of wind in the garden.*

Given that the toddler wants—in fact, needs—to make decisions for himself, it is inevitable that the toddler will also experience a range of negative emotions. If toddlers want something, they want it now; they are not capable of delayed gratification. If the parent says no to the toddler, thwarting the toddler's desire in some way, but also allowing the toddler to protest, he learns a valuable lesson. Being able to have a range of emotions is healthy for the toddler. However, the toddler will only be able to give expression to the range of emotions if the caregiving adults can tolerate the range. If the caregiver disapproves of negative emotions then those emotions will be inhibited.

Lieberman (1994) sees a parallel between the physical secure base behaviour of the toddler, whose parent is able to let the toddler explore, simultaneously keeping a watchful eye on the toddler and letting the toddler return for comfort or reassurance as required, and the parent allowing the toddler to give expression to a range of emotions, including frustration, disappointment, anger, defiance and despair. The toddler learns that he is separate from the parent, that disagreements are inevitable in separate people and that the expression of negative feelings can be lived through, experienced and overcome.

Lieberman (1994) says that 'when the adults manage to remain emotionally available even while firm in their position, they also teach the child that he will not be abandoned during difficult moments, that momentary rage will not result in lasting alienation, and that there is calm after the storm. This experience of a well-managed tantrum is the emotional equivalent of secure base behaviour' (p. 3). Over time, and many well-managed tantrums later, the toddler gradually internalises the loving, accepting image of his parents.

Language and symbolic capacity

From 18 months, most toddlers use a number of single words, although they may not be spoken clearly. They understand a lot of what is said to them, and start using two- to three-word sentences. Between two and three years of age the quantity of speech increases. At this age, toddlers can talk about events in the 'here and now', becoming quite skilled at conversation. Now the toddler takes turns, speaking and listening, and responds to directions and questions. By three years, people unfamiliar with the child can understand the child most of the time, although errors are still made with sounds. During this fourth year, the child makes sentences, tells stories and has a vocabulary of 1500 words.

Between 18 months and two years toddlers begin to use pronouns—'I', 'me', 'mine'—to refer to the self. They know their own name and can point to themselves when their names are called. For example:

> *Harper, at 18 months, when asked 'where is Harper?' would point to herself with a huge smile on her face, and imitate, 'Harper'.*

Perhaps more importantly, even before 18 months, toddlers have learnt 'no' and can use it effectively, often when their behaviour means 'yes'. Stern (1985) discusses the meaning and acquisition of language as new ways of 'being-with' (p. 170). Meaning results from interpersonal negotiation between the toddler and the parent, around what can be agreed upon as shared. 'And such mutually negotiated meanings (the relation of thought to word) grow, change, develop and are struggled over by two people and thus ultimately owned by us' (Stern, 1985, p. 170).

In conceptualising the toddler's acquisition of language as a new way of being with the parent, rather than solely a major step in the direction of separation and individuation, the acquisition of language is powerful in facilitating togetherness (Stern, 1985). Developmentally, the thought or knowledge is already in the toddler's mind ready to be linked to a word given to the child by the parent. Thus, language provides new experiences in togetherness, a mental relatedness through shared meaning.

Having language means feelings can be labelled and identified. Words acting as symbols for objects and activities are a means of sharing one's experience with others.

Development of empathy

As the toddler's internal sense of a loving protective parent grows he takes on the qualities that the mother or father has demonstrated and the infant has experienced. The toddler develops empathy, an understanding of how an experience is for the other, a reliable sense of right and wrong, and, eventually, the toddler identifies with the values and morals of the particular family and community. For example:

> *Maaike at 21 months was being minded by her grandmother. After feeding and changing Maaike, her grandmother sat down beside her and yawned. Looking up into her grandmother's face Maaike asked, 'Tired Nanna?'*

Development in the toddler years has an ebb and flow around the two primary challenges of exploration and intimacy, and doing what pleases the toddler and approval of the parents. For example, once mobile, the toddler focuses on exploration, perfecting the skills required. Often around 18–20 months there is a period when the toddler displays heightened separation anxiety, wanting closeness to the parent, resenting being separated, as if being able to explore has made the toddler aware of the dangers involved. The toddler wants the reassurance of the parent's availability and protection as the experience of separation becomes reality.

The toddler's intrinsic need for the approval of those he is dependent on and loves is how the toddler is socialised into the family and social context. With a quiet 'no' and serious look many toddlers will stop doing what they have been told not to do, move away or return to the parent for a cuddle and comfort. As stated previously, it is the cycle of disagreement–resolution–reconciliation, which occurs repeatedly in the daily life of the toddler to a greater or lesser extent, that is the cornerstone of the toddler's psychological development (Lieberman, 1993).

Of course, as the toddler grows and is challenged in different ways, for example, the birth of a sibling, the need to assert himself may intensify. However, it is always on the basis of relationship that the toddler will most effectively learn to inhibit inappropriate behaviour and impulsive physical urges.

Essential tasks of parenting in the toddler period

Parenting a toddler is a challenge to any parent. Parents who find the high demands but dependency of the baby enjoyable and rewarding are often nonplussed with the energy, determination and contrariness of the toddler. The common characteristics of the toddler are developmentally determined, not a factor of personality. In several studies where toddlers and mothers were observed in natural settings, mild to moderate conflicts took place once every three minutes, with major conflicts three per hour (Forehand, King, Peed & Yoder, 1975; Minton, Kagan & Levine, 1971; Patterson, 1980). The conflicts reduced as age increased with two to three year olds having twice as many conflicts as four to five year olds.

Perhaps essential to successfully parenting a toddler is being able to see the situation from the toddler's point of view, the challenges the toddler is trying to resolve. It is inevitable there will be conflict as the toddler strives to become his own person, attempting to meet his own needs while learning to be mindful of the needs of others. Optimally, a dynamic partnership emerges from the secure base of infancy, where the parent is aware of his own needs and responsibilities yet holds in mind those of his toddler.

Common factors in disagreements between parents and toddlers include: different perceptions about what is safe and what is not; the toddler's desire to have or do, 'right now'; the negativism and determination as the toddler's sense of self gains voice; and the seeming inevitable temper tantrum when the parent says no. Attempting to gain an understanding of how the toddler views things, and respecting his developmental needs, while at times being lovingly firm, is the basis of the effective partnership. (See Lieberman, 1993, for a discussion of these factors, and how they can be understood and worked through.)

Many parents may be affected by factors that make parenting a toddler difficult; for example, doing it in isolation, no previous experience, many different demands at any given time and no-one available to assist or help them understand why it is so difficult. In addition, parents also vary in their own experience of parenting. This will influence how they will parent. The automatic experience is that parents will parent in the same way they were parented unless they are seriously determined not to do so, and have done something about making sure that doesn't happen.

Parents who remember strict or harsh parenting are often determined to do it differently. The pendulum swings to the other extreme. Terrified of repeating the harshness, they are loath to say no to the toddler, denying the toddler reasonable limits. When they do attempt to set limits, the toddler's defiance and temper tantrum touches the memory of the harsh parent and the victim child. The current parent, in self-defence, becomes the authoritarian parent meting out punishment. Alternatively, the parent gives in to the child, determined not to repeat his childhood, but does so reluctantly, even angrily, so neither child nor parent feels good about the outcome.

A parent with a history of neglect and deprivation also has an internal model of parenting that is not conducive to a dynamic partnership of negotiating conflict, finding resolution or agreeing to differ. Often these parents have struggled to be there for their infant to enable the infant to develop a secure base from which to explore the world physically and emotionally. These parents can feel overwhelmed by the emotional energy and negativism of the toddler and feel that the toddler is targeting them specifically. They feel disappointed that their child doesn't like them. They fail to set appropriate limits as they try to gain the toddler's affection and are confused when it doesn't work. Very often they are trying to be good parents. When conflict arises, and the parent acquiesces, the toddler may have been successful in asserting himself in the short term, but the parent is frustrated, and the child feels uneasy.

In situations of necessity, if parents are able to be quietly and gently firm, the child has a sense of security, trusting that the parents he loves know what is best for him. It is the repetition of this experience dozens of times in the toddler years that is the development of the dynamic partnership of cooperation. Remaining calm in the face of strong opposition and demonstrating control of one's emotions and feelings is a model for the toddler. This is particularly so when it is followed by warm reconciliation or respectful acknowledgement of difference.

CLINICAL PRESENTATIONS

Common clinical presentations of toddlers are regulation issues, behavioural problems (in particular, aggressive behaviour) and developmental problems (for example, delay or language difficulties). Clinical presentations of infants and toddlers require that the relational environment also be taken into account, even when there is a physical or medical diagnosis. The instance of earlier trauma should not be overlooked in toddlers. In these cases, focused and comprehensive assessment needs to occur (see Chapter 10). The healthier the relationship between the parents and the infant, the better the outcome for the child.

Regulatory disorders

Regulatory disorders are characterised by the infant's difficulties in regulating behaviour and physiological, sensory, attentional, motor or affective processes, and in organising a calm, alert or affectively positive state. Common difficulties involve feeding, sleeping and emotional control; for example, a toddler may be fearful or anxious. Parents may be concerned that their child is irritable, intolerant of change, easily distressed and hypersensitive. Others are seen as inhibited and withdrawn, slow to engage and react. These characteristics are often seen as inborn or 'temperamental' variables, but a comprehensive assessment includes seeing how parental handling of the infant either reduces or contributes to the infant's difficulties. The diagnosis of a regulatory disorder involves both a distinct behavioural pattern and a sensory, sensory-motor or organisational processing difficulty (Zero to Three, 1995). The use of Axis II, Relationship Classification (Zero to Three, 1995), will provide information about the relationship context in which the problems are occurring.

Disruptive behaviour and aggression

A common presentation in the toddler period is the child who is seen as 'difficult to control', with frequent and prolonged tantrums, aggressive outbursts (particularly when frustrated), poor impulse control and overactivity. These toddlers may be fussy eaters and poor sleepers. They may show disturbances of secure base behaviour, with running away in a fearless fashion or angry outbursts towards the parents.

Aggression in toddlerhood occurs as a consequence of social, emotional, cognitive and linguistic development, within the context of the family relationships. Aggressive children develop habitual ways of perceiving and responding to their environment, usually in a hostile manner, and will continue to do so if the aggression is not checked (Tremblay, 2004). From a large selection of longitudinal studies Tremblay found that the peak age for physical aggression was between 24 and 42 months and that most children will learn to use more socially acceptable alternatives when angry or frustrated before they enter school. Thus, rather than learning to become aggressive, children are socialised out of aggression. Dionne, Tremblay, Boivin, Laplante and Perusse (2003), from a large sample of twins, established that genetic factors had the greater contribution to the variation in frequency of aggression at age 18 months. Given that genetics plays such an important part in the expression of aggression, there are significant environmental factors that affect learning to use alternate ways of managing frustration.

Tremblay et al. (2004) found aspects of the prenatal environment and the early post-natal environment to be predictors of frequency of physical aggression. Among the best predictors in the ante-natal period were: young age of mother, low maternal education, maternal history of problem behaviours, maternal smoking during pregnancy, single parenthood and low income. The best predictors in the early post-natal period include the mother's coercive behaviour towards her child and poor relations between parents. Of course, some of these factors may be confounded with genetic factors and some of them will have a direct effect on the developing brain and its capacity to regulate emotions. However, the interactions the infant has with his parents, siblings and peers will also influence the developing brain (Cynader & Frost, 1999). Thus, parents' ability to regulate their emotions, as observed by the quality of their marital relations and their interactions with the child, will have an effect on the child's ability to learn to control his own emotions.

Given the weighting of environmental variables that are associated with aggressive behaviour, early identification of risk factors and intervention could reduce the incidence of aggression in toddlers and its long-term consequences.

Language

Approximately 20 per cent of the preschool population have some degree of speech or language impairment (Beitchman, Nair, Clegg & Patel, 1986). These children are at risk of developing mental health problems, especially if they have receptive language difficulties (that is, difficulty comprehending simple language or instruction). Beitchman et al. (1986) and Baker and Cantwell (1987) both found that about 50 per cent of children with a communication difficulty also had behavioural, emotional or social problems.

Developmental milestones are a useful guide when screening speech and language development, keeping in mind that a bilingual child takes longer to achieve the same language level as that of a monolingual child. It is recommended that if there is concern about a child's speech or language development the child be referred to a speech pathologist. After careful assessment including developmental history, observation, transcription of expressive language and standardised tests, a provisional diagnosis of the type and severity of the problem will be made. The speech pathologist will work with the parents and relevant carers to plan out a suitable program of intervention.

ASSESSMENT, FORMULATION AND INTERVENTION

Assessment and formulation of behavioural and emotional difficulties in toddlers requires a very careful developmental history of the toddler, a description of the problem and the context of the problem, observation and recording of behaviour and in some circumstances a developmental assessment of the toddler. It is also of value to have an appreciation of the parents' perception of their parenting, and the meaning attributed to the behaviour by the parents.

Before agreeing on an intervention plan it is important to know how the parents have addressed the problem and why it hasn't worked. It is preferable to work within a framework that is acceptable to the parents, to achieve goals that they have identified. A full assessment usually requires a minimum of three to five sessions of 45 minutes or more.

Factors in assessment and formulation

A comprehensive assessment is based on an understanding of the developmental tasks of the period of toddlerhood and observations of the infant–carer relationship. Factors to include in assessment of disorders in toddlers include:

- developmental history
- factors in the caretaking environment
- intrinsic toddler factors
- relationship or interactional variables.

Developmental history

You are interested in the history of the problem and the parents' responses to it, plus a full developmental history. It is important to listen to the way the parents speak about their child and conceptualise the problem:
- Was the pregnancy planned or wanted?
- the birth and parents' responses to it
- the child's achievements of milestones, in particular, hearing, vision and language
- separations from the child, including any hospitalisations
- When did the behaviour begin?
- circumstances around the behaviour.

Factors in the caretaking environment

Assessment includes characteristics of the parents such as:
- age of mother
- marital status
- mental health of mother and father
- parents' education and knowledge of child development
- parents' capacity to regulate feelings, particularly negative ones, marital conflict and family violence
- parents' capacity to recognise the child's needs.

The characteristics of the environment are also important:
- family functioning and cultural and community patterns
- Is there opportunity for exploration and play?
- supports available, both familial and community.

Intrinsic toddler factors

The characteristics of the toddler will reflect both developmental tasks of this age group as well as the individual personality and life experience of this particular child, including:
- temperament
- developmental level—past and current affective, language, cognitive, motor, sensory and interactive functioning
- predisposing medical conditions
- fears, anxieties
- mobility.

Relationship or interactional variables

Consider:
- What does this baby mean to the parents?
- parents' expectations of child's functioning
- parents' capacity to welcome the child close for comfort when the child seeks it
- parents' capacity to allow the child to explore within a safe distance
- the fit between parent and infant
- how the parents meet the challenge of matching mobility with safety.

Intervention principles

The assessment of the toddler and family will have enabled the clinician to make a formulation and to have identified the exact nature of the problem and its complexity, and the protective factors in the child and the family. In addition, the clinician and family will have come to a new shared understanding of the difficulties and the way forward.

The intervention will depend on the age of the child, the specific problem and the family context. If a physical or medical problem or developmental delay is suspected, referral to a specific practitioner or paediatric assessment team would be in order. However, there could be mental health issues that could develop or may need to be addressed.

EXAMPLE: TASMINA

Tasmina, two years, commenced day care after being looked after by her mother and her two Croatian-speaking grandmothers for the previous two years. Her mother, Renata, sought help when the day-care worker expressed concern that Tasmina would not talk to them. Tasmina was happy at child care but didn't speak much and they had difficulty understanding her. Tasmina talked within her family circle and it hadn't occurred to her parents that there could be a problem. Renata felt that because Tasmina was tall for her age adults expected more of her.

Tasmina was an attractive child with big brown eyes, who was inclined to quietly focus on people when she first met them without comment. It was explained to Renata that rather than being a behavioural issue, bilingual children were often slower with expressive language. It was suggested to Renata that she and her husband and extended family decide which language each would use with Tasmina, either English or Croatian, as it would be helpful for Tasmina to hear good English and good Croatian rather than a hybrid of both. Perhaps the grandmothers could speak only Croatian and at least one of her parents only English. Although a referral to a speech pathologist could be made it was probably wise to wait a few months to allow time for Tasmina to settle into the day care. Renata was relieved, and decided to wait before proceeding further.

When Tasmina was three, Renata asked for the name of a speech pathologist. She wanted to be sure Tasmina's language development was proceeding normally as Tasmina had a lisp. The speech pathologist met with Tasmina and Renata, and assessed Tasmina at home and in the day-care centre. Tasmina enjoyed the subsequent five visits of the speech pathologist to her home and the games they played. The speech pathologist also gave Renata exercises to do with Tasmina.

Renata reported an increase in Tasmina's expressive language and her confidence, although she still had a slight lisp. The day-care staff were amazed at how quickly Tasmina became more confident in talking with the staff and her peers.

1 CLARIFYING UNDERSTANDING OF NORMAL TODDLER BEHAVIOUR— LANGUAGE, COGNITION AND ATTACHMENT

A thorough explanation of what to expect from a toddler needs to be given to the parents. Very often, the toddler's behaviour is normal, which is often a relief, and it is the fit of that behaviour with the parents' expectations that is the problem. Attachment behaviour and its meaning to the child is often an area that is not understood, particularly the back and forth of intimacy and separation.

If the child has been ill or hospitalised the parent would find it helpful to understand how that experience could influence the toddler's behaviour.

EXAMPLE: MAAIKE

Maaike was born with tracheo-oesophageal fistula and tetralogy of Fallot, which required surgery on the oesophagus within 12 hours of birth, open-heart surgery at eight months, further surgery at 17 months and over a hundred visits and admissions to hospital for dilations and pneumonia over the first 24 months. Maaike's parents were exhausted. She still did not sleep through the night as her peers were able to do. The parents, Marie and Hans, sought help. They were still getting up to Maaike when she woke in the night, and wondered whether they should not get up and let her 'cry it out'. Maaike was in her own room but slept very restlessly, often calling out at night even as she slept. Maaike was developing well in all other respects, and her parents wondered if they were spoiling her by being so attentive during the night, as she seemed to have become more bossy with her language.

The parents were encouraged to tell their story, how hard the two years had been for them, the strain on their relationship and their ongoing concerns for Maaike's well-being. The discussion turned to what the two years might have been like for Maaike, the constant disruptions of hospitalisation even though there was always someone with her, and the repeated experience of being anaesthetised, of being completely out of control.

BEHAVIOURAL AND EMOTIONAL DIFFICULTIES IN TODDLERS

There seemed to be at least three issues that Maaike struggled with, which were typical of two year olds but exacerbated for Maaike because of her medical condition: a terrifying fear of separation, needing reassurance of the parents' availability, and a need for a sense of control. The parents could see how these typical toddler issues were being expressed by Maaike. They were reassured that her behaviour was normal and agreed to look at alternative ways to get uninterrupted sleep, by taking turns getting up to Maaike and calling in grandparents whenever available.

2 WORKING WITH THE PARENTS, TO HELP THEM GAIN AN UNDERSTANDING OF WHY THEIR CHILD'S BEHAVIOUR AT THIS AGE MIGHT BE DIFFICULT FOR THEM

Sometimes it is a misfit of temperament expectations. Many mothers without brothers and perhaps without living with their father, who have only experienced female children, are challenged by the energy and intensity of emotional expression of a boy toddler. Sometimes the child's temperament may play an important part in the situation. The child may indeed be a difficult child and it is how the parent reacts and responds that exacerbates the situation.

EXAMPLE: HENRY AND REBECCA

Rebecca, the eldest of three daughters in a family where her father was a quietly spoken academic, had a full-term, 4 kilogram boy, Henry, at 37 years. She had been a successful architect and enjoyed her work but chose to leave work to be a full-time mother. From day one Henry was a delight, but also a mystery to Rebecca. She was able to breastfeed but sometimes felt she could not satisfy her growing boy. Henry crawled early at five months, by eight months pulled himself up to stand and was walking at 10 months. Henry enjoyed being mobile, but Rebecca had to be vigilant as Henry seemed not to understand 'no', or to have any fear. Rebecca herself was a rather cautious person and found it difficult to understand Henry's bravado. She felt constantly exhausted and overwhelmed.

When Henry was 26 months he was enrolled at day care for one day per week to enable Rebecca to have some respite. After a few weeks at day care Rebecca sought help, for Henry had bitten one of the other children on two occasions. This was the final straw for Rebecca; she was mortified that her child could do such a thing. She didn't understand how Henry could be so energetic, why he was so intense (he was throwing tantrums if she tried to restrict his movements), and where the aggression was coming from. When she tried to discuss it with her husband, he laughed it off saying Henry was just a normal boy.

In this situation, it was a case of empathically listening to Rebecca's story and her lack of preparedness for Henry's gender and personality. Henry's behaviour was normalised, and strategies worked out together for how Rebecca could more empathically deal with Henry's intense expression of negative emotions.

Sometimes the problem relates to the parenting experienced by the parent, especially her understanding of her experience when she was a small child.

EXAMPLE: ELIZABETH

> Elizabeth sought therapy for the abusive background she suffered for most of her childhood and adolescence. After 10 years of therapy she felt she could put her past behind her. It was not until some years later when she had her own children that she realised it hadn't gone away. Elizabeth felt she successfully mothered her two little girls. It was Matthew, two and a half years, with whom she was having difficulties. As a relatively small child, Elizabeth was made responsible for her brother who was only 15 months younger, and then the subsequent four children who followed. It was the brother immediately following her that she always had difficulty relating to. When Matthew became negative and aggressive towards his sisters or herself Elizabeth found herself grabbing Matthew angrily and forcibly moving him to one side. Elizabeth was immediately ashamed of her lack of control. In discussion Elizabeth identified the feeling of being overwhelmed by the responsibility of this boy. Memories of a little girl being responsible long before she was ready to be were awakened. Elizabeth was able to separate her little boy Matthew from her brother, and also as an adult to develop skills in responding to Matthew's energy, aggression and negativism in a calm manner, which enabled both to emerge from the conflict feeling better about themselves.

3   EXPLORING THE PARENT'S ATTACHMENT HISTORY TO IDENTIFY WHY ATTACHMENT NEEDS OF THE TODDLER MAY NOT BE BEING MET AND ENCOURAGING BEHAVIOURAL CHANGE

An exploration of the parents' attachment history may enable the parents to make sense of what is happening in their present-day situation. We saw earlier that the attachment status of the adults is predictive of that of their infant (Chapter 2). When parents are sensitively supported to understand how their own experience may be affecting their behaviour and that of their toddler, it is possible for these insights to enable behavioural changes to occur. Intervening and acting on one factor of the system will change the system; that is, if the mother changes her representations of her toddler, her behaviour will change and so will her toddler's (see Stern, 1995, described in Chapter 7).

EXAMPLE: SUSAN

> Mrs Jones, was referred by the Early Childhood Nurse because she was depressed and struggling to manage her two little girls, Kathryn, 11 months, and Bronte, three years. Mrs Jones, Susan, was a petite, dark-haired woman, who sat with her shoulders hunched, not looking at the therapist as she told her story of her difficulty meeting the needs of her two girls.
>
> She said she struggled to divide her time between the two of them. When Bronte was around she couldn't talk with other people. Bronte wanted her to play

with her all the time, followed her around the house and kept making 'phenomenal demands'. Her partner, Peter, was supportive, but he worked long hours, often leaving before the children were awake in the morning and getting home in the evening after the girls were in bed. At the weekend he offered to do things sometimes, but Bronte resisted him and would say, no she wants mummy to do them, and then Peter would feel rejected and reluctant to offer.

Bronte had always been a demanding child, but had become more difficult since Kathryn's birth. Susan and the therapist wondered how much time there had been for Susan as a baby. Susan felt she should give equal time to both of them and that was very difficult because of how much time Bronte demanded. She also felt guilty that she was *'just telling Bronte no, no, no all of the time'*.

Susan was the middle child of three girls, with a sister twelve months older and one three years younger. Susan and the therapist wondered how much time there had been for Susan as a baby. She got along reasonably well with her sisters but they had little in common now because neither sister had children. Her mother was in another country and not very supportive. Her mother's attitude seemed to be that it was very difficult, but it was *'worse for me with three of you'*, and she would tell Susan that *'one just has to get on with it'*. She didn't really offer Susan much sympathy for how difficult it really was. On the two days in the week that Bronte was not in day care Susan woke up with a sense of dread about how she was going to manage the incessant demands. The therapist suggested that Bronte's behaviour told us how it was for Bronte, that she seemed to be a little girl who was feeling a bit insecure about her relationship with her mum and was showing lots of signs of needing to be reassured. Susan was encouraged to initiate activities with Bronte, to put her at her ease, to invite Bronte to join her as she moved around the house completing chores. For example, *'mummy's going to do the vacuuming now, you can come and join me and help me, or else you can play with your dollies'*. Susan was encouraged to be more decisive about what was happening and to initiate positive things with her.

Susan spoke about being riddled by a sense of guilt if the children were watching television; she felt she should be interacting. The therapist explained that watching television for an hour a day was within normal limits. The suggestion was made that she and Bronte could choose which program they were going to watch, and then at the end of that program, the television was to be switched off to give Bronte a bit of a sense of control over it as well.

Susan spoke of finding Bronte's difficulties with social situations challenging and described how Bronte would put her thumb in her mouth and carry her blanket around with her when visitors came, even Susan's sister. It was explained how young children often had fears that were difficult for adults to understand but it was important to respect the fears and allow the child time to work through them. Bronte needed to be allowed to be close to her mother at times when she was afraid to separate in the company of someone she did not feel completely comfortable with, and allowed to separate in her own time.

Susan was conscious that Kathryn was beginning to show signs of clinginess in some situations. Her fear was that she was going to make Kathryn into a shy little girl like her sister. Susan was encouraged to be as available as possible to her daughters and to say clearly when she needed to have a break and do other things.

It was apparent that Susan did not like the shy, sociably inhibited part of herself. This part of herself was projected onto Bronte and Bronte became a mirror image of that part of herself that she disliked.

Over the following weeks Susan found that by being available to Bronte, Bronte was able to play on her own as her mother went about her chores. As the therapist and Susan worked together discussing Susan's past and its impact on her parenting, Susan was able to see that she was doing it differently to what she experienced and to be less critical of herself, and gradually she began to enjoy her daughters and parenting.

SUMMARY

Toddlerhood can be described as the rapid awakening of a separate life from the protective mantle of the close relationship within the family. With mobility and language there is an explosion of energy, activity, intensity, and a will to do and be one's own person, which can be baffling to parents and carers, and at times threatening to the parent–child relationship.

Understanding the development of toddlers and their two primary challenges balancing the security of being close to one's parents with the exhilaration of discovery and exploration, and pleasing the parents and having their approval with asserting oneself while experiencing their disapproval. This can help parents to appreciate the toddler's position. The goal of the toddler years is to develop a dynamic partnership where disagreements can be resolved, or at least both parties can agree to differ. By its very nature, toddlerhood means conflict. As the toddler experiences conflict followed by resolution and restoration with the parent, he is learning valuable psychological lessons about conflict resolution, and how he can go to emotional depths and come out of it wiser.

ADDITIONAL READING

Barton, M. L., & Robins, D. (2000). Regulatory disorders. In C. H. Zeanah (Ed.), *Handbook of infant mental health* (2nd ed., pp. 311–325). New York: Guilford Press.

Steiner, H., & Yalom, I. D. (1997). *Treating preschool children*. San Francisco: Jossey-Bass.

Zeanah C. H., & Boris, N. W. (2000). Disturbances and disorders of attachment in early childhood. In C. H. Zeanah (Ed.), *Handbook of infant mental health* (2nd ed., pp. 353–368). New York: Guilford Press.

CHAPTER 10

Consequences of trauma

KEY CONCEPTS

- Experience-dependent brain development
- Effects of stress hormones on brain development
- Implications of early trauma for later functioning and adaptation

---
FACTORS IN ASSESSMENT AND FORMULATION

- Range of diagnosis that may be related to trauma
- Clinical syndromes associated with trauma in infancy

Trauma can be broadly defined as experiences that threaten the individual's psychological or physical well-being or physical existence and that overwhelm the individual's coping mechanisms. Chronic or enduring stressors are likely to result in attempts at adaptation and will produce significant organisational change at both psychological and neurobiological levels.

In infants, traumatic experiences are frequently related to threats to their attachment relationships and sense of security. Infants can experience significant indirect trauma such as witnessing harm or threat to their mother, usually the primary attachment figure, or threats of abandonment.

Infants may experience a range of inadequate, inappropriate and inconsistent caretaking and communication. Such environments do not allow the infant to develop secure attachment relationships with their parents.

In situations of traumatising care involving maltreatment, abuse and neglect, infants show features of disorganised attachment (as discussed in Chapter 2). These infants show poor capacity to self-regulate, modulate anxiety and process emotional information. They show high levels of arousal and a persistent stress response. This category of attachment is a predictor for ongoing developmental difficulties and behavioural and emotional disturbances.

Extreme trauma in infancy involves direct and indirect maltreatment and abuse. Traumatic experiences and interactions are directly inscribed in the fabric of the developing brain as they influence development of particular pathways. Perry, Pollard, Blakely, Baker and Vigilante (1995) describe this as the brain 'organising' itself around traumatic experiences. Extreme or chronic trauma results in long-term dysregulation of stress and emotional systems and brain structure and functioning may be permanently altered.

This chapter will discuss the basic processes of brain development in infancy and a model of brain–environment interaction. It will highlight the importance of the caretaking and affective environment for optimal neurobiological development and the adverse effects of trauma, maltreatment and neglect on brain development. The implications of early trauma for later mental health will be discussed.

EXPERIENCE-DEPENDENT BRAIN DEVELOPMENT

Rapid brain growth occurs during the first three years of life via synaptogenesis and the development of neuronal pathways. Synaptogenesis refers to this process of laying down of connections between brain cells and leads to the development of specific pathways. Connections between neurons develop in response to stimulation and sensory input and are therefore 'experience-dependent'. Repeated activation of particular connections strengthens those pathways and increases the likelihood that they will persist into later life. Following this period of rapid pathway development, those pathways that are not used are deleted via the process of 'pruning'.

Early experience is crucial in determining the development of brain structures—pathways and networks—and also brain functioning, the operation of these same pathways and networks. Chemical connections between neurons (synapses) rapidly develop during the first three years of life. More synapses and connections are produced than are used in later life and a process of deletion or 'pruning' begins around six or seven years of age. Rapid brain development during infancy establishes crucial pathways needed for neuropsychological processes such as:
- attention
- learning
- memory
- affect recognition and regulation
- impulse control.

Infants are initially unable to regulate their own feeling states and level of arousal, and these capacities develop gradually. The infant is dependent on her mother or other primary caretaker to regulate the overall amount of stimulation and input that she is exposed to. The quality of the caretaking relationship is crucial for early brain development. This model sees the brain as a socially responsive organ and stresses that biological development is sensitive to the social and emotional context of development. Techniques that allow visualisation or imaging of the working brain show how active the brain is from birth. In fact, the brain in infancy is more active than the adult brain as a result of rapid growth.

Attachment and brain development

Sensitive care promotes growth and the development of self-regulation. Early brain development is promoted by secure attachment. Infants in well-regulated relationships that involve the sharing of positive affective states show optimal brain growth and development.

From a neurodevelopmental point of view, the infant's primary caretaker, usually the mother, and to a lesser extent other attachment figures, play a crucial role in helping to regulate the overall amount of neurophysiological arousal the infant experiences. Extremes of over- and under-arousal are aversive to the infant and will produce a stress response and release of stress hormones such as cortisol and adrenaline.

Neglect and overstimulation will both produce stress and have potential effects on neurodevelopment. Neglect results in a diminution of crucial organising experiences for the brain. If these are not provided in the infant–parent relationship during critical periods, normal developmental processes can be damaged permanently.

Attachment theory stresses that responsive, attuned care helps the infant to maintain an optimal range of arousal. The secure infant gradually develops her own capacity to self-regulate as she develops limbic pathways (the system involved in control of emotional states) needed for understanding and regulation of emotional states. Insecure infants experience higher levels of stress and may be less competent in affect regulation.

As discussed in Chapter 2, insecure infants show varying patterns of processing emotional information ranging from avoidance (down playing of emotional reactivity) to anxiety (heightened emotional display). These patterns are developed in infancy in the context of the relationship between the mother or caretaker and the infant and set the pattern for ongoing handling of emotions and stress. They form part of what becomes the individual's characteristic personality style and are based on differing patterns of neurological development. The effects of the attachment relationship on emotional development are summarised below:
- secure attachment—optimal level of arousal; flexible emotional responses
- insecure/avoidant attachment—down-play emotional responses
- insecure/ambivalent attachment—heightened emotional display.

The 'good-enough mother' modulates the infant's level of physiological arousal. The poorly parented infant experiences extremes of under- and over-arousal that are aversive and stressful. Chronic exposure to stress in infancy with high levels of circulating stress hormones, such as cortisol, has direct effects on the developing brain.

The sensitive parent is able to regulate or 'fine-tune' his or her engagement with the infant according to the signals the infant communicates. For example, if the infant signals tiredness or a move away from interaction, the parent responds to this by reducing the level of stimulation, such as by speaking softly or darkening the room.

EFFECT OF TRAUMATIC EXPERIENCES

Trauma in infancy can have a range of immediate and long-term effects on development: These include:
- direct trauma responses—dissociation and immediate effects of withdrawal
- changes in biological stress systems
- effects on brain structure and function
- effects on social and emotional development
- attachment disorganisation
- ongoing vulnerability to stress and a range of mental health problems.

Dissociation and trauma

Dissociation refers to a neurologically based protective mechanism of withdrawal or distancing from trauma. Dissociation has been described as a defence mechanism involving distancing or lack of integration of parts of consciousness. It is a mechanism employed in acute trauma in both adults and children and performs an important function of protecting the individual from the full impact of the event so she can continue to function.

Infants and the young of many species are known to respond to trauma with a dissociative response. This is thought to underlie the 'freeze or play dead' response seen in many young animals and is mediated via the dopamine and endogenous opioid systems.

If used excessively in early life, dissociation may become a persistent and maladaptive coping strategy. Excessive dissociation prevents the individual from integrating or 'overcoming' the trauma and may produce difficulties in memory and sense of self.

Ongoing use of dissociation as a defence mechanism appears to be a key feature of more severe adult disturbances such as personality disorders and complex Post-Traumatic Stress Disorder.

Changes in biological stress systems

Infants are particularly vulnerable to the effects of trauma both as a result of having underdeveloped stress-adaptation mechanisms, and being dependent on adult support for processing traumatic experiences. The adult HPA (hypothalamic pituitary adrenal) axis that regulates the stress response is in the process of development during infancy, leaving the stressed infant vulnerable to high levels of stress hormones.

Infants are also not able to 'escape' from many traumatic events particularly when the source of trauma is their attachment figure on whom they are dependent for survival. This has been described as the 'paradox' of child maltreatment—the infant has no choice but to approach for security the very person who frightens them—an approach–avoidance conflict.

As discussed in Chapter 1, human infants are extremely sensitive to the quality, timing and tone of emotional communication. They have been described as being pre-programmed for social interaction with an innate capacity to seek and form a primary emotional relationship with another person, usually the infant's mother. This sensitivity implies that the infant will detect subtle disturbances of interaction, such as the carer with depression, with potential long-term developmental effects. Treatment for depression that commences early and focuses on the infant–parent relationship leads to a much improved outcome for infant development (perinatal mental illness is discussed further in Chapter 12).

Effects on brain structure and function

In high-risk situations of neglect and maltreatment, the infant appears to be chronically stressed and raised corticosteroid levels and neurochemical effects mediate developmental problems. Research has demonstrated persistent changes in neurological functioning in children who have been severely traumatised (De Bellis et al., 1999).

Several mechanisms of potential damage may be involved:
- neurotoxic effects of cortisol—particularly on the hippocampus, which has a high number of cortisol receptors. The hippocampus is involved in memory processes.
- dysregulation of the developing HPA axis and ongoing vulnerability to stress—a reactive and inefficient stress adaptation.
- disruption of limbic system regulation—the limbic system is involved in control of emotional states.
- effects on neurotransmitter systems—dopaminergic, serotonergic and opioid. These chemicals are involved in multiple brain processes and in the regulation of mood.

The effects of trauma on brain development may result in difficulties in tolerating stress, managing emotions and impulses, regulating mood states and interpersonal functioning. These problems may be first evident in the toddler period, when children may present with problems around frustration tolerance, impulse control and mood, and may be slow in developing emotional regulation. Some of these problems in toddlers may have other causes and careful formulation is required (see Chapter 9).

Effect on social and emotional development

Trauma, particularly involving attachment relationships, will disrupt the development of the infant's emotional understanding and social competence. Traumatised infants have difficulty processing emotional information and learning the complexities of emotional interaction. They tend to focus on negative and aggressive aspects of interaction and are angered by signs of distress in others. This is thought to underlie the problems in empathy that are an important feature of the longer term impact of trauma on personality functioning. Traumatised children will frequently show ongoing problems with forming trusting relationships with others. They may develop patterns of attachment disorder as described in Chapter 2. Those who have been extremely neglected are likely to be avoidant in their interaction with others and this leads to unsatisfactory relationships.

Attachment disorganisation

The disorganised pattern of attachment (described in Chapter 2) is clearly associated with traumatic attachment experiences and reflects the infant's ongoing fear and confusion about her attachment figures. Disorganised attachment involves features of dissociation and withdrawal, ambivalence and confusion and lack of an effective strategy for managing anxiety. The infant with disorganised attachment tries in various ways to understand and regulate her attachment figure. Later attempts at controlling behaviours towards the parent may emerge.

Vulnerability to stress and mental health disorders

In terms of later mental health, early trauma may damage the capacity to:
- relate to others
- regulate and understand emotions
- manage anger and frustration.

This cluster of difficulties is central to the severe personality disorders, which may be seen as the outcome of the effects of early trauma on development (Gunderson & Sabo, 1993).

ASSESSMENT, FORMULATION AND INTERVENTION

Infants and toddlers who have experienced trauma can present in a variety of different ways. It is important to ask parents about stressful experiences or exposure, even with young infants. Indirect exposure to trauma is common and includes exposure to conflict and domestic violence and can have as significant effects on the infant as direct exposure.

Infants may react to trauma with withdrawal and emotional 'flattening' and become poorly interactive. They may be alert and concentrate on the environment but not engage with adults. This has been described as 'frozen watchfulness' and suggests that the infant is scanning the environment for a potential threat. Feeding can be affected and a syndrome of 'failure-to-thrive' can develop in severe cases (see Chapter 8).

Older infants may also be withdrawn, fearful and avoidant. Ongoing exposure to conflict and fearful events may result in angry and disruptive behaviour in some toddlers as well as clingy and needy behaviours. The toddler feels simultaneously angry towards and in need of the parent, who is also the source of the threat. Toddlers will express and communicate traumatic experiences in play (so-called post-traumatic play) and in behaviour with peers. Prior to the development of language, traumatic experiences may be 'remembered' in sensory systems such as smell and vision as unintegrated images or memories (see implicit or procedural memory in glossary).

Assessment and formulation principles

Traumatised infants may present clinically with a syndrome characterised by:
- over-reaction to trauma-associated stimuli
- poor modulation of aggression
- disorganised attachment behaviours and anger towards attachment figures
- poor regulation of moods
- poor tolerance of negative affect.

It is important that clinical assessment consider the possibility of trauma when infants present with this pattern of difficulties.

Acute responses to trauma in infancy vary according to the age of the child but may involve:
- withdrawal and poor responsivity
- feeding difficulties and failure to thrive in persistent trauma
- loss of developmental achievements and 'regression' to earlier forms of behaviour and emotional communication
- preoccupation with the trauma and re-enactment of the trauma in play in toddlers and preschoolers
- aggression and behavioural disturbance.

Post-Traumatic Stress Disorder

Young children may develop features of Post-Traumatic Stress Disorder (PTSD) and will avoid situations reminiscent of the trauma. Recovery from the effects of trauma is very much dependent on the parent's emotional availability and capacity to support the child (assessment of parenting capacity is discussed in Chapter 4).

Acute stress responses in infants

Acute responses to trauma in the very young include withdrawal and dissociation. Infants may become emotionally 'flat' and unresponsive and interact poorly. With sensitive care, these acute responses should resolve.

Disruptive behaviour disorders

Aggressive and disruptive behaviours are common in older infants who have experienced trauma, particularly physical abuse and exposure to violence. These infants are often anxious and have difficulties in attention and focus. They may show features of over-reaction and stress in the face of situations and events that remind them of traumatic experiences. These infants may be diagnosed with a disruptive behaviour disorder but this does not address the underlying trauma.

EXAMPLE: PAUL

Paul, aged 24 months, has been placed in foster-care having been urgently removed from the care of his mother. Paul has been physically abused and hospital examination found evidence of old fractures as well as more recent bruising and hitting. Paul's mother describes a series of violent male partners and alleges that Paul was assaulted by her current de facto. She admits that she has desperately tried to please her partners at the expense of caring for and protecting Paul. Paul has been in respite care on an irregular basis since the age of four months. On occasion, he has been left with friends. Paul has witnessed his mother being assaulted and reacts with screaming and distress in situations where there are arguments or raised voices.

Paul, in his foster placement, is virtually silent and withdrawn. He eats rapidly and hoards food. In play he re-enacts violence towards a baby doll and between adults repeatedly. He has been noted to become distressed when any violence appears on television.

Paul shows features of acute stress reaction. He is likely to have experienced multiple traumas with attachment disruptions, neglect, and both direct and indirect exposure to violence. He has witnessed assaults on his mother, which are particularly stressful. Paul is likely to have signs of chronic stress and be hypervigilant and highly anxious. His play shows features of traumatic preoccupation.

Intervention principles

The first priority in cases of trauma is to ensure the safety of the infant and to prevent further exposure to trauma. If possible, the infant's relationship with the primary attachment figure (usually the mother) should be protected. In situations where the mother or other primary caregiver is the source of the trauma, a thorough assessment of her capacity to support her infant and the risk to the infant should be undertaken.

The second stage is an assessment of the infant's development and the effects of traumatic exposure. (Development can be assessed using tools such as the Bayley Scales of Infant Development or the Griffiths Mental Development Scales, described in Chapter 7.) Intervention focused on reducing anxiety and promoting attachment security can be done with primary or alternative attachment figures. Children placed in alternative care need support in re-establishing relationships and mourning the loss of previous relationships.

EXAMPLE: MELANIE

> Melanie witnessed the murder of her mother by her father at 18 months of age. Her father was gaoled and Melanie placed in the care of her maternal grandmother. The grandmother was being treated for depression as she blamed herself for her daughter's choice of abusive partner, leading to a complex bereavement reaction. Melanie had witnessed chronic conflict and violence between her parents and had poor language development. With her grandmother she alternated between being clingy and wanting to be bottle fed, and being oppositional and angry. She slept poorly and refused most food, which caused a lot of anxiety for her grandmother.
>
> Intervention needed to focus on supporting the grandmother in her new role and treating her depression. In play therapy, Melanie used dolls to act out or communicate her story about the murder and she needed ongoing reassurance about her safety and protection from her father. Melanie had many features of Post-Traumatic Stress Disorder that gradually resolved over a 12-month period. Melanie's anxiety decreased as her grandmother felt better able to support her. Melanie's eating and sleeping improved gradually and she developed more language skills, although still below expected developmental levels. While supporting Melanie's adjustment in the short term was vital, there was a need for longer term support and therapeutic intervention in order for her to be able to understand the details of the event and adapt to the loss of her mother over time.

SUMMARY

The effects of trauma on brain development are significant and there are implications for future mental health. Brain development in infancy is experience-dependent in an emotional sense. The quality of the emotional relationship between infant and parent determines the nature of the attachment relationship the infant will develop with that parent. When the attachment relationship is traumatising, the infant's brain development is directly affected, with significant implications for social and emotional development through infancy and into later life.

Trauma can also occur outside of the attachment relationship, for example, when an infant witnesses violence. This is particularly traumatising when the violence is directed at the infant's mother or other primary carer. Post-traumatic stress reactions can occur in these instances.

Indications that an infant has experienced trauma can include stress reactions, withdrawal, regression, delayed development, feeding difficulties or aggression and other behavioural disturbances. Consideration of trauma should always be made in infant assessments, given the wide array of possible reactions to trauma and clinical presentations.

ADDITIONAL READING

De Bellis, M., Baum, A., Birmaher, B., Matcheri S., Keshavan, C. H., Eccard, A. M., et al. (1999). Developmental traumatology part 1: Biological stress systems. *Biological Psychiatry, 45*(10), 1259–1270.

Glaser, D. (2000). Child abuse and neglect and the brain: A review. *Journal of Child Psychology and Psychiatry, 41*(1), 97–116.

Gunderson, J. G., & Sabo, A. (1993). The phenomenological and conceptual interface between borderline personality disorder and PTSD. *American Journal of Psychiatry, 150*(1), 19–27.

Nelson, C., & Bosquet, M. (2000). Neurobiology of fetal and infant development: Implications for infant mental health. In C. H. Zeanah (Ed.), *Handbook of infant mental health* (2nd ed., pp. 37–59). New York: Guilford Press.

Perry, B. D., Pollard, R. A., Blakely, T. L., Baker, W., & Vigilante, D. (1995). Childhood trauma, the neurobiology of adaptation and 'use-dependent' development of the brain: How 'states' become 'traits'. *Infant Mental Health Journal, 16*(4), 271–291.

Teicher, M. H. (2002). Scars that won't heal: The neurobiology of child abuse. *Scientific American, 286*(3), 68–75.

CHAPTER 11

Gender development and identity

KEY CONCEPTS

- Distinction between sex and gender
- Biological, psychological and sociocultural components of gender identity
- Early development of gender identity
- Gender identity disorder and cross-gender identifications

FACTORS IN ASSESSMENT AND FORMULATION

- Family and cultural assessment of models of sex and gender development
- The infant's gender identity development
- The infant's peer relationships and social functioning

When infants are born with 'intersex disorders', such as ambiguous genitalia, the effects on the infant and family can be profound. There are difficult decisions to be faced by parents about assigning biological sex to their baby, and there can be later psychological difficulties related to this. Many intersex infants have surgery to assign a sex, and this decision is usually based on the physical presentation of the infant. Psychological issues can emerge in infancy related to the development of 'gender identity' and the concern for some infants is an expressed discomfort with their gender (gender dysphoria). This occurs in infants with normal sexual differentiation. It is usually only in later infancy that these concerns become apparent and parents at this time may seek help and advice. Parents who have had to deal with issues of assigning sex from the birth of their infant may have ongoing concerns about their infant's sexuality and gender behaviour and often require ongoing support.

In working with parents and infants where there are issues about sexuality and gender it is important to understand the parents' ideas and expectations of sexual differences and the attendant gender-related behaviour and the way this influences their relationship with their infant. Cultural expectations about gender behaviour have a powerful influence on parental expectations of infant behaviour, and working in a culturally sensitive manner is necessary in order to understand and respond to concerns.

In this chapter we will consider what contributes to our cultural understanding of 'sex' and 'gender'. We will consider the idea that sex is biologically determined (and perhaps not limited to two sexes), and that gender is socially and culturally determined, although influenced by underlying genetic traits. We will review problems of gender identity found in infancy and look at ways of responding to these issues within a cultural context. Factors in cross-cultural assessment and intervention will be discussed.

CONCEPTS OF SEX AND GENDER

Infant mental health has had surprisingly little to say about gender. While infant researchers may observe and comment on 'sex differences' there has been little analysis of this, and even less analysis of underlying assumptions of models of gender development.

The retrospective psychoanalytic accounts by Freud, while they may be criticised on other grounds, have at least taken gender as a fundamental category of analysis. In some ways, infant mental health shows remnants of Freud's early one-sex model—a model of male development with the female defined only in relation to this. More recently, interests have turned to understanding the complex interactions of biology and social experiences or culture that are involved in creating gender.

Concepts of sex and gender exemplify the tensions between biology and culture, and old and newer models of development. In older models, sex is usually seen as genetically influenced and innate, and results in psychological or social differences in males and females or gender roles. Contemporary theories point out that biology always interacts with environment. Biological sex differences are influenced by culture and language and differing social expectations of males and females. Cultural expectations also influence parenting and the earliest interactions with male and female infants.

Biological sex and infant development

The majority of neonates are designated either male or female at birth, or prenatally with the use of ultrasound technology. Biological sex has profound implications for infant development for complex reasons. First, there is increasing evidence of *difference in male and female brain differentiation*, although the extent to which this directly influences observable sex differences in behaviour and psychological functioning is unclear. Second, *caregivers* have their own sets of *beliefs and expectations* about male and female infants, which influence their perceptions of and interactions with their infants. Finally, different *social and cultural* groups have complex and variable *expectations* and definitions of masculinity and femininity, which define appropriate behaviours, personality attributes and social roles. These definitions change over time. Infants develop a sense of gender identity or a self-definition as male or female in the first two to three years of life, and this is influenced by biological, psychological and sociocultural factors. There are ongoing debates over the relative importance of these factors in producing observable differences between males and females but it is clear that differences are evident in infancy.

Definitions

Contemporary theories distinguish sex from gender:

Sex refers to anatomical and biological (genetic and hormonal) categories of male and female, but even biology is complex and subject to interpretation. In nature, there may well be more than two sexes or at least variability in male and female sexual characteristics.

Gender refers to a prevailing sociocultural model that defines social expectations of masculinity and femininity. These expectations encompass sociocultural models of personality, attitudes and behaviours that are seen as linked to each sex. Gender also refers to the social performance indicative of an internal sexed identity—the outward behaviours of masculinity or femininity as they are socially defined.

Gender identity is a complex mixture of biology, socialisation, psychological identification and sexuality. It refers to the individual's sense of himself as a biological, psychological and social male or female.

Gender role refers to the behaviours, attitudes and personality traits designated socioculturally as masculine or feminine. Gender role is incorporated in the self as a set of behaviours, attitudes and personality traits designated socioculturally as masculine or feminine. In children, this is measured by such variables as affiliative preference for same-sex peers, fantasy and play roles and type of play. There is an ongoing controversy over the influence of biological variables such as prenatal sex hormones on observable gender-role behaviour.

Sexual orientation is defined by response to sexual stimuli and sexual identity refers to the definitions of oneself in terms of sexual preference. Sexual orientation emerges after puberty but is not necessarily congruent with sexual identity. For example, it is possible for a male to be primarily aroused by homosexual stimuli but to have a gender identify of himself as a heterosexual.

Male and female sex differentiation

Biological sex may be defined on many levels—ex-determining genes, sex chromosomes, HY sex-determining antigen, gonads, hormones, internal reproductive structures or external genitalia. In some infants, sex cannot be determined as exclusively male or female and complex decisions must be made about sex assignment and surgical intervention.

Genetic sex is established at fertilisation when the genetic material of sperm and ovum are united. The ovum contains 22 chromosomes and a single X sex chromosome. The sperm contains 22 chromosomes and either an X or Y sex chromosome. The normal combination patterns are:
- male—46 XY
- female—46 XX.

There are several variants of this pattern, some of which are associated with problems of biological sex development and infertility. For example:
- Turner's Syndrome 45 X—missing X chromosome in a female
- Klinefelter's Syndrome 47 XXY—additional X chromosome in a male.

The Y chromosome is necessary for the development of male sexual characteristics. A gene on the Y chromosome known as the 'sex-determining region' (SRY gene) codes for the production of 'testes determining factor', which promotes the development of testes and seminiferous tubules. The testis produces the male hormones testosterone and androstenedione and a substance that works to inhibit the development of female (Mullerian) structures, known as 'antimullerian substance'. The X chromosome contains genes for ovarian development and in the absence of male hormones, the course of foetal development is female.

SEXUAL DIFFERENTIATION

The process of sexual differentiation begins with an undifferentiated gonad, that is, tissue that has the potential to develop as either male or female. Before eight weeks gestation no differences exist in internal or external genitalia of male and female embryos. The external genitalia are initially identical in both males and females. The penis and clitoris both develop from the genital tubercle.

INTERSEXUALITY

Deviations in the normal steps of sexual differentiation can result in so-called 'intersex disorders' with disruption of internal and/or external sexual structures. There are a variety of conditions, some with unusual external genitalia and others with poorly developed internal sexual structures. Some neonates have 'ambiguous genitalia', most commonly masculinisation of the external genitals of a female infant due to exposure to male hormones in utero where an excess of androgen is produced by the adrenal glands. Other conditions include hemaphroditism or coexistence of both male and female structures, and testicular feminisation—a condition where a chromosomally male infant has female-appearing external genitalia.

The clinical question involved with intersexuals is how to decide to what sex the intersexed infant should be assigned. Money and Ehrhardt (1972) studied the rearing of intersex children in the 1950s, and concluded that sex of rearing—upbringing—was the most important factor in producing a 'successful' outcome as male or female. They also stated that attempting to change gender after the age of two and a half years was not likely to be successful.

EXAMPLE: MARY

Mary, aged two years, was born with multiple pelvic abnormalities including an imperforate anus, ambiguous external genitalia and penile agenesis and urinary system abnormalities. Examination of chromosomes showed the infant to be male 46 XY and an ultrasound examination showed internal undescended testes. Mary needed emergency surgery to the urinary system and bowel and was raised as female, having later genital surgery. At two, Mary is a secure child with female appearance who enjoys 'female type play' but also 'rough and tumble' activities. While there is some evidence that male and female brains develop differently in utero, socialisation is a very important influence on gender identity.

Caregivers' beliefs and expectations

Core gender identity was defined by Stoller (1968) as the fundamental sense of belonging to one sex. This is an emotionally valued sense of identity and develops between the ages of 18 months and three years. This process will be affected by biological factors and the infant's interactions with carers. For both male and female infants, the first experience of intimacy and sexual feelings is with the primary carer. Within the family, the infant learns about the experience, expression and control of sexual feelings, and about sexual difference. The attitudes of carers about sex, sexuality and gender will have a significant effect on the child's gender development. Infants appear to develop a sense of their own gender and an understanding of gender as a fundamental aspect of the self and others in three stages:

Gender labelling—from about 18 months the infant is able to label individuals as male or female according to external appearance. Infants do not see gender as fixed, and if appearance changes, they think gender may have changed.

Gender constancy—by three years of age gender is part of the self-concept. The child is interested in same-sex peers and activities. He is aware that changing appearance or activity does not change gender.

Gender stability—by four to five years gender is seen as an unchangeable, stable attitude of the self and others.

According to psychoanalytic theorists, such as Fast (1984) and Stoller (1968), the acquisition of gender identity occurs as a component of separation and individuation and the development of self-identity. The attachment relationship is the context in which sense of identity and gender identity both develop.

Social and cultural expectations

In the west, gender is used to distinguish socially constructed roles and cultural representations from biological sex. What we call gender is seen as social, and biological sex is seen as its point of origin and natural limit. In this model, gender should conform to sex.

CULTURAL VARIANCE IN ATTITUDES TOWARDS GENDER

Anthropological and sociological studies have identified significant cultural variation in gender systems and attitudes towards gender variance. Wide variations exist in beliefs about the nature of biology and what constitutes sex, and physical difference per se is not always seen as sufficient to produce gender. The Zuni tribe of North American Indians, for example, do not allocate sex at birth regardless of the appearance of external genitalia, as there is a belief that it may change. Complex rituals are used to 'discover' the sex of the infant and determine sex of rearing. In this situation culture is used to 'interpret' biology that is not self-evident and is not automatically linked to gender identity (Laqueur, 1990).

In some cultural contexts, ambivalent and non-stable gender roles and identities are accepted and not necessarily seen as pathological or disordered. It is possible for gender to be neither male nor female, and for gender transformation to occur well after the age at which psychoanalytic and social learning models would see it as 'irreversible' (Herdt, 1994). The most studied example of culturally understood gender change is the 'Penis at 12' syndrome in the Dominican Republic and equivalent conditions in Papua New Guinea and the South Pacific. In these examples, children with an enzymatic deficiency (5-alpha-reductase needed to convert testosterone to dihydrotestosterone) are born with ambiguous external genitalia and raised in many cases as female. Virilisation (that is, the activation of the deficient enzyme) may occur at puberty and many 'change gender' and successfully adopt a male identity. This change is usually unproblematic and this may well reflect the social acceptance of the phenomenon and challenges the concept of a fixed and unalterable 'Core Gender Identity' (Stoller, 1968).

Similarly, the social acceptance and position of gender-variant individuals shows great cultural variation. Among North American Indians, cross-gendered individuals known as Berdaches have been documented in over 150 groups. Berdaches are assigned a position of high social status within a spiritual system and are seen as a 'third gender', transcending male and female categories. In several religious traditions, deities are seen as hermaphroditic or capable of gender change, which enhances rather than diminishes spiritual power. In the Hindu tradition, for example, the Lord Krishna frequently changes sex and male transvestism is used in Tantric devotions. The Hijras of contemporary India are a diverse group of ceremonially castrated males, intersex individuals and 'feminine males' and are again seen as 'alternative' genders within the Hindu context (Newman, 2002).

SIGNIFICANCE OF CULTURAL VARIATIONS

The significance of these cultural variations is that they raise the possibility of alternative models of the relation between sex and gender and suggest that there is no fixed relation between the body, psychological identification and the social manifestations of gender. It has also been argued that cultural context determines whether gender variation is seen as a 'disorder' needing treatment or an understood and tolerated variation. For the clinician it is important that adoption of a western model and formulation of gender identity and development do not preclude an understanding of possible alternative frameworks, and that a particular normative model of gender development is not rigidly imposed on children and families seeking to understand gender variation.

It is clear that whether gender variability is an 'infant mental health issue' is strongly influenced by cultural expectations of gender behaviour. What is seen in one culture as problematic, may not be seen in the same way by another culture. The important consideration is whether concerns about gender behaviour have an effect on the infant's social relationships and functioning.

PROBLEMS OF GENDER IDENTITY

Diagnostic categories related to problems of gender identity have emerged in a particular historical context after the development of the model of sex and gender.

Two categories will be discussed here—gender dysphoria and Gender Identity Disorder. The origin of these problems in infancy is unclear, and, as we have seen, the complex effect of cultural and social expectations about sex and gender is one reason for this. Factors that may be involved in the development of gender dysphoria or Gender Identity Disorder include biological development, infant–parent relationship issues, or the effect of being born intersex. It is unclear, of course, whether any of these factors tell us anything about biology or nature, however, it is useful to consider the range of thought about gender disorders as they influence approaches to assessment and intervention.

Gender dysphoria

Gender dysphoria is defined as unease about one's biological sex. It refers to the individual's experience of the inappropriateness of or discomfort with his gender, despite having typical male or female chromosomal and anatomical sexual configurations. This may be evident in infants from two years of age who express excessive desire to be the other sex or who have an aversion to their own sexual anatomy. In the preschool period this may be consolidated as a psychological identification with the opposite sex or cross-gender identification. In 'normal' development young children may express the wish to have the genitals of the other sex but do not usually dislike their own bodies. Children born with ambiguous genitalia or intersex conditions may have confusion about their gender, depending upon how easily the child can be assigned to a gender category and how parents are able to support the child.

Gender Identity Disorder

Gender Identity Disorder (GID) in the DSM-IV (American Psychiatric Association [APA], 1994) classification system refers to a strong identification with and preference for the gender role characteristics of the other sex. This is expressed through play, behaviour and verbal statements of a desire to be the other sex. Most young children receiving this diagnosis correctly label their own sex but have a desire to be the other sex. This desire may be articulated as early as two or three years of age. Children may intensely dislike their own genitals and refuse to wear typical male or female clothes. This disorder occurs in children with normal anatomical/chromosomal sex.

As a diagnostic category, GID remains a focus of much contemporary debate. Polarised views abound and essentially revolve around issues of nature versus nurture in the creation of gender identity. In *biological determinist models*, gender identity is seen as founded in prenatal brain development in response to hormonal exposure (Swaab & Fliers, 1985), and largely determines gender role development. In *sociocultural models*, gender identity is seen as a complex internalisation of cultural systems of meaning and subject to variation across cultures and historical periods (Mead, 1949). Biological models see GID as a brain development disorder largely uninfluenced by socialisation.

These very different models lead to different understandings of gender dysphoria and opposing views regarding intervention.

Biological determinist models

Biological models, in simplified terms, see GID as the result of abnormal brain sex differentiation, with subsequent gender development occurring along predetermined lines and in conflict with the assigned gender role. Sex, and in particular 'brain-sex', is seen as the foundation of gender in its social and cultural forms. Intervention for GID then becomes a matter of either changing gender identity to fit the body, or using sex-modifying procedures to align the body with the sense of subjective gender. Given the determining nature of brain processes, the latter approach of aligning the body with the person's sense of gender is favoured. Paradoxically, it also follows from this approach that intersex infants with ambiguous external genitalia should not automatically be assigned to a particular sex (usually female), as their prenatal sexual differentiation will influence gender identity in the same way. There have been several intersex individuals unhappy in their assigned gender role and their experiences are used to discredit a purely social constructionist account of gender identity development (Butler, 1990).

In this binary model, where there are two sexes and two genders, gender should conform to sex and 'normality' is defined as congruence between sexual anatomy and gender identity. To be gendered in opposition to sex is to have a disorder, despite the fact that sex and gender are analytically distinct. Biological accounts suggest that biological treatments should be the major approach.

Sociocultural models

Constructionists argue that gender is not the result of essential biological sexual difference, but rather gender is an elaborate social construct within which biology is interpreted. Gender is seen as causally prior to biological sex differences (Colapinto, 2000). These accounts emphasise the social practices that reinforce a particular culture's gender categorisation and see nothing intrinsic and fixed about a binary gender system. At their most extreme, these accounts argue that 'gender dysphoria' is the response of an individual who does not conform to defined gender role and that GID is a psychiatric label used to pathologise those experiences of gender non-conformity. While an individual with gender dysphoria may suffer distress, social discrimination and secondary emotional problems, it is argued that sociocultural change and the dismantling of rigid gender categories is the level of needed intervention rather than individual 'treatment' for a 'disorder'.

Social constructionists may not see the role for individual intervention and argue for much more social flexibility in the interpretation of gender. In practice, the majority of parents of an intersex infant support some intervention and find it difficult to raise their infant when uncertain about gender. Factors such as the family's tolerance of this uncertainty, the 'degree' of difference in the child's appearance and the family's beliefs about gender should be taken into account in decision making.

Understandings of gender dysphoria and GID

A number of factors contribute to our understanding of gender dysphoria and GID. Biological development, infant–parent relationship issues and the experiences of people born intersex are all areas of study that have contributed to knowledge in this area.

Biological development

Biological theories have looked at possible genetic influences, the effects of prenatal sex hormones and studies of children for evidence of possible sex-related differences in cognitive abilities and noted that as a group, GID boys are considered physically attractive when assessed by independent raters (Zucker & Bradley, 1995). On the whole there is no clear evidence for a simple biological course of GID. Current models of brain-sex differentiation hypothesise that in-utero development, possibly in response to hormones, may result in a 'cross-gendered' development of certain brain structures. While there is some limited evidence for structural brain differences in adult transsexuals, little work has yet been done on infant brain-sex development.

A complicating issue is that adults interact very differently with male and female infants, which may in itself affect the way the brain develops.

Infant–parent relationship issues

Stoller (1968), from a psychoanalytic point of view, comments on an overly close relationship with the mother—an excessively symbiotic physical relationship—and the absence of a psychological father in boys with GID. Mothers, Stoller thought, had their own conflicts over femininity, penis-envy, and were excessively masculine in their own childhoods and bisexual. For Stoller, the little boy with GID cannot separate from his mother or identify with his father so he 'becomes' his mother.

In assessment of families with concerns about a child's gender development it is important to examine the parents' acceptance of their child's sex, and a history of any gender confusion in the parents' own childhood. Assessment should also focus on the parent's practices of gender socialisation, such as choice of toys and games activities.

Effect of being born intersex

Intersex infants are known to their parents as being ambiguously sexed from birth. Ambiguity about gender is not very well tolerated in our culture, by parents or surgeons, and the demand is to operate to fix the body. Parents therefore have to go through the decision-making process about which sex their child will be and this clearly influences their relationship with their child. The focus on genitals and the often protracted multiple operations needed to correct

GENDER DEVELOPMENT AND IDENTITY

them must mean that parents are sensitised to possible gender deviance. That is, parents expect there might not be congruence between the assigned sex and the gender behaviour that emerges, and are therefore more likely to notice behaviour that is not consistent with gender norms.

EXAMPLE: MARY, CONTINUED

Mary (described earlier in this chapter) was adopted at birth with new parents being fully informed about her chromosomal (male) sex. The parents were advised to raise Mary as a girl as 'clearly' as possible but describe themselves observing her for 'signs' of excessive male behaviour. Mary's parents tended to encourage her towards stereotypically female toys and games and dressed Mary in a very feminine style. Some families in this situation may be anxious and excessively limit the child's behaviour and activities.

ASSESSMENT, FORMULATION AND INTERVENTION

Increasingly, there have been challenges both to the notion of the purely social construction of gender identity and to the idea that 'nature' only knows two sexes. This increasing complexity allows for the development of a biopsychosocial understanding that can take into account interactions between biological and psychosocial factors in mediating gender identity.

In clinical practice and the assessment of children and young people with gender dysphoria and their families, these debates are frequently a focus of discussion. Parents in particular are often concerned with understanding their child's experiences and creating their own aetiological model. Adolescents presenting with requests for sex-modifying procedures are often familiar with contemporary debates and have a particular account of their own condition. The situation becomes more complex when working with families and individuals in a multicultural context where there are various specific cultural understandings of gender systems, gender development and degrees of tolerance for atypical gender behaviours. Clinicians in multicultural contexts need to be aware that definitions of GID have developed within a particular cultural framework and contain within them assumptions about gender systems that may not be shared by families presenting for assessment. In these situations exploration of the families' understandings of gender and sex within their own context is an essential component of comprehensive formulation.

Cross-cultural assessment

A major issue in the assessment of gender dysphoria in multicultural contexts is how best to establish the particular model of sex-gender and gender deviance held by the child and family. Planning appropriate intervention can only occur when it is seen how the family understand gender variation and how it will be managed within the cultural framework of the family. It is also important that the child be supported in his overall social context and in managing what may be a 'cultural gap' between the family and mainstream social values.

The following examples illustrate some of the complexities of cross-cultural assessment.

EXAMPLE 1: MICHAEL

Michael is a three-year-old boy referred by his preschool for assessment as he has clear cross-gender identification and behaviours. Michael's family are from Thailand and they have been resident in Australia for 12 months. The parents are non-English-speaking Buddhists and describe a belief system ascribing positive value to gender transition and an acceptance that some children are born as a 'third gender'. Michael's parents are aware that he is being teased at preschool and is having difficulties with his peers. There are adult transsexuals in the extended family. Michael is not discouraged from cross-gendered behaviour and the school has found it difficult to discuss issues with Michael's parents.

Several issues and dilemmas are raised in this situation. Should Michael's family be encouraged to view Michael's development as disturbed and his cross-gender identification as pathological, even though they currently do not see it as such? Should the school environment be one that discourages Michael from expressing his cross-gendered interests even though he can express these at home? How is it possible to 'change' Michael's family's understanding of gender identity and is it ethical to attempt to do this? In practice, a key issue is working with Michael's stated difficulties with his peers and academic performance. Regardless of his family's acceptance of him, Michael is attempting to adapt to a peer group and community in which his experience is unusual and his position as cross-gendered may have negative effects on his ongoing development.

EXAMPLE 2: SAM

Sam is a four-year-old boy from an Arabic family who present with concerns that he is effeminate and 'homosexual'. Sam has some cross-gender interests but does not meet diagnostic criteria for GID. The family culture is one of significant homophobia and rigid models of gender-role behaviour. Sam's father is seeking genetic and hormonal investigation of Sam believing that he has a biological disorder. He has been physically punishing Sam for his behaviour.

In this situation Sam is exhibiting gender-aberrant behaviour as defined by his family's cultural understanding of appropriate male behaviour. The immediate clinical concern is the degree of hostility directed towards Sam and the difficulty of engaging Sam's father. It may be necessary to involve culturally representative clinicians if available and to encourage involvement of all family members in initial negotiations in relation to an intervention framework. It is important to acknowledge and respect the family's concerns about Sam's development, and to contain immediate anxiety by offering appropriate support and to be cautious in 'challenging' the family's understanding of Sam's 'disorder' as biological in origin.

As these examples illustrate, cultural context influences both the presentation and understanding of gender dysphoria and gender-aberrant behaviour. Non-normative gender-role behaviour may in one context be seen as an unproblematic variation (Example 1), while in another it may be defined as a disorder (Example 2). Different cultures will formulate any concept of 'gender disorder' according to varying models of sex-gender and the development of gender identity. They will also vary in concepts of the fixity or fluidity of gender identity and degrees of accommodation of gender transition. In some contexts it will be possible to adopt alternative or additional gender positions.

Assessment principles

Initially, it is important to explore the family members' particular understanding of gender and gender variation and to introduce the concept of cultural relativity. This is crucial in families where there are conflicting views between the child/adolescent and parents.

In clinical practice, in addition to standard assessment of the child's gender development and behaviour, it is important to explore the family's cultural and spiritual context and models of gender.

Issues in cross-cultural assessment of GID

1 How does the culture understand the differences between male and female?
2 What account is given of the development of male and female individuals? Are differences and roles 'innate' or 'learned'?
3 Are all individuals male or female, or are alternative positions possible?
4 What does the religious/spiritual context say about gender roles and positions? Are there taboos against the violation of gender roles and gender change?
5 Does the culture separate questions of sexual orientation from gender, or is gender variation seen as signifying potential homosexuality?
6 What are the cultural attitudes towards homosexuality and gender variation?
7 Does the culture have an assigned place for gender-variant individuals?
8 What attitudes exist about sex-modifying procedures and the involvement of medical/surgical systems in interventions aimed at gender change?

Variations in models of gender also occur within majority culture and within families. The clinician can use a multicultural frame to avoid the assumption of the dominant model and explore the specific model(s) of the child and family in an open manner.

The aim of cross-cultural assessment is to understand the system of gender attribution within which the child's development is situated. This system determines the meaning given to the child's behaviour or wishes regarding gender and also influences the intervention approach. The child's development, however, also needs to be seen in the context of the dominant gender system, school, peer group and other groups beyond the family. Regardless of family and subcultural belief systems, the child is also immersed in a conventional western model of gender and must come to some accommodation of this.

Intervention principles

Children with aberrant gender-role behaviours distress their families, schools and peers, and certainly are distressed by this themselves. And yet, there is little evidence of the effectiveness of interventions and serious questions about the ethics of intervention.

Those who believe that the therapeutic interventions should focus on eliminating the cross-gender behaviour argue that this is the ethical choice for several reasons—reduction of social ostracism, treatment of underlying psychopathology and prevention of transsexualism and, more controversially, the prevention of homosexuality.

Others argue that attempting to change the behaviour will not eliminate the 'disorder' and will further damage the individual. In this view, the strategy becomes one of increasing social acceptance and helping the child live in a culture that is stigmatising and punitive to those who cross gender categories.

Ethnomethodological approach

An ethnomethodological approach suggests that the social construction of systems of gender attribution is of major importance in the conceptualisation of gender development and its disorders. Gender systems show cultural and historical variation and current debates about the nature of GID reflect a general move towards acknowledgement of cultural relativity and questioning of western normative developmental models. In a multicultural context, families will present with widely divergent views on these issues. Some will see deviation from typical gender behaviour as problematic and others will not, and developmental understanding may be influenced by particular religious beliefs. The difficulty for clinicians is that the child may be experiencing mental health problems such as gender dysphoria and secondary difficulties such as separation anxiety and peer problems, to the extent that intervention is warranted.

Similar principles apply here as in many cross-cultural clinical situations where the professional is not of the family's cultural background:
1. appropriate use of interpreters and cultural representatives
2. assessment of the family's understanding and attributions
3. advocacy for the needs of the child to accommodate to the social environment
4. sensitivity and tolerance of frameworks that are incommensurate with western ideals
5. engaging with the family within their own cultural framework.

Developmental approach

The focus of clinical intervention may be best centred on the developmental needs of the child and promotion of an integrated sense of identity, rather than on challenging the family's views on gender development and disorder. While psychoeducation may be useful, particularly regarding the child's overall emotional development, an overly confrontational stance risks alienating the family and further placing the child in an untenable position. Cultural relativity, that is, the acceptance of multiple models of gender, is a difficult clinical position to maintain but is essential in assessment.

EXAMPLE: DAVID

David is brought for assessment by his mother following concerns being raised at preschool about his expressed wish to be a girl. David is four years old and presents as an attractive child who is quiet and withdrawn. David tells you that he has 'a secret wish to be a girl'. He has an elaborate fantasy life centred on an image of himself as a 'fairy girl'. He draws fairies and always role plays the female in games. At home he likes to dress as a fairy or in his mother's clothes and shoes. He is interested in makeup and brushing his older sister's hair. He says he dreams that he will turn into a girl and says he will be a mother when he grows up.

David meets the criteria for GID and his family become involved in a program aimed at broadening his interests and exposing him to some positive aspects of being male. David spends time with his father and is introduced to gender-neutral games and activities, which he enjoys. Intervention aims at reducing David's anxiety about male gender in a non-punitive way and supporting his development and peer relations.

Over a 12-month period, David persists in his preference for female identity but makes a better adaptation to the school environment. His teachers in primary school are supported in providing a range of activities and David's parents are supported in coping with their anxiety about his development.

SUMMARY

GID is a condition placed at the interface of culture and nature. The debates about the relative contributions of biology and psychosocial factors reflect the ongoing tensions inherent in our models of sex and gender. Working with culturally diverse populations gives some insight into the complex systems surrounding gender and its disorders, and encourages clinicians to reflect on their own particular cultural biases and models. Advocating for improved social tolerance and understanding of gender variation, in the broader community and other institutions such as schools, extends the clinical role but is an important component of social reform in reducing distress and developmental risk for gender-variant children/adolescents.

The clinician who can avoid imposition of a particular gender model can more effectively assist the child/adolescent to facilitate his individual development of an uncomplicated sense of gender identity and to facilitate family acceptance and understanding of the child's developmental needs.

PART D

Parents and society

CHAPTER 12

Perinatal mental illness

KEY CONCEPTS

- Increased risk of psychiatric disorder during the perinatal period
- A range of difficulties and disorders present at this time
- Potential effect on relationships including the infant–parent relationship and infant development

FACTORS IN ASSESSMENT AND FORMULATION

- Necessity for accurate assessment and diagnosis
- Consideration of safety issues for infant and parent
- Assessment of the effect of the illness on parenting capacity
- Relationship-based interventions may be indicated

The term 'perinatal mental illness' covers a variety of mood and behaviour disturbances that a woman may experience during pregnancy and the post-partum period. There has been an ongoing debate about whether the perinatal period, the time immediately before and after birth, represents a time of increased risk for mental illness in women, and whether there are disorders particular to this period of life. The question of why pregnancy and childbirth might act as triggers for the onset of the range of psychiatric illness in otherwise healthy women is an area of ongoing research and debate. Current evidence is that women are diagnosed with depression about twice as often as men, and that there is a peak of first episodes in the childbearing years, with onset more frequent after childbirth. Half of these episodes develop within three months and about three-quarters develop within six months of giving birth (Cooper, Campbell, Day, Kennerley & Bond, 1998; Cooper & Murray, 1995; Cox, Murray & Chapman, 1993).

'Post-natal depression' is a commonly used term that describes a range of mental health problems occurring in the post-partum period. In many ways it is a misleading term because it is used to cover a range of mood and anxiety disorders of varying severity, and does not represent a clear diagnosis of the maternal mental health problem. This chapter will explore the range of difficulties often included under this terminology in order to think more carefully about the diagnostic and treatment issues that arise with maternal mental illness. The major points to consider in assessment and intervention will be explored, including ways to minimise any potential effect on the infant–parent relationship and therefore on infant development.

This chapter will also review factors that increase vulnerability to mental illness at this time of transition and upheaval, consider the implications for assessment and intervention and discuss the evidence that exists for parental mental illness as a risk factor with a potential effect on optimal infant development.

THE CONTEXT OF PERINATAL MENTAL ILLNESS

There is ample evidence available to confirm that many women experience mental health problems in the perinatal period. What is not understood clearly is why this period is a vulnerable time for women, or, rather, what factors interact to create vulnerability to mental disorders at this time. Understanding the biopsychosocial context for mental illness means acknowledging both the social pressures women face during this time as well as the possible effect of changes in body chemistry.

Occurrence of perinatal mental illness

Studies suggest that up to 40 per cent of women experience psychological distress after having a baby. Not only the mother, but also her partner and children may be affected by this and the effects may be transient or long lasting. This distress does not always fit easily into traditional psychiatric or illness (medical) definitions. Only about 10–15 per cent of women will meet diagnostic criteria (American Psychiatric Association [APA], 1994) for Major Depression, while other women may fulfil criteria for a range of other psychiatric disorders (Cooper et al., 1988; Cox et al., 1993). Whatever diagnostic or classificatory system is used, it is clear that assessment and intervention with women and families presenting with mental distress or illness in the perinatal period must take the following factors into account:
- that the woman is pregnant or has recently given birth

- that she has a vulnerable infant whose need for care and protection must be kept in mind
- that psychiatric illness at this time has a potential effect on all family members and relationships.

In urban situations, significant depression has been reported in 25 per cent of British mothers with school-aged children and 40 per cent of working-class mothers. Post-natal depression is commonly cited as occurring in 10-15 per cent of new mothers. The incidence is reported to increase three-fold within five weeks of delivery (Cooper & Murray, 1995; Cox et al., 1993; Cross-National Collaborative Group, 1992).

Mental illness or adjustment difficulties?

The transition to parenthood, which occurs at a biological, psychological and social level, and the range of factors that influence the ability of an individual or couple to adjust to the many changes associated with parenthood, have been discussed (see Chapter 5). Many, but not all, of those who have difficulties at this transitional stage were already vulnerable or mentally ill, or had long-standing, interpersonal difficulties (personality disorders) before they became parents.

Parenthood brings with it a range of contradictory social expectations and attitudes. Men, as well as women, make many adjustments and may experience losses in the transition to parenthood, but do not have the enormous bodily and hormonal changes experienced by women at this time. Societal attitudes to women who choose to either work or parent full-time remain ambivalent and the many women who attempt to combine both often struggle to get the right balance for themselves and their families.

There is an argument that mental health and adjustment difficulties are best understood as a normal part of adjustment to parenthood. Arguments are made against 'medicalising' emotional distress at this time on the grounds that this further stigmatises the woman having difficulties at a time widely regarded and represented as one of joy and celebration. The argument is made that this disregards the effect of unrealistic and contradictory social expectations of, and attitudes to, mothers and mothering and the evidence, for example, that a lack of social support increases the risk of depression post-natally.

The counter argument is that if the reality of perinatal mental illness is not recognised, many women and their infants suffer without adequate intervention and treatment. Severe mental illness at this time has implications for the immediate safety of the parent and the infant as well as a potential longer term effect on infant development. In summary then, the argument against medicalising perinatal distress and disorders highlights the importance of the social and interpersonal factors that contribute to vulnerability. It must also be acknowledged that a range of disorders occur at this time, some of which are best understood and managed as 'adjustment disorders', while some women will fulfil criteria for significant psychiatric illness and lasting disability. Appropriate management will include what can be considered 'medical' approaches in combination with a range of psychological and social strategies.

Early identification

An important aspect of mental health problems occurring perinatally is that this is a time when most women are in regular contact with obstetric and later paediatric health services. Thus, there is an opportunity for early identification and, potentially, intervention with women at risk of perinatal mental health problems. Most obstetric services now incorporate psychosocial questions into antenatal screening procedures to try to identify women at high risk of ongoing difficulties, and early childhood staff are increasingly trained to screen for and identify problems post-natally. Ideally, early referral to appropriate supports and other services can follow. As women regularly visit health workers for care over this time this may be their main avenue for receiving care of both a preventive and therapeutic nature.

Assessment tools

Careful assessment of the psychological and social well-being of all pregnant women or mothers with infants or young children should be part of routine health care. There are, for example, several assessment skills and tools that allow early detection of distress and depression, with the aim of minimising the effects on the woman and her family. The Edinburgh Postnatal Depression Scale (EPDS or ES) is a simple, well-validated screening tool, easy to apply in primary care settings. It can also be used ante-natally and well beyond the post-natal period, with some minor adjustment to the instructions. Results correlate closely with formal extended psychiatric evaluation. For further information about the scale and its use see Cox, Holden and Sagovsky (1987). Other assessment tools are discussed further, later in this chapter.

THE SPECTRUM OF DISORDER

Mental illness occurring in the perinatal period includes a spectrum of mild to severe problems from the 'baby blues' through to florid psychotic illnesses. In between lies what is often called 'post-natal depression' (PND), that is, all the depressive disorders that do not fall within the category of the 'blues' or psychosis.

Thus, the clinical picture includes a wide array of presentations, ranging from adjustment disorders and dysthymia to severe depression and psychosis. Anxiety and/or obsessive-compulsive symptoms are common and may be a prominent component of PND, but anxiety disorders (Generalised Anxiety Disorder; Agoraphobia, Panic Disorder; Obsessive Compulsive Disorder, Post-Traumatic Stress Disorder) may also diagnosed in their own right at this time. Depressive symptoms are often 'atypical'. Sleep disturbance, a common symptom of depression, is hard to assess in new parents who often have a degree of sleep deprivation. Inability to sleep even when the baby sleeps is an important sign of distress. Inability to enjoy the baby or fear of the baby may also be present.

The 'blues'

The 'baby blues' are common, transient symptoms occurring in 50–80 per cent of new mothers (Cooper & Murray, 1995). Symptoms include: mood swings from sadness to elation, with tears likely either way; increased sensitivity; irritability, exhaustion and a variety of aches and pains. Some experts believe that if the predominant mood is positive, the 'blues' should be described as the 'pinks' or the 'highs'. These symptoms may last from a few hours to 10 days and usually peak on the third or fifth day after delivery, the time for most women when their 'milk comes in'. The timing and frequency with which these symptoms occur has led to general acceptance that physiological changes play a large part in the symptoms associated with the 'blues' although no particular hormonal or other physiological marker has been identified as causal. During delivery and in the immediate post-partum period there are dramatic falls in the hormonal levels associated with pregnancy and further changes with the onset of lactation.

Support and encouragement combined with the information that these symptoms are likely to be short-lived, constitute sufficient management in most instances. Severe 'blues' or 'pinks' are considered to indicate a higher risk of subsequent clinical depression or other psychiatric disorder and indicate a need for ongoing monitoring if the mood lability and other symptoms persist.

Psychosis

Post-partum or puerperal psychosis (PPP) is a serious, but fortunately rare disorder, occurring after about 0.1–0.2 per cent of deliveries (Kendell, Chalmers & Platz, 1987). The onset is commonly within the first three weeks after delivery, but it may sometimes begin with a prodromal mood disturbance (usually unrecognised) during pregnancy. PPP is usually a diagnosis of affective or mood disorder, that is, a manic or depressive episode or a mixed picture. The onset of schizophrenia and recurrence of previously diagnosed psychotic illness also occurs post-partum. Within the DSM-IV system there is the option of indicating post-partum onset of mood disorders, including manic and depressive psychosis, but this option is not available within the DSM-IV classificatory system if schizophrenia is the primary diagnosis (APA, 1994; Castle, McGrath & Kulkarni, 2000).

The clinical picture includes a combination of mood and thought disorder, which may manifest as: loss of contact with reality; confusion; disorganised thinking; strange ideas; delusions; hallucinations; extremes, or rapid swings of activity and mood, which may be confident, aggressive, talkative, grandiose, extravagant, elated, withdrawn, anxious, quiet, miserable, numb, agitated or immobilised; and/or insomnia and anorexia. In comparison with psychotic disorders occurring at other times there is often greater fluctuation in mood and mental state and episodes of confusion or disorientation that may resemble a delirium or disorder secondary to a medical illness. Assessment needs to exclude an organic or medical explanation for the symptoms and this is discussed further below.

The predominant risk factors for puerperal psychosis are a family history of psychosis, and/or a prior history of psychiatric disorder (Jones & Craddock, 2001). Other risk factors include a first baby, having no partner at the time of delivery, undergoing caesarean section delivery or the baby being very sick or dying.

Assessment must always include consideration of maternal and infant safety. In the acute stage of the illness, the mother may not be able to care for the baby without supervision, and alternative care for the baby may need to be arranged in the short term. Management usually includes hospital admission (with the baby as appropriate), medication and sometimes electro-convulsive therapy (ECT), in addition to counselling and support for all concerned.

Recovery from a particular episode is usually good, although there is a high risk of recurrence, particularly with later pregnancies, and for some women a post-partum psychotic episode may herald ongoing episodes of illness independent of pregnancy. Psychiatric support is helpful in decision making about the risk of recurrence with subsequent pregnancies, and active management and intervention to prevent recurrence is advisable.

Post-natal depression and anxiety (or non-psychotic depression)

As discussed above, symptoms constituting illness must be distinguished from 'normal' reactions to the multiple physiological, psychological and social stresses accompanying the arrival of a baby. A new mother is almost inevitably exhausted, preoccupied with and concerned about herself and the baby, and may be overwhelmed at times with worries about the infant or the marital relationship while coming to terms with the adjustments entailed in becoming a mother. Nevertheless, chronic stress and sleep deprivation are a health hazard, and a diagnosis of clinically significant depression should be considered when the mood changes or persistent anxiety are of more than two weeks' duration and result in physical, psychological and/or significant social dysfunction. Conservatively estimated, anxiety/depression is suffered by some 15 per cent of new mothers and, since it frequently goes unrecognised and untreated, can become a chronic problem (O'Hara, 1997).

Most women who suffer significant perinatal mental illness have a combination of general risk factors contributing to their vulnerability. These factors include:

- *past history of psychiatric disorder*, especially depression (including post-natal depression) and psychosis, or a significant family history of psychiatric illness. These factors may indicate a genetic or constitutional vulnerability.
- *lack of personal and/or social support*, in particular, an unsupportive or absent partner but also limited social supports, for example, refugee or immigrant families.
- *current stressful life events*, trauma or adversity including any complications for mother or infant such as premature or post-mature delivery, current or recent bereavement, multiple birth; premature or sick baby; and 'abnormal' appearance of baby.
- *personality factors*, in particular, obsessionality or difficulties maintaining relationships and limited sense of self, for example, in people with Borderline Personality traits (APA, 1994; also see Chapter 15).
- *previous or early trauma* including a history of physical, emotional or sexual abuse or problematic relationships with family of origin. Some studies also suggest previous obstetric or gynaecological difficulties.

Some studies also indicate that maternal age (<18 or >32 years) and marked ambivalence about the pregnancy are also contributing risk factors (O'Hara, 1997).

Women who fail to attend for ante-natal care or who are identified during pregnancy as suffering significant anxiety or depression are at risk of increased difficulties after delivery. As mentioned above, women who have no partner or support person in attendance, suffer severe 'blues' or 'pinks' ('highs') or experience breastfeeding problems also need careful monitoring in relation to their mental health and well-being (Brockington, 1996).

Effect of perinatal mental illness on the infant and family

As has been discussed in earlier chapters, the infant is extremely dependent on the sensitivity and responsiveness of her primary caregivers. Depression and/or significant social or personal adversity interferes with social functioning and emotional availability, and may make parents less contingent and sensitive in interaction with their babies.

Australian studies (for example, McMahon, Barnett, Kowalenko, Tennant & Don, 2001) have found a close association between maternal mood and unsettled infant behaviour in their sample of women admitted to residential parent-craft hospitals. Their study confirms the interactional nature of relationship difficulties in this period, that is, mothers are also dependent to an extent on the responses they receive or perceive from their infants for a sense of their own competence and effectiveness as parents. Post-natal mood disorder can interfere with accurate interpretation of infant cues and increase the risk of depressive or negative attribution of infant behaviour and responses. Both the parent and the infant bring strengths and vulnerabilities to the new relationship and the 'fit' between them in the context of other supports and stressors determines how the new relationship develops.

Several studies have now indicated that maternal depression, especially in combination with other risk factors, can decrease the security of infant attachment at 12 months and affect the infant's social and short-term cognitive development.

Cooper and Murray (1997) conducted a longitudinal study examining the effect of PND on infant development in a low-risk British sample. They found that maternal depression at two months post-partum did affect the sensitivity and attunement of mothers to their babies, who used less affirming language and were more negating of their infants' experience. This had an effect on cognitive development at 18 months. Social and personal adversity had an effect on the security of infant attachment.

Other researchers (for example, Kurstjens & Wolke, 2001) found a significant effect on cognitive development in boys associated with chronicity of maternal depression—particularly in low-socioeconomic-status families, or in infants with other perinatal risk factors. Boys may also be more vulnerable generally to the effect of maternal depression (Hay, 1997).

Post-natal psychiatric illness also affects partners and the quality of the marital interaction. Because lack of a supportive partner is a clear risk factor for post-natal mental illness, the direction of these associations is not always clear. Rarely, men are also diagnosed as suffering the range of perinatal psychiatric disorders that occur in women. More significantly, men were found to be at much greater risk of depression post-partum if their partner was also depressed. Lovestone and Kumar (1993) found depression in male partners followed admission of their spouse to a mother–baby unit. The effect of parental mental illness on other children in the family also needs to be considered (Seifer & Dickstein, 2000).

ASSESSMENT, FORMULATION AND INTERVENTION

The general principles of assessment outlined in Chapters 3 and 4 apply to families where one or both parents suffer a mental illness in the perinatal period. Clearly, it is important that an accurate assessment and diagnosis of the parent's illness is made and that he or she receive appropriate treatment and support in his or her own right if this is indicated.

Diagnostic efforts at this time include consideration of whether the situation is suggestive of difficulty adjusting to parenthood in otherwise well-functioning adults, an episode of mental illness in a previously well person, or recurrence of illness in someone with previous or ongoing mental health problems. Perinatal presentation may also be an indication of decompensation in a person with personality dysfunction or disorder, who may give a history of long-term problems with relationships, intimacy and emotional regulation. Drug or alcohol misuse need to be excluded as factors contributing to the presentation and medical illness, for example, post-partum infection, thyroid malfunction, uncorrected anaemia or viral illness also need to be excluded. Clear diagnosis of the nature and duration of the parental illness is important prognostically and in assessing immediate and ongoing risk to parent and infant.

Assessment and formulation principles

Particular issues arise in considering the implications for infant mental health and well-being of parental mental illness in the perinatal period. Each family needs to be assessed individually with careful attention to identifying the risk and protective factors affecting their relationships and potentially the infant's well-being.

Screening tools

As discussed above, a number of screening tools exist for use in the perinatal period, the most well known and commonly used being the Edinburgh Postnatal Depression Scale or EPNDS. This simple self-report scale, developed initially for use at six weeks post-partum, is now used in a variety of settings and is validated against structured diagnostic instruments and questionnaires as useful in identifying women (usual cut-off score >12 on the EPNDS) who are suffering significant psychiatric illness and need further assessment and intervention.

This is no substitute for a thorough assessment, but the EPNDS is a useful tool for identifying those at risk and currently suffering.

A thorough assessment includes the immediate effect of the illness on the parent's capacity to provide adequate care and protection for her infant. This is assessed in the context of the availability of other social supports and relationships. For example, an episode of mania in an otherwise well-functioning woman with good supports raises immediate concerns about her capacity to care for the baby in the short term, particularly if her psychosis includes bizarre or grandiose ideas about the infant (for example, that he is the messiah). However, if she is compliant with and responsive to treatment, other family members are able to care for the infant in the short term, and she develops insight into her illness and returns home to a supportive family and treatment network, the outcome for the infant–parent relationship and the infant's development is likely to be good.

EXAMPLE: KIM

Kim was referred for assessment eight days after delivery of her first child with elevated but irritable mood, insomnia and rapid speech. She had been discharged from hospital two days after delivery and followed up at home under the early discharge program. Her husband had become concerned because she was up all night and appeared increasingly disorganised in relation to caring for herself and the baby. At times she was saying what he thought were 'peculiar things', for example, that the baby was a reincarnation of her grandmother, was 'very special' and 'a timeless soul' and that her name should be changed to reflect this. Her husband said this was not consistent with Kim's previous beliefs or with the family's cultural and religious beliefs.

Kim had no previous psychiatric history but her sister and a maternal aunt have bipolar disorder. Although the couple had recently moved to the city they had extended family who were available to provide support after the baby's birth, and her mother was already living with them. Kim had not yet established breast-feeding although she was attempting it inconsistently.

Although Kim did not agree she was unwell, she was compliant with the assessment process, and agreed to a two-week hospital admission. Initially, she was quite confused and disorganised in her behaviour with marked fluctuations in her mood and mental state over the course of a day. Investigations were undertaken to exclude an organic cause for her symptoms. No facilities were available to allow admission of the baby with her, so her husband and mother cared for the baby during this time. Kim responded to treatment with anti-psychotic medication, a mood stabiliser and education about the nature of her illness. Once she had recovered she expressed some sorrow that she had not been able to breastfeed because she was admitted to hospital and her behaviour was too disorganised, but she also acknowledged that her family had cared for the baby well during this time and that she hadn't had to worry about the effect of the medication on the baby. Kim and her family were able to use information about her illness to comply with treatment. Husband and wife expressed some sadness and concern about the risk of recurrence of the illness, especially if they were to consider another baby. Although the longer term prognosis of her illness was not predictable, there were clear protective factors for the baby, and the family had strengths and resources that modified the impact of her illness on their relationships.

In a much less florid or bizarre presentation where a single mother with few supports presents with depression and gives a long history of difficulty in intimate relationships, unstable mood and poor self-esteem, and expresses hostility and resentment towards her baby, then concerns are likely to be greater in the long term for the quality of the relationship and the infant's well-being.

EXAMPLE: LAKSHMI

Lakshmi was a 24-year-old single woman with a history of unstable relationships. She had had two terminations before giving birth to Jai. The delivery was uncomplicated. Lakshmi was estranged from her family, who were critical of her lifestyle and told her she had brought shame upon the family by having a child outside of marriage. Although she had a history of high academic achievement in the early years of high school, she had become 'rebellious' in her mid-teens. She had first suffered depression aged 17 years and had several trials of anti-depressant medication and various attempts at developing a therapeutic relationship with mental health services. She had become more depressed during the pregnancy after breaking up with the baby's father, whom she had only known for a few months. When seen at the six-week check up, she appeared flat in her mood, expressed little enjoyment in the baby, calling him 'pest' and 'fuss bucket'. She was slow to respond to his cues, including his distress. She was socially and personally isolated, with features to suggest a major depression. She was reluctant to see her GP or a psychiatrist and when she did, refused medication on the grounds that 'I've tried it before and it doesn't help'.

The risk factors for this family are predominantly social in that they are isolated with few supports and Lakshmi has a history of difficulty in intimate relationships, ongoing conflict with her own family, ambivalence about the baby and his effect on her life and lifestyle, as well as trouble establishing supportive relationships with treatment services.

In this scenario, the psychiatric illness is less florid and acute than in the case of Kim above, yet the ongoing risks to the infant–parent relationship and those impacting on Jai developmentally are greater. In assessing families presenting with perinatal psychiatric illness, it is never enough to determine parental diagnosis, the whole picture must always be considered so that appropriate interventions and supports can be provided.

Risk and protective factors for consideration include:
- severity of current parental mental illness, insight, response to treatment and prognosis
- availability of social and therapeutic supports
- capacity and willingness of the parent to use available supports and resources
- effect of illness on parenting capacity in the short and longer term.

In terms of immediate risk to the infant, it is of particular concern if the infant is included or incorporated into the delusions or bizarre belief systems of the psychotic parent, even if the beliefs appear positive. Clearly, when beliefs about the infant are overtly negative or bizarre, for example, 'I, his mother am evil and have given birth to the devil incarnate', particular care to protect the infant must also occur. Situations where the infant is included in delusional belief systems, or parental hallucinations, for example, 'she is talking to me and telling me what to do, how to live my life', must be treated as an emergency and steps taken to ensure that the infant is provided with the care and protection that she needs until the parent has recovered enough to resume the infant's day-to-day care. Maintaining some supervised contact between parent and infant during this time is important. Supporting the establishment and maintenance of breast-feeding during parental hospitalisation should also be prioritised if possible and appropriate. Mother–baby units are discussed below as one option for supporting the infant–parent relationship even when the parent is acutely mentally ill.

Equally worrying if sustained in the longer term, although usually presenting less dramatically than in parental psychotic illness, is overt or covert hostility expressed by the parent towards the infant. This may occur when the parent perceives the infant as aggressive or intentionally difficult. For example, in a comment like, 'He is crying again to get at me, he always cries just when I'm trying to have a sleep', or 'Typical, selfish male, only wants what he wants and it has to be right now, just like his father'. This may be associated with parental depression, her beliefs about the baby, or the circumstances of the baby's conception, or may be a reflection of parental personality, and her capacity to put aside her own needs in order to meet those of the baby. A degree of parental ambivalence is inevitable and a normal part of the transition to parenthood, but sustained or pervasive hostility, even when physical needs are appropriately met, must raise concerns about the infant's well-being.

For example, a young mother was heard to say to her toddler, 'Let's go home for lunch, Breanna. What shall I give you to eat, maybe the dog food, that's about what you deserve, isn't it?' It is up to the clinician in these circumstances to determine the significance of this kind of remark and the context in which the family are being seen will determine how and when parental hostility is addressed. A thorough assessment will enable a decision to be made about parental depression and isolation and how this might be contributing to the parent's difficulties in enjoying her baby.

Formulation needs to include consideration of the biological, psychological and social factors that contribute to this family's presentation at this time, as well as the predisposing, precipitating and perpetuating factors in their presentation and protective factors or strengths upon which an intervention can be built.

Formulation

As in all presentations where the focus is on infant as well as parental mental health, the formulation must include more than diagnosis of parental mental illness, and more than diagnosis of infant developmental or health issues. A full understanding of the family situation includes consideration of the range of biological, social and psychological factors that contribute to the family's presentation at this time, in this manner. As the examples described above indicate, prognosis is about much more than diagnosis and adequate intervention will address a range of family, personal and social issues in order to optimise infant and parent development and well-being.

Intervention principles

Perinatal psychiatric disorders are a heterogeneous group of presentations and disorders, and interventions need to be tailored to fit the needs of a particular family. Different management strategies are indicated for different situations and many families will benefit from more than one approach to their problems. For example, it is rarely if ever enough to prescribe anti-depressant medication to a woman suffering depression in the post-partum period without also developing her support network, involving partner or family members in psycho-education and support, perhaps suggesting a PND group program to reduce her isolation and develop her cognitive and behavioural strategies for managing the symptoms of depression, and considering whether an intervention aimed at improving her interaction with her baby is indicated.

Optimal management of families presenting at this time is a team effort that requires coordination and targeted interventions that address the range and intensity of the family's needs and difficulties.

Ideally, intervention at this time includes:
- early recognition
- accurate assessment of the issues for parent and infant and extended family
- adequate individually tailored intervention
- consideration of relationship factors (infant and partner).

Effective detection and adequate management of these disorders require coordination of a wide variety of primary and secondary care services, including midwives, health visitors, clinical psychologists, community psychiatric services, general practitioners, pharmacists, obstetricians and psychiatrists, with other community agencies, such as voluntary organisations and social services, providing further support.

Range of interventions that may be useful

The evidence base for management strategies for post-natal depression is summarised by Kowalenko, Barnett, Fowler and Matthey (2000). They found evidence in treatment of post-natal depression to support the use of home-based interventions including:

- non-directive counselling (Cooper & Murray, 1997; Holden, Sagovsky & Cox, 1989)
- cognitive therapy (Cooper & Murray, 1997)
- dynamic psychotherapy focused on the mother–baby relationship (Cooper & Murray, 1997).

Anti-depressant medication has also been found to be an effective intervention for this group (Appelby, Warner, Whitton & Faragher, 1997). Group treatment that incorporated psychotherapeutic, supportive and cognitive strategies was also an effective treatment for women with PND, and fathers were also invited to attend (Morgan, Matthey, Barnett & Richardson, 1997).

Women with severe mood disorders or psychotic illness are likely to need more intensive interventions including hospitalisation and intensive community follow up. The identified benefits of admitting babies to hospital with their mothers include minimised disruption to the development of the mother–baby relationship and increased likelihood of the establishment and maintenance of breastfeeding. Disadvantages include consideration of risk to the infant not only from the mother but also from other acutely ill inpatients. The limited availability of specialist mother–baby units and services is also a significant factor (Milgrom, Burrows, Snellen, Stamboulakis & Burrows, 1998).

The use of psychotropic medication during pregnancy and lactation

This is by necessity a brief introduction and overview of a complex and ever-changing area of knowledge and practice. All medications approved by Therapeutic Goods administrations in developed countries are rated according to evidence for their safety of use in pregnancy and lactation. These ratings are regularly updated as evidence about safety and efficacy of medications prescribed to the mother at this time becomes available. Because information about current evidence and safety of any particular drug or class of medication changes constantly, it is necessary to consult up-to-date prescribing guidelines or hospital-based information services (for example, Royal Women's Hospital, 2001).

It is wise to be cautious about prescribing drugs during pregnancy or when a mother is breastfeeding because most medications cross the placenta into the foetal circulation and are also metabolised and excreted to varying degrees in breastmilk. In early pregnancy the main concern is the risk of teratogenesis or foetal malformation. In the third trimester the main risks are neonatal toxicity or withdrawal syndromes following delivery. There is also concern about the possibility of a long-term effect on infant neurological and psychological development that may not be evident at birth (Field, 1998). During breastfeeding many drugs taken by the mother are excreted in the milk and ingested by the infant, with consequent concerns about their effect on the infant with regard to both short-term toxicity and longer term neurodevelopment (Yoshida, Smith & Kumar, 1999). Also, ethical issues restrict the ability to trial medications on women during pregnancy and lactation, and so inevitably incomplete safety information is often obtained from animal studies.

GENERAL PRINCIPLES

The following general principles should guide the prescription of new medication or the continuation of established therapy during pregnancy and in breastfeeding (adapted from Scottish Intercollegiate Guidelines Network [SIGN], 2002):

- establish a clear indication for drug treatment (that is, the presence of significant illness in the absence of acceptable or effective alternatives)
- use treatments in the lowest effective dose for the shortest period necessary
- drugs with a better evidence base (generally more established drugs) are preferable
- assess the benefit/risk ratio of the illness and treatment for both mother and baby/foetus.

While the potential risks to the infant of prescription of psychotropic medications in pregnancy and lactation are clear, there is increasing evidence too that untreated or under-treated maternal psychiatric illness is not without side effects for the baby. Maternal risks include suicidal behaviour, poor ante-natal care and self-care, inadequate nutrition and self-medication with drugs or alcohol, all of which present risks to the foetus (Austin & Mitchell, 1998). There is also evidence of increased obstetric and foetal complications in children born to women with mental illness (Orr & Miller 1995; Sacker, Done & Crow, 1996; Wisner et al., 2000).

Perinatal mental illness and breastfeeding

Women who develop mental illness following childbirth have lower rates of breastfeeding than the general population. There are many reasons for this, including:

- they are group at risk of reduced social and personal support

- depression can interfere with the ability to persevere if breastfeeding is hard to establish
- if they need psychotropic medication, they are likely to be discouraged from breastfeeding because of the potential risks to the infant. (However, the risk of breastfeeding in this situation may be over-estimated and the advantages under-estimated (Wisner, Perel & Findling, 1996.)

The process of metabolising and excreting psychotropic medication is complex, with variation in milk/maternal plasma ratios for different individuals and different medications and between foremilk and hind milk. The physical maturity and health of the baby will also influence any effect of drugs taken by the mother. Premature or sick infants are likely to be more vulnerable to the effects of exposure to maternal medications. The evidence base and information about this topic are limited by the small number of adequately conducted trials and the lack of any systematic approach to monitoring and registering information about the use of psychotropic medication in breastfeeding women. Also, the constantly changing availability of medications for treating psychiatric illness means that infants are exposed to medications about which little information is available.

Medications prescribed to breastfeeding mothers are best taken as a single dose where possible and should be administered before the baby's longest sleep period. Breastfeeding is best done immediately before administering the dose and should be avoided for one to two hours after any dose of medication (the time of highest plasma concentrations).

SUMMARY

The perinatal period represents a time of increased risk of mental illness for women, and disorders occurring at this time range in nature and severity, from transient adjustment disorders to the psychiatric emergency of puerperal psychosis. The term 'post-natal depression' or PND is used to cover a variety of non-psychotic, usually mood or anxiety, disorders occurring at this time. All families presenting with parental mental illness during this period require a thorough individualised assessment. Mental illness occurring at this time has a potential impact not only on the parent but also on family and couple relationships as well as on optimal infant development. Assessment and intervention must include consideration of safety of the parent and infant. Interventions need to be tailored to the needs of the family, but can include a range of strategies. Guidelines for the use of psychotropic medications in pregnancy and lactation are included. All clinicians are advised to be familiar with local, up-to-date resources about prescription of psychotropics during pregnancy and lactation.

CHAPTER 13

Parents abused as children

KEY CONCEPTS

- Developmental effects of abuse and neglect
- Impact of childhood abuse on subsequent parenting
- Transgenerational issues in parenting and trauma

FACTORS IN ASSESSMENT AND FORMULATION

- Balancing risk and protective factors
- Parental capacity for self-reflection
- Sources of stress and support
- Protective factors against repetition

Parenthood is a major test of psychological maturity and parents who experienced maltreatment in any form are a very disadvantaged group with multiple vulnerabilities. Child abuse and neglect have a major effect on development, with lifelong consequences, and the effect of neglect may be more pervasive than that of isolated episodes of physical abuse. Those children who are both abused and neglected are particularly at risk of lifelong difficulties. Fonagy, Steele, Steele, Higgitt and Target (1994) state: 'parents with a history of deprivation, neglect or abuse are more likely to encounter problems at all stages of family life, including behavioural difficulties, health, educational and psychiatric problems in their children and relationship problems between family members' (p. 233).

This chapter will explore the effect of child maltreatment, and what this means for the child grown up, attempting to parent. This chapter will also consider what enables some people with awful histories to 'break the cycle' and do it differently. Many parents who have been maltreated as children are able to become effective parents. The implications for clinical work with these families are considered.

THE MALTREATED CHILD AS PARENT

Not all abused children become abusing parents. Estimates of the percentage who do repeat their abusive or neglectful experiences with their own children vary enormously. Kaufman and Zigler in 1987 estimated that 90 per cent of abusing parents give history of being abused, but only about 30 per cent of those who are abused will become abusers. They review studies that vary in this estimate from 18 to 70 per cent, and discuss the difficulties in obtaining more accurate estimates. They also note that environmental factors such as poverty, lack of social support and marital problems further increase the risk of child abuse.

McGloin and Widom (2001), in their study of resilience in abused and neglected children grown up, using stringent criteria (a good outcome in spite of high risk, sustained competence under stress, across several key areas of functioning) found that 22 per cent met strict criteria for resilience. These abused children grown up demonstrated competence, not just survival. Females were more likely to be resilient and to be so across a number of domains. Sexual abuse and neglect were negative indicators, but physical abuse was less so.

The consequences of child abuse and neglect

Children's normal emotional reactions are undermined by maltreatment, leading to an atypical organisation of emotions and their expression. There is increased risk of insecure or disorganised attachment relationships with caregivers, and a significant effect on social and emotional development and competence. Childhood maltreatment is a significant risk factor for later social, emotional and behavioural problems.

Maltreated children:
- are more often avoided or rejected by peers
- show more under-controlled and aggressive behaviour
- have difficulty interpreting and responding to emotions in others
- are delayed in development of internal state language (language about feelings)
- are more vigilant and distracted by aggressive stimuli
- are more likely to attribute hostile intent to actions or events that are ambiguous or neutral
- show greater arousal and anxiety in response to aggression between adults
- have problems organising, regulating and responding to emotional experience (Rogosch, Cicchetti & Aber, 1995).

Relationship problems in the family are generalised to other interactions and circumstances. There is a cumulative negative effect on competence, and with increasing age children become more aware of their deficiencies, particularly socially.

Maltreated children grown up

If we think about these children, now grown up, we begin to get a picture of how difficult intimate relationships including parenting might be. Early parenting involves interpretation of non-verbal social cues from the infant and child both during attempts at connection and communication and times of distress. The issues for the maltreated child now attempting to parent are discussed below.

ATTACHMENT CLASSIFICATION

Internalised models of caregiving relationships are more likely to be insecure or disorganised (see Chapter 2 for a description of attachment classifications). This has long-term implications for social relationships, sense of self and capacity for intimate relationships.

EMOTIONAL REGULATION AND PERSONALITY DEVELOPMENT

There is evidence that exposure to violence or neglect in early childhood affects the development of brain pathways involved in emotional self-regulation and the capacity to interpret social cues (Glasser, 2000; Perry, Pollard, Blakely, Baker & Vigilante, 1995). These are central aspects of social and emotional functioning and affect the capacity for managing stress and relating to others.

DISRUPTED RELATIONSHIPS

Difficulties in establishing secure and supportive relationships are clearly a consequence of the above points. Successful parenting is much easier in the context of a network of satisfying and supportive relationships.

VULNERABILITY TO PSYCHIATRIC DISORDER

Parents abused as children are at increased risk of psychiatric disorder, substance abuse and personality dysfunction. This also contributes to the risk of parenting difficulties (Belsky, 1993). Belsky and Vondra (1989) write: 'personality can function to support or undermine his or her parenting ability' (p. 166). The impact of abuse and neglect in childhood on personality development is likely to be more significant than the impact of modelled abusive behaviour.

CUMULATIVE DISADVANTAGE

The disadvantage becomes cumulative for abused children grown up and attempting to parent. They are more likely to be alone, socially isolated or in conflicted relationships. The nature of their history means that the appropriate support available from extended family is likely to be limited.

Transgenerational issues

For everyone who becomes a parent, there is a necessary review of and re-engagement with the experiences of growing up in one's family of origin (see Chapter 5). Evidence for the powerful way in which very early, often unconscious or procedural memories are communicated to infants by their parents is found in the correlation of about 70 per cent between Adult Attachment Interview classifications of prospective parents and the subsequent security of their relationship with their infant (Lyons-Ruth, Bronfman & Atwood, 1999; van IJzendoorn, 1995).

Transgenerational communication of traumatic experiences and the ongoing effect of parental trauma on parenting capacity and infant development are demonstrated in the association between infant attachment disorganisation and lack of parental resolution of loss or trauma (Main & Hesse, 1990). This is discussed in more detail in the remainder of this chapter.

CLINICAL PRESENTATIONS

Parents with histories of maltreatment will present in a variety of ways to services concerned with infant and child health and welfare, or to mental health services. For example, the parent may present to psychiatric services with post-natal anxiety or depression. These parents are at increased risk of a range of mental health difficulties including substance abuse. Parenthood brings with it the reactivation of memories and feelings about their own experience as children. This can lead to depression, anxiety and conflict as they face the realities of parenting and struggle to 'do it differently'. Parents may also present because of concerns about infant safety and well-being. Child protection services may already be involved. The infant may be the focus of the assessment if there are difficulties with sleeping, feeding or other aspects of self-regulation or development.

In all clinical settings, simple questions during the assessment process can alert the clinician to factors from the parent's own childhood that may be contributing to the current difficulties, for example:
- What do you remember as important about your own childhood?
- Are there things your parents did with you that you are happy to repeat?
- Are there things you would like to do differently?

Each parent and family will have different risk and protective factors related to their experience of maltreatment, and therefore their capacity to parent, and an individualised assessment is always necessary.

Risk and protective factors

There are general factors that convey resilience, including genetic, temperamental and intelligence variables and being good at something, but what else contributes and is protective? What interaction of genetics, experience, hard work and good fortune enables some parents to do it differently, to struggle so hard not to repeat the parenting they experienced? What enables them to tolerate the intimacy of a nurturing relationship with their children and what implications does this have for therapeutic interventions with these families?

Egeland, Jacobovitz and Sroufe (1988) identified factors in the background of abused parents in their high-risk sample that were associated with repetition of abusive parenting. Abusing parents were likely to score higher on measures of anxiety and depression, and to experience more current life adversity.

Discontinuity

The strongest association with discontinuity or 'breaking the cycle' was found in what Egeland et al. (1988) termed 'Relationship Variables'.

These were:
- the availability of an emotionally supportive relationship—in addition to the abusing relationship—during the parent's early childhood
- an ongoing therapeutic relationship of at least 12 months with a professional during any period of the parent's life
- the formation of a stable and satisfying relationship with a partner during adulthood.

These factors describe situations that allow the child or adult to develop alternative or transformed models of relationships apart from the abusive one. This suggests the transformative capacity of secure adult relationships, and gives life to the notion of developmental possibility across the lifespan. It is also a reminder of the intense developmental impetus provided by the transition to parenthood. The momentum of this developmental challenge brings with it enormous potential for change in work with adults who have just become parents.

The other aspect of this is the extent to which the child provides the parent with an opportunity for a 'second chance'. Most parents want to do the best for their children and there is the potential for a transformative experience in parenting, given sufficient support.

EXAMPLE 1: CAITLIN AND GEMMA

Caitlin is in her early thirties. She was referred for urgent psychiatric assessment when her daughter, Gemma, was three months old. Her father-in-law had died the week before and her husband had just started a new and demanding job. He was preoccupied, but not with his new family.

She was unable to close her eyes without intense flashbacks of childhood beatings by her father and if she did sleep, she was troubled by repetitive dreams in which she survived but a young girl did not. Her mood alternated between weepy despair and rage directed at her husband and the doctors involved during her labour. About her daughter she said, 'The only time I feel close to her is when I breastfeed, then tears just run down my cheeks. The rest of the time she could be anyone's child.'

She met the criteria for a diagnosis of Major Depression and also had symptoms of Post-Traumatic Stress Disorder.

Her experience of childbirth was part of the trigger for the return of the memories of physical abuse. She said, 'I hadn't forgotten the beatings, I just hadn't remembered them either'. There was a connection for her between the pain, helplessness and humiliation associated with the childhood beatings and her labour, which had been prolonged and difficult. She had felt abandoned and unprotected by her husband when the forceps delivery went ahead with incomplete epidural block.

Her father was a teacher. The beatings with a belt and occasionally deliberate burns with a cigarette began when she was three, after her parents' return from two years overseas for the father's career. Caitlin had been left in the care of grandparents. The departure of her parents when she was nine months old and at the peak of attachment behaviour left her with an insecure attachment to them. Her grandparents had fallen out with her parents in arguments about their treatment and care of Caitlin and had little contact with the family. Her grandparents had died during her adolescence, which was a turbulent time, and she felt she had achieved less academically than she was capable of. She had also had a series of volatile relationships before marrying. Their marriage had been settled until their daughter's birth. Her relationship with her parents remained difficult, with frequent contact but equally frequent arguments. They were supportive of Caitlin and her husband in practical and financial ways.

When describing the abuse from her parents, Caitlin said, 'Sometimes he'd hit me a few times. Other times he'd just lose control. I could tell he wanted to kill me then. My mother was just as bad but abused me with her tongue, not with a belt. We still have arguments that are so vicious they leave everyone speechless'. She said, 'My identity was formed in surviving. I was so determined they wouldn't destroy me. How could they have done it to me? Why did they? Was I so bad? The bastard. I feel he's still beating me now. I can't get away from it'.

Caitlin did not feel likely to hurt Gemma, frequently saying, in fact, 'She is to die for', but as Gemma grew up Caitlin had difficulty knowing how to interpret her behaviour and communications, and to set limits on her behaviour.

When Gemma was nine months old, the age at which Caitlin was left with her grandparents, Caitlin expressed amazement that Gemma knew the difference between her mother and father. It had become impossible for her to experience her daughter as vulnerable to separation and loss.

In Caitlin's case it is possible to speculate that the separation from her parents, which had contributed to their long-standing, volatile relationship, might also have allowed her to internalise a nurturing experience with her grandparents. Initially, she described thinking very little of them. It was as if they had been pushed into the back of her mind along with the abuse. Questions about her memories and knowledge of them led to floods of tears, and some relief, and a sudden strong memory of running to her grandmother and burying her face in her skirt. The memory was associated with a feeling of safety and warmth.

EXAMPLE 2: BEE AND JASON

Bee and Jason are in their late twenties and have two children, Jesse, three, and Amy, eight months. Their early lives, compared with Caitlin's wealthy home, were characterised by poverty, deprivation and uncertainty. Bee's father never lived with the family and her mother alternately abused her or expected her to run the household. From the age of seven, when her younger brother was born, Bee was often left to care for him alone for days at a time. She has a distressingly clear memory of hitting and shaking him in desperation, when she was about 10, and of seeing one of her mother's de factos burn him with a cigarette. She regularly saw her mother sexually assaulted, beaten up and, once, shot. Bee was living on the streets by the age of 13, homeless but not prostituting. She spent periods of her adolescence in foster care or children's homes.

Jason was abandoned by his mother as a child and he was brought up variously by his grandfather, his alcoholic father and in multiple brief foster placements. His early life was characterised primarily by neglect.

They had been married about eight years before their first child was born, having met through involvement with a church community in their teens. They had ongoing significant financial difficulties, but refused welfare or housing commission support.

Bee is very articulate about the conflict she is presented with in her struggle to provide a different experience for her children. She has never physically abused her children but has had significant depression after each birth, and has twice asked for the children to be fostered. It is more difficult in Bee's history to identify the person who cared for her, although she talks fondly of her grandfather who lived with them when she was small. She has also formed an enduring marital partnership and both have had a range of therapeutic input over some years. They also have a strong Christian faith and their involvement with the church community is an important aspect of their lives.

Self-reflective capacity

Fonagy, Steele, Steele, Moran and Higgitt (1991) identify 'the capacity to self reflect' as a variable that has a major effect on quality of parenting. They write:

> The reflective self plays a central role in parenting. The infant is as helpless mentally as physically...Attunement requires an awareness of the infant as a psychological entity with mental experience. It presumes a capacity on the part of the caregiver to reflect on the infant's mental experience and re-present it to the infant translated into the language of actions the infant can understand. The baby is, thus, provided with the illusion that the process of reflection of psychological processes was performed within its own mental boundaries. This is the necessary background to the evolution of a firmly established reflective self...The child's reflective self develops in response to the psychic capacity of the caregiver (Fonagy et al., 1991, p. 207).

The reflective self is an aspect of self-development that is likely to be significantly impaired by childhood experiences of abuse and neglect. In Fonagy's research, parental capacity for self-reflection is associated with increased infant security of attachment and 'theory of mind' development in the infant.

Parents' unresolved issues

> Parental attachment representations determine the way parents are inclined to communicate about emotions in intimate relationships, in particular the attachment relationship with their children (van IJzendoorn & Bakermans-Kranenburg, 1997, p. 153).

Rates of disorganised infant attachment are found to be higher in families where parents are 'frightened or frightening' (Main & Hesse, 1990). In these families children are exposed not only to direct abuse or to domestic violence, but to parents who are 'judged unresolved with respect to trauma' and loss (Main & Hesse, 1990, p. 167). For an infant, a parent preoccupied with or responding to memories of past abuse is frightening because her behaviour and responses are 'non-contingent'. To the infant the parent and her reactions are unpredictable. A lack of parental resolution of trauma may be associated with parental fear in response to infant distress (Main & Hesse, 1990). For the parent, the infant or his behaviour acts as a trigger for memories or re-experiencing of past trauma and loss.

These parents have a limited capacity to regulate themselves and therefore to assist their infant in this. Rather than mirroring infant distress (transforming and processing it for the infant), they may be overwhelmed so that distinctions between parent and infant (self/other) are lost or not developed.

One aspect of a disorganised attachment pattern then, is an inability to predict the other's behaviour, the lack of a strategy for interpreting interpersonal cues and attributing intent. This echoes the social and emotional difficulties described in abused and neglected children.

Recollections of the abuse and neglect

In parents abused as children the capacity to reflect on and think about the experiences of childhood seems also to have an effect on the risk of repetition of abuse. Parents who are able to recall their childhood experiences and the associated emotions are less likely to repeat the abuse than those who have no recall or recall without emotions.

Fraiberg, Adelson and Shapiro, in their seminal paper 'Ghosts in the Nursery' (1975), say this about parents who are likely to repeat their own abuse:

> these are the parents who, earlier, in the extremity of childhood terror, formed a pathological identification with the dangerous and assaultative enemies of the ego...identification with the aggressor (p. 419).

> What was not remembered was the associated affective experience...The original affects had undergone repression (p. 419).

> Our hypothesis is that access to childhood pain becomes a powerful deterrent against repetition in parenting (p. 420).

Herzog, Gara and Rosenberg (1992) also suggest that those abused parents in the most psychological pain are those likely to provide the best care for their children. Easily written, but not so easily lived! The extent to which adults abused as children use dissociation, splitting and projective identification has a huge effect on the capacity to balance the difficult memories and feelings associated with their own childhood experiences, and the needs of their infants and children for care in the here and now.

John Briere (1989) talks about this as the extent to which the capacities of the self are overwhelmed by recollection of the trauma, just as the effect of the trauma itself is linked to the extent that the child's emerging sense of self was overwhelmed or disrupted.

Empathy (for the child now and in the past) is proposed as a resource that the parent can draw on to counter abusive impulses.

Remembering context

Stern in *The motherhood constellation* (1995) writes about what he calls 'The Remembering Context', that is, the day-to-day interactions between parent and infant that evoke or trigger memories: 'the experiences on both sides of the interaction—the mother's and the baby's—across a generation...These constantly evoked memories seem to act mostly at a preconscious level…In this remembering context, the old schemas-of-being-with-mother will tumble out and pervade the new mother's experiences' (pp. 182–3).

For parents with abuse history this may generate distress, re-experience of trauma or conflict, and anxiety about how to do things differently. As discussed above, infants exposed to dissociated parents suffer trauma and distress when parents are 'frightened or frightening'. Lack of resolution of trauma and loss, not exposure to trauma and loss per se, is predictive of infant disorganisation in attachment.

EXAMPLE 2, CONTINUED: BEE AND JASON

Bee describes the remembering context very clearly. 'I remember the first time it happened. He stopped being my darling little Jesse. We had no money, he was sick. I was upset and alone with him in the car. He was crying. Suddenly he just turned into this black, awful thing. I just wanted to kill him to shut him up. I felt I lost everything. She's inside me. I can never get rid of her.'

Another time she said, 'I can understand the satisfaction she (Mum) must have felt just belting and belting into me. I can understand that. It's awful isn't it? Sometimes I almost envy her that she could do that. It feels so unfair. Here I am struggling with it, living with it my whole life trying so hard to be different. She's never even said sorry or even tried to change'.

Bee can describe so clearly something like the experience her mother might have had abusing her yet she does not act on it. She can even envy her mother the release of feeling this abuse would allow.

Bee's mother continues to deny that the abuse was damaging. She shows no remorse, and asserts that 'children don't remember things accurately'. This may not just be denial, but a demonstration of her inability either to reflect on her own experience or behaviour, or to acknowledge her children as 'experiencing'.

Perhaps the recognition of another as experiencing and observing might reduce abuse not only through a mechanism involving empathy with the infant's experience, but also perhaps by something more simply related to the experience of being observed. Recognition that an infant has experiences of his own might act to inhibit abuse by evoking shame.

Parenting difficulties

Abusive parents are more likely to have unrealistic expectations of their children, based on distorted perceptions of their needs, feelings and abilities (Gara, Rosenberg & Herzog, 1996; Herrenkohl, Herrenkohl & Toedter, 1983; Putallaz, Costanzo, Grimes & Sherman, 1998). They are more likely to attribute adult qualities to their infant, and to presume motives beyond the child's ability.

Sometimes the provision of basic developmental information can be very helpful.

These parents have difficulty defining appropriate limits for their infants and hate to see them upset. Bee's husband, Jason (Example 2), who experienced more neglect than abuse, tended to set firm limits and use physical discipline with their children. Bee attempted to meet their every need, finding it difficult to be firm or unrewarding. This conflict and difference in parenting style arose from the link, and therefore the confusion for them, between their own experiences and their wish to 'do it differently'. Distress or anger in the child in response to a limit-setting parent evoked for Bee her experience of distress caused by a parent, so overwhelming that at times she feared for her life. A good parent is so idealised for Bee that she imagines she should never be anything but gratifying; she should always 'get it right' in her interactions with their children. Both parents want to protect their children not just from repetition of the actual physical abuse but from the lack of recognition, fragile sense of self and punitive internalised images that make their own lives so difficult. They are also at risk of requiring their children to provide constant reassurance that they are 'getting it right'.

The awareness, too, of what they are providing for their children makes the sense of lack about their own experience acutely painful and sometimes generates envious and attacking feelings towards their children when they are perceived as insufficiently grateful.

ASSESSMENT, FORMULATION AND INTERVENTION

As mentioned above, these families present to a range of settings with a range of difficulties. Once the transgenerational issues are assessed as contributing to the presentation, risk and protective factors for repetition of maltreatment in this generation must be assessed.

Identifiable risk factors in a parent for repetition of abuse include:
- an attitude that parenting is a right rather than a responsibility
- lack of acceptance of responsibility for past difficulties with their own child
- no affective acknowledgement of the impact of their own abuse
- current psychiatric illness or substance abuse
- unstable, chaotic and/or violent domestic circumstances.

Protective factors against repetition of abuse can be summarised as:
- stable socioeconomic circumstances
- an internalised alternative or nurturing working model developed through the experience of being nurtured
- self-reflective capacity
- affective recall of the abuse (Egeland, Bosquet & Chung, 2002; Reder, 2003).

Assessment and formulation principles

As a clinician:
- it is important to set realistic therapeutic goals for the family and yourself
- the clinical material, past and present, is difficult, cognitively and emotionally
- it is necessary to maintain a supportive relationship with the parents without condoning abusive or neglectful behaviour, and this balance can be difficult
- there may be competition for your care and attention—the parents and infant both have high needs
- working collaboratively with other services and agencies is essential.

Intervention principles

- There is a constant need to assess the potential and actual risks to both infant and parent.
- It can be difficult to engage high-risk families, in part because of their previous experiences in child and adulthood with welfare and health services.
- It can be difficult to assess and consider the parents' issues without losing sight of the infant's needs and vulnerabilities.
- There is often conflict between the time the parents need to get themselves sorted out, and the infant's need for safe, adequate parenting now, and this needs to be included in assessing risk.
- Knowing when to act and when to wait and in order to give the parent time to respond and change requires clinical judgement.

Goals of intervention

The goals of intervention become clearer when based on what is known to be protective against repetition of child abuse.
- **Maintaining safety**—It is essential to think about the actual infant's safety even though the parent's issues can be so preoccupying. Maintaining the safety of all family members is a priority.
- **Practical support**—Identifying practical and emotional obstacles to adequate parenting is important. Practical support where possible for families with high levels of stress related to poverty or other environmental problems recognises these contextual factors as real contributors to continuing abuse. Domiciliary-based services increase access for many families and allow intervention at a very immediate level in the home.
- **Diagnosis and appropriate treatment** of psychosis, depression, anxiety and substance abuse are essential. All interfere with the ability to respond appropriately to the infant, but also reduce the capacity to be self-reflective, and therefore to work through and integrate past experience.

- **Keeping the infant in mind** and, as appropriate, speaking for the infant's experience gives the parent the opportunity to recognise and interpret it. Making clear your belief that most parents want the best for their children as well as your mandatory reporting obligations—modelling an ability to think about the well-being of both parent and infant.
- **Therapeutic relationship**—Providing sustained, non-judgemental and supportive input over at least 12 months.

There is the tantalising possibility of providing the parent with a therapeutic relationship that allows her to internalise or strengthen an alternative or nurturing model. This takes time to establish, and meanwhile the infant may be at risk. Unfortunately, the factors that determine those most at risk of abusing also identify those likely to have the most difficulty developing a therapeutic or supportive relationship.

The aversive nature of the parent's childhood memories and the extent to which avoidance and dissociation are used will determine how much of the abuse experience can be recalled. Aspects of it may remain too overwhelming or require significant time and the development of therapeutic trust, or the parent may need to develop more adaptive strategies, apart from dissociation, for example, as ways of dealing with intrusive or overwhelming memories and experiences.

Part of integrating aspects of childhood and self into a more coherent whole may involve conscious recognition of the importance of those people who were nurturing. Rediscovering these aspects of childhood experience may be as important as affective recall of the abuse but cannot occur until a secure therapeutic relationship is established.

Initially, the clinician should aim to:
- identify risk and protective factors in parent and infant, and use knowledge of the difficulties abused children grown up experience, to help deal with parents who are inevitably needy and difficult
- help the parent or parents articulate and understand feelings about their own childhoods and what they want to do differently.

The absence of physical abuse is no guarantee of good enough parenting, but the capacity to accurately enough interpret and reflect the infant's experience may be. Relationship-based interventions, for example, dyadic parent–infant or family work, can be aimed very directly at this. Interventions may need to include:
- developmental information and psycho-education, including parent training and skill development.
- relationship-based intervention—dyadic or family therapies. The use of video-tape can be very helpful for some families in providing a practical way of reflecting on their behaviours and interactions.
- notification and/or arranging respite care.

SUMMARY

Therapeutic involvement with families where a parent has been abused as a child unfolds over years and often follows an unconventional course. Strengthening the self-reflective capacity of the parent through therapy aimed at recall of the feelings associated with the abuse is likely to protect the infant. This work is exhausting and painful, not just for the parent. It is hard for clinicians to relinquish the desire for them to be really good parents, let alone not abusive, and difficult not to feel disheartened or overwhelmed at times. As a clinician, tolerating the material both from the parent's past and in the present, including intense feelings of emptiness, distress and at times malevolence, and working in a context where risks to the infant may be high is difficult.

Survival strategies for clinicians include:
- identifying your own professional strengths, weaknesses and availability
- assessing accurately what your role is to be with the family (for example, case manager, individual, dyadic or family therapist)
- setting realistic therapeutic goals for the family and one's self
- regular communication with a network of services/supports for each of these families
- clear definition of your role as part of this
- setting realistic therapeutic goals for the family
- a balanced clinical load
- adequate time and support/supervision to reflect on your own feelings and interventions
- a balanced life.

ADDITIONAL READING

Browne, K., Hanks, P., Stratton, P., & Hamilton, C. (Eds.). (2002). *Early prediction and prevention of child abuse: A handbook*. New York: Wiley and Sons.

Kaufman, J., & Henrich, C. (2000). Exposure to violence and early childhood trauma. In C. H. Zeanah (Ed.), *Handbook of infant mental health* (2nd ed., pp. 195–207). New York: Guilford Press.

Newcombe, M. D., & Locke, T. F. (2001). Intergenerational cycle of maltreatment: A popular concept obscured by methodological limitations. *Child Abuse and Neglect, 25*(9), 1219–1240.

CHAPTER 14

Parents with personality disorder

KEY CONCEPTS

- Influences on personality development
- Personality dysfunction and disorder—implications for parenting
- Attachment trauma
- Transgenerational effects
- Borderline personality disorder

FACTORS IN ASSESSMENT AND FORMULATION

- Motivation for parenting
- Conflicts and challenges associated with parenting
- Parental history of trauma and abuse
- Infant mental state and developmental outcome

The conflicts, challenges and types of interaction that parents with personality disorder bring to their relationships affect their children's psychological development. Personality development commences in infancy and is affected by a range of biopsychosocial factors. Infants with a primary caregiver with personality dysfunction experience disruptions to the usual development of personality. These disruptions can lead to personality dysfunction in later life, creating a transgenerational effect.

The term 'borderline personality disorder' refers to a severe type of personality dysfunction, and describes a group of individuals with long-term difficulties in relationships and adaptation. The diagnosis of borderline personality disorder is made more often in women and reflects the higher rates of childhood sexual abuse of girls and the socially influenced ways in which males and females express distress. Men with severe personality disorder are more likely than women to be behaviourally disruptive and may be diagnosed with antisocial personality disorder. Women with personality disorder are more

[CLINICAL SKILLS IN INFANT MENTAL HEALTH

likely to be distressed and to self-harm. For both men and women, personality disorder affects interpersonal relationships, stress tolerance and parenting capacity.

This chapter will describe personality development and personality dysfunction, in particular, relating to mothers with borderline personality disorder, the interactional patterns they establish with children and the effects on infant mental health and development. Implications for assessment and intervention are discussed.

PERSONALITY DEVELOPMENT

Personality refers to ingrained or habitual ways of psychological functioning that emerge from the individual's developmental history and which, over time, come to characterise the child's and then the adult's style. There are numerous theories on the development of personality style or 'self', but there is ongoing debate about the relative contributions of heredity and environment to personality. Genetic factors influence an individual's temperament or pattern of neurophysiological reactivity and may be involved in some individual differences in personality. Environmental factors influencing personality development include child-rearing practices, family relationship patterns, and family encouragement of particular patterns of emotional expression, thinking and social behaviour. In practice, while genetic predispositions may be involved, these are difficult to quantify. Nature and nurture interact in personality development and influence a person's personality traits and functioning.

Influences on personality development

As we have seen in earlier chapters, most theories agree that psychological and social experiences in infancy and early childhood are foundational. These experiences, particularly the quality of emotional care an infant receives and infant biological predisposition, are the basis for the individual's mode of psychological functioning. Infancy is seen as a critical development period during which the basis of personality functioning is established. The infant period is one where models of relationships and the self develop in the context of the caregiving relationship. Infancy is also a period where the ability to regulate emotions and impulses and to tolerate stress is formed. These functions set the foundations for emotional and psychological health.

Biological, psychological and social factors all interact to influence personality development. In addition to genetic predisposition and biological make-up, social experiences themselves influence biological and neurological development. For example, the developing brain is affected by the type and intensity of stimulation and input it receives and is shaped by the quality of care and interaction the infant experiences.

Biological and genetic influences

Biological or innate predisposition can influence personality and includes individual differences in temperament, neurophysiological reactivity and self-regulation. There is likely to be a genetic contribution to some personality traits. This is unlikely to be a single gene inheritance, but rather a genetic influence on the biochemical substrate of traits such as impulsivity and reactivity.

TEMPERAMENT

Temperament refers to individual differences in neurophysiological reactivity and adaptation. Differences in temperament may account for the variation seen in newborns in patterns of environmental adaptation and may affect parents' perceptions of an infant's character. While temperament is not equivalent to personality, innate factors may contribute to the emerging personality style. (For further discussion of temperament, see Chapter 1.)

NEUROLOGICAL FUNCTIONING

Individual differences in neurological functioning may contribute to personality development. For example, there are variations in the speed of information processing, reaction times and attention span that are evident from birth. Most parents adapt to the characteristics of their particular infant and moderate the overall amount of stimulation and input the infant receives.

Experience and stimulation shape the infant's developing brain and set up patterns of self-regulation and functioning. An infant in a well-structured family environment—that is, an environment that provides love and reasonably consistent caregiving routines—is likely to develop appropriate capacities for focused attention and concentration. Infants responded to in a sensitive and emotionally attuned way will develop the capacity to regulate their own emotional states.

Key neurological pathways involved in the control of emotional states are found in the limbic system. The limbic system is a group of brain structures that forms a network vital to the control and expression of emotional states. It includes the amygdala, the hippocampus, the hypothalamus and the cingulate cortex. The limbic structures have important connections to the frontal cortex and the systems operate to regulate emotional states and emotional interactions. These complex structures and pathways develop during infancy and their development is dependent on the caregiver's interaction with the infant. The brain requires the appropriate input during critical periods of development if these networks are to develop optimally. An infant who is neglected or cared for in a traumatising way may have impaired brain development and/or neurological pathways that do not function optimally.

As we have seen in previous chapters, the infant–parent relationship is important for the development of many functions and abilities, but perhaps the development of brain pathways is the most important basis of all. Unseen by parents, their daily caregiving interactions are helping to shape and mould those parts of the brain that respond to experiences after birth. Early brain development lays the important foundations and is shaped by ongoing experience. The fact that the cortical area of the brain develops after birth means that this part of the brain develops in relationship to the primary caregiver. There is a risk, as with all developments in understanding about infants, that this fact will lead to increased pressure on carers, particularly women, to be perfect parents. In 'good enough' infant–parent relationships, where infant needs are generally responded to sensitively and with the infant's needs in mind, then brain development occurs naturally and without the requirement of any added stimulation.

Psychological influences

The psychological domains of personality include the individual's model or representation of herself, her understanding of relationships and ways of managing emotions and stress. The infant comes to develop a model of the self and others as a direct result of her interactions with her primary caregiver. Infants are initially dependent on the carer to act as a buffer, or regulator, of intense feeling states and then gradually they develop their own abilities to tolerate emotional states. The infant experiences the carer as available and responsive and, as Winnicott (1960) describes, she needs to feel 'omnipotent' or that the world is at her command. This feeling of omnipotence is gradually given up, as the infant becomes able to tolerate increasing delay and frustration. The infant who experiences the social world as supportive and responsive develops a core sense of the world as predictable and safe and of herself as good and worthy of love. The infant in a secure attachment relationship experiences the primary carer as sensitive and responsive, and can rely on her for feelings of safety and comfort, that is, she is experienced as a 'secure base' (Bowlby, 1988). This provides a basic sense of security and the core of self-esteem.

MODEL OF THE SELF

During infancy a key developmental task is the development of a sense of self and internal models of representation of self and others. Bowlby (1988) describes these as 'inner representational models' and they emerge from the patterns of interaction with the primary carer—usually the mother. Infants with organised patterns of attachment develop strategies for managing the availability of the carer and positive ways of dealing with emotions. They develop a model of relationships that is functional and supports social interaction. Organised infants can use the attachment figure for support and even if insecure can manage their anxiety about the caregiver's availability. Disorganised infants are those with confusing, unpredictable and sometimes frightening carers who fail to develop an internal experience of their parent as a 'secure base'. They remain anxious and may have a poor understanding of the self and social relationships. (Patterns of attachment are described in Chapter 2.)

UNDERSTANDING OF RELATIONSHIPS

All relationships are based on the development of emotional understanding. Emotional capacity is the ability to understand emotional communication, regulate or control emotional states and to share emotional interaction with others. This is the basis for empathy and the development of trusting reciprocal relationships.

Infancy is a crucial period for the development of emotional capacity. The infant cannot tolerate strong feeling states and is dependent on the primary carer for control of emotions. The parent, right from birth, helps the infant tolerate anxiety and strong feelings and begins the process of providing an emotional vocabulary or words that describe feeling states. The infant in a well-attached relationship experiences fluctuations of emotional intensity in a contained and safe way and the parent maintains the infant within an optimal range of arousal. The infant gradually comes to develop her own capacities to tolerate feelings and regulate emotional states, representing a move from external regulation by the parent to internal self-regulation from the infant. This is dependent on the development of brain circuitry in the limbic system and orbito-frontal cortex.

MANAGING EMOTIONS AND STRESS

Infants develop ongoing and characteristic ways of managing stress and negative feelings. These are variously called adaptive and defence mechanisms and refer to various strategies that an individual uses to manage anxiety and feelings. Parents may directly influence an infant's defence style by discouraging or encouraging certain behaviours. For example, strong displays of emotion may be encouraged in some families but not in others. Expression of anger, emotionality and expression of dependency needs are also socialised in variable ways.

Stress tolerance develops along with the functioning of neurological and endocrinological pathways needed to tolerate high levels of stress hormones and to help the body respond to stressful situations. The hypothalamic pituitary adrenal axis (the HPA axis) is the neurological and hormonal system that develops during infancy and is vital for the response to stress and trauma.

In response to a frightening event, the system releases stress hormones, such as cortisol, adrenaline and noradrenaline, from the adrenal glands. These hormones prime the body for defence—the so-called 'fight or flight' reaction', in which glucose is released for energy and blood is sent to the large muscles. This system is not functioning fully at birth but develops over the first two years of life—hence, the importance of a parent who can modulate the infant's emotional distress. The young infant has an additional protective system that is used initially—the 'freeze or play dead response'—which is observed in many mammalian species. In the face of trauma a young infant will freeze or remain still rather than prepare for 'fight'. This response appears to have developed over the course of evolution and to be programmed into the human infant. (See Chapter 10 for discussion of the effects of trauma in infancy.)

Social influences

Family environment and patterns of relationship, as well as social and community functioning, affect personality development. Factors such as family cohesion, conflict and the quality of sibling relationships can act as protective or risk factors to healthy development. Infants raised in chaotic, unstructured and disadvantaged families are more likely to experience neglect and insensitive care. In these circumstances, the development of optimal self-regulation is at risk.

Personality dysfunction

Personality dysfunction occurs in adults when there has been a disruption to personality development. This has its origin in the early years during crucial periods of personality development, and becomes ingrained as a chronically maladaptive style during adolescence. Personality dysfunction frequently involves disturbed self-experiences, disturbed interpersonal behaviour and maladaptive coping mechanisms. Current classifications of personality disorder focus on the interpersonal disturbances experienced by individuals with dysfunctional or maladaptive models of self and others, that is, the effect of their personality dysfunction on their relationships with others.

Major factors contributing to personality dysfunction include adverse early experiences, attachment disruption, trauma and abuse. Some individuals may also be biologically vulnerable and less resistant to adversity. Severe personality disorder has been linked with child maltreatment and emotional neglect.

Individuals with severe personality disorder have frequently experienced failure of the caretaking environment, with no alternate attachment figures to provide some protection and a secure base, and patterns of care that are confusing and unpredictable. In many cases, these dysfunctional patterns of relationships are transgenerational. That is, parents who themselves have experienced early abuse and adversity find it difficult to parent and are at risk of replicating disturbing infant–parent interactions with their own children. Early trauma has disrupted these parents' own personality development and has limited their understanding of their infant's needs and their capacity to tolerate the emotional demands of nurturing an infant.

Types of personality dysfunction

Characteristic aspects of personality dysfunction are grouped into types of personality disorder. The symptoms of different personality disorders listed in systems, such as the DSM-IV (American Psychiatric Association [APA], 1994), describe behaviours used by individuals to manage or control severe anxieties. The personality disorders are grouped into three clusters based on descriptive similarities. This clustering system is useful in some research and educational situations, but has serious limitations in clinical situations because individuals frequently present with co-occurring personality disorders from different clusters. The clustering system has not been consistently validated.

- Cluster A includes the Paranoid, Schizoid, and Schizotypical Personality Disorders. Individuals with these disorders often appear odd or eccentric.
- Cluster B includes the Antisocial, Borderline, Histrionic and Narcissistic Personality Disorders. Individuals with these disorders often appear dramatic, emotional or erratic.
- Cluster C includes the Avoidant, Dependent and Obsessive-Compulsive Personality Disorders. Individuals with these disorders often appear anxious or fearful.

Personality Disorder Not Otherwise Specified is a category provided for two situations: (1) the individual's personality pattern meets the general criteria for personality disorder and traits of several different personality disorders are present, but the criteria for any specific personality disorder are not met; or (2) the individual's personality pattern meets the general criteria for a personality disorder, but the individual is considered to have a personality disorder that is not included in the classification (for example, passive-aggressive personality disorder).

Where there is a personality disorder, one can say that a catastrophe has occurred in early life, so that the individual's development has been compromised, leaving her vulnerable to stress and anxiety, that is, with a poor capacity for self-regulation of affect. This pattern has serious implications for infants when adults with personality disorder become parents.

GENERAL DIAGNOSTIC CRITERIA FOR PERSONALITY DISORDER

Personality disorder refers to an enduring pattern of inner experience and behaviour that deviates markedly from expectations of the individual's culture.

This pattern is manifested in two (or more) of the following areas:
- cognition, that is, ways of perceiving and interpreting self, other people, and events
- affectivity, meaning, the range, intensity, lability and appropriateness of emotional response
- interpersonal functioning and relationship disturbances
- impulse control difficulties
- the enduring pattern leads to clinically significant distress or impairment in social, occupational or other areas of functioning, such as relationships with family and friends, ability to get and keep jobs, and the ability to deal with day-to-day interactions within society
- the pattern of behaviour is stable and of long duration and its onset can be traced back at least to adolescence or early adulthood; early traumatic experiences can often be recalled by those with personality disorder
- the enduring pattern is not better accounted for as a manifestation or consequence of another mental disorder.

BORDERLINE PERSONALITY DISORDER

The diagnosis of borderline personality disorder refers to a severe disturbance of personality function with a range of identifiable features, rather than a description of a person with challenging behaviours. Borderline personality disorder is characterised by disturbed attachment relationships, impulsivity, poor anger control, mood instability and self-defeating behaviours that impair social functioning and cause individual distress. People with borderline personality disorder shift rapidly between trying to be too close in relationships (idealising) and rejecting contact (devaluing). This behaviour is detrimental to all interpersonal relationships and reflects a deficit in the person's sense of self and identity. The person may over-identify with others in an attempt to anchor herself, but then become anxious and overwhelmed by this intimacy. This unstable sense of identity is unpleasant and disturbing to the sufferer and may result in substance abuse and self-harm as a way of attempting to manage negative feelings (APA, 2001). The term 'borderline personality disorder' is often used as a general term to refer to severe personality disorder.

As the following vignettes show, people with borderline personality disorder can experience extreme frustration in trying to get appropriate help and to have their problem recognised.

> *Each day is hard to determine what it will be like. Some can be great, depending on what goes on (just like everyone else), but little things can set you off even if you start out OK. Little things can turn it into a nightmare. I would find I might be working and someone will say something to me that upsets me; a little criticism perhaps, and I will think, 'I hate them', hate the job and think about leaving on*

the spot when really it was over nothing and could easily be resolved. I have had a shocking childhood with feeling rejected and worthless. I have had difficult relationships, one with abuse, one with an alcoholic, and just many failed ones due to their being very wrong and I just was with them for fear of being alone. I've lost boyfriends because I've pushed them away with my behaviour. I've had many lost jobs, been fired and quit many times, and feel very unsure of my future in terms of what I want to do. All in all it makes you feel very scared and confused. At times I feel like I'm almost on the edge of insanity and even now think of suicide regularly. I have attempted that a fair few times in my life. Sometimes for attention but other times for just a way out and as a cry for help. (Jodie, 35.)

I've had a lot of people say it's an excuse I use in life to not work and that things that go wrong in my life are because of me, not it. I find not many people have heard of it and those that have either have their own reasons for what they believe, that is, a label for many people that are hard to diagnose. I've come across many counsellors and GPs that haven't heard of it. I even had a GP ask me to explain to him what it meant—very confusing and humiliating, really, because I could tell he found it hard to believe. My own parents, who I believe caused this, deny that I have a problem but use this term in my face if I say something about anything they don't like me talking about. If I get upset my mother will say, 'Oh Ben, that's just your illness talking'. (Ben, 43.)

> The DSM-IV criteria define borderline personality disorder as a severe disturbance of personality functioning characterised by affective dysregulation, identity problems, poor impulse control and persistent difficulties in interpersonal functioning (APA, 1994). There is probably a larger group who do not meet these criteria but who still have significant interpersonal difficulties and problems in parenting and may be described as having 'borderline traits'. In community samples, up to 4 per cent meet the criteria for borderline personality disorder and in clinical samples, up to 25 per cent (APA, 2001). Significantly, in clinical samples, up to 90 per cent recall traumatic early experiences and report sexual and emotional abuse that occurred in the context of disturbed relationships with caretakers (Ogata et al., 1990).

As in many other disorders, a number of aetiological factors appear to contribute to the development of borderline personality disorder including genetic/neurobiological, family environment and personality/cognitive factors (Trull, Stepp & Durrett, 2003). (An integrated model has been outlined by Hoffman-Judd and McGlashan, 2003.) The majority of individuals with severe personality disorder have experienced multiple adversity and failure of the caretaking environment. Abuse and early trauma, particularly during the infant period, disrupt the crucial brain pathways needed for control of impulses and emotions and for an understanding of social relationships (see Chapter 10).

Severe personality disorder involves disturbances of self and relationships and the ability to maintain stable attachments. These individuals have maladaptive coping styles and are often seen as 'difficult' or self-defeating. They may experience current and ongoing distress related to early trauma similar to Post-Traumatic Stress Disorder. All have features that affect parenting capacity.

Disturbed self-experiences

Individuals with borderline personality disorder are often lacking a firm centre of identity and may appear fragmented or lacking in coherence. They may find it hard to describe their inner experiences and lack a vocabulary for talking about emotional issues. They may experience anxiety, intolerance of being alone and fear of abandonment. They may attempt to cope with this anxiety by seeking out intense experiences or risk-taking, and they are at risk of substance misuse. Risk-taking and potentially self-damaging behaviours are ways that the individual distracts herself from painful feelings and avoids reality.

Disturbed interpersonal behaviour

Attachment behaviours are disturbed in individuals with severe borderline personality disorder, who find it difficult to maintain an appropriate distance in relationships. They may wish that a relationship can meet all their needs and be overly close, or may alternate this desire with feeling abandoned and rejecting contact. Relationships are often unstable and chaotic. Fears of being alone and of abandonment can be intense.

Maladaptive coping mechanisms

Individuals with personality disorder have limited ways of managing anxiety and feelings and may use inappropriate and self-defeating coping strategies, such as blaming others or 'acting out'—that is, acting impulsively without thinking. These mechanisms are often ways of denying, or of getting rid of, intolerable feelings. In some very disturbed individuals self-harm can be a maladaptive way to seek help and to express negative feelings.

Post-traumatic symptoms

Borderline personality disorder has many features in common with Post-Traumatic Stress Disorder as these are described in the DSM-IV (APA, 1994). Individuals who have experienced early abuse may be continue to be distressed by these events into adult life and experience reliving of these episodes in the form of nightmares and intrusive recollections. They may experience fear and anxiety in situations that remind them of the abuse. These post-traumatic features can be particularly intense when the individual becomes a parent, as the presence of the infant brings back feelings related to the parent's own childhood. Some parents may avoid the infant, or become anxious or depressed as they struggle with memories of their own abuse by caregivers.

PRIMARY CARERS WITH BORDERLINE PERSONALITY DISORDER

There is little research on parenting among individuals with borderline personality disorder. However, problems with parenting in this group are often seen clinically, and affect infant development, in particular, the development of infant attachment and later behaviour problems.

Mothers with personality disorder face specific issues when they attempt to nurture their infant. Many are anxious and others experience a sense of lack of understanding of their baby. These parents who have experienced neglect or trauma may be desperately hoping to establish a caring relationship with their infant and hope to have their own emotional needs met by the infant. Mothers with borderline personality disorder are at high risk of attachment and relationship difficulties with their children and tend to have high rates of child abuse, and consequent referral to child protection services.

Common clinical presentations

Mothers with personality disorder may present at various times including during pregnancy, the perinatal period and during infancy. Pregnancy may be a difficult experience for the woman who is unsure how she will tolerate becoming a parent, and ambivalent or mixed feelings are common. Some women, particularly those who have experienced severe abuse, may find the physical sensations of pregnancy unpleasant and find it hard to tolerate intimate examinations. Delivery can also be very stressful experience. Mothers with histories of neglect and abuse may find it hard to nurture their infant and may have difficulties in understanding their infant's communication. They find negative emotions in the infant overwhelming and can find it hard to deal with their own frustration and anxiety. Mothers with BPD are also likely to have unstable partner relationships and dysfunctional relationships.

Experience of pregnancy

For a woman with borderline personality disorder, the transition to parenthood, already a challenging process for most women (see Chapter 5), can be a traumatic experience. Pregnancy may occur as a result of impulsive sexual acts and in the context of unstable or abusive relationships. The desire to become a parent may be ambivalent and may involve conflicting motivations, such as the desire to care, the need to be cared for and a compulsion to re-enact, or rework, early traumatic attachment experiences.

Effect of unresolved trauma on parenting

For parents with borderline personality disorder, child rearing is difficult and threatening, because of their own frightening experiences of the infant–parent relationship. Many recall an early life characterised by rejection, devaluation and inappropriate intrusion and insecurity (Ludolph et al., 1990; Zanarini, Gunderson, Marino, Schwartz & Frankenburg, 1989). Many have experienced trauma and abuse at the hands of attachment figures. Frequently, these early traumas have not been resolved or processed, even in a rudimentary fashion, and continue to affect all relationships, through either direct re-enactments of earlier trauma, or reparative attempts to change disturbing relationship dynamics.

Relationship and attachment with the infant

The parent may find it difficult to promote attachment security in their infant through consistent and empathic care. These parents find understanding and responding to the infant's emotional state difficult, and may misinterpret or avoid the infant's emotional communication. They may have a fundamental difficulty in acknowledging the independent psychological existence of the infant and be motivated by their own unresolved and traumatic attachment issues.

Risk of child abuse

The traumatised parent may retraumatise her infant through insensitive, inconsistent, frightening and confusing interactions (Beebe & Lachmann, 2002). The parent is often unable to put these difficulties into words, is rapidly overcome by frustration and anger, and has difficulty with the range and intensity of emotions aroused in a relationship with a dependent infant.

Several patterns are observed in early infant–parent relationships. The infant may be perceived as a good part of the parent's self, to be protected from abuse, or as the 'bad' part of self that deserves to be abused. At other times, the infant becomes the persecutor, the original bad parent, and is attacked. These psychological mechanisms are not conscious and the end result is a confusing pattern of abuse, rejection and attempts at nurture. These parents show a lack of empathy for the child—a failure to conceive of the infant as an individual being with her own emotional experiences.

Effect of parental disorder on infant mental health

Disturbances in early relationships, and interaction between parents with borderline personality disorder and their children, begin in infancy, because of inappropriate reading of infant cues. Some mothers describe feeling estranged, anxious, overwhelmed or even angry with infants from birth. Mothers who have experienced early abuse may be fearful of abusing the infant and become withdrawn. Others want to protect the infant and appear intrusive and anxious.

For the infant, the interactions with the parent may be confusing or inconsistent. The infant may be distressed by this and find it difficult to predict the parent's response or to feel that her communications are validated. Infants may develop various clinical syndromes and types of emotional disturbance and, while a number of factors may contribute (genetic influences, temperament and protective environmental factors), the disturbances all involve a disorganised attachment relationship with the parent, and its subsequent effects on self-development, including difficulties understanding and processing feelings, and poor tolerance of anxiety. Many of the children show several characteristic features: anxiety and anger directed towards the parent, increased aggression, poor ability to name and modulate affect, internalised negative self-attributions and disorders of empathy (Newman & Stevenson, in press). Others may become fearful, depressed and withdrawn, particularly if the parent is frightening and aggressive.

Disorganised attachment

Unresolved trauma in a parent with personality disorder directly influences the relationship with the infant and produces attachment disorganisation (Fonagy et al., 1995). When the parent is unempathic, inconsistently responsive and confusing or frightening, infants are unable to organise a strategy to deal with the parent's behaviour (Solomon & George, 1999). The pattern of infant and child difficulties, or behaviours, resulting from abusive/traumatic parenting is based on neurophysiological effects, as well as on insecure attachment. Problems such as poor affect modulation and impulsivity may reflect the effects of a traumatic environment on the developing nervous system (Perry & Pollard, 1998; Schore, 2001). The infant with disorganised attachment may develop patterns of punitive and controlling interactions with the parent in the preschool years. Disorganised attachment has also been linked with the development of disruptive behaviours and conduct disorders. Infants and young children with disorganised attachment behaviours may present with problems of emotional and behavioural dysregulation and have difficulties in peer relationships.

Effects on self-development

Children of parents with borderline personality disorder show many features of disturbed self-development and poor emotional regulation. They have experienced traumatising attachment behaviours and parenting, and this produces ongoing stress. These children are often highly anxious and have limited understanding of emotional interaction and of relationships. Behavioural and impulse control, frustration tolerance and stress adaptation can all be affected. Severely traumatised children will also have difficulties with attention, language development and aggression. This particular cluster of difficulties may receive various diagnoses by clinicians but it is always important to look at attachment history and history of trauma.

ASSESSMENT, FORMULATION AND INTERVENTION

Assessing situations where a mother with a personality disorder has an infant in her care requires a careful consideration of issues of risk. As we have seen, these parents have a very limited ability to respond to their infant's needs, despite often being highly motivated to be a 'good parent'. Issues involved in risk assessment discussed in Chapter 4 are very relevant when a parent has a personality disorder. An important clinical role is determining what type of parenting capacity exists, and this can be difficult to ascertain when seeing an infant–parent dyad briefly in a clinical situation. Seeing the mother and baby at home as well as in a clinical setting will provide the most information about how the dyad functions together and the effect of the infant's environment, including other people who may be involved in her care. Principles of assessment in this chapter are primarily about assessing parenting capacity given the high level of risk to the infant for disturbed interaction. Formulation involves the challenging question of whether an infant is at significant enough risk to warrant separation from her caregiver. Intervention principles centre on the need to assist the parent to perceive the needs of the infant, and there have been some programs designed with this specific focus in mind.

Assessing parenting capacity

Assessment of parenting capacity for the parent with personality disorder should focus on the nature of developmental risk to the infant and the capacity of the parent to recognise the emotional needs of the infant. Various assessment tools can be used to assist in the assessment of parenting capacity, and these are discussed below.

Parental attachment history

It is important to assess the effect of the borderline mother's unresolved early trauma and mental state with respect to attachment and the manner in which this is reflected in her relationship with and interaction with the infant. Maternal attachment history and state of mind regarding attachment may be assessed using the Adult Attachment Interview (AAI) (George, Kaplan & Main, 1996). Adults with borderline personality disorder have been found to be unresolved with respect to attachment trauma using the Adult Attachment Interview Classification System (Main & Goldwyn, 1991). This means that their own experiences of early trauma continue to trouble them in the present and affect relationships. (The AAI is described in Chapter 2.)

Infant–parent interaction assessment

In terms of interactional assessment, there are a number of established methods that can be helpful in eliciting information about infant–parent dyads. The Working Model of the Child Interview (WMCI) (Zeanah, Benoit, Hirshberg & Barton, 1993) has excellent face validity. The WMCI examines the mother's perception of the infant and her representational model of the infant in terms of her own attachment history.

Analysis of video-taped free play and interaction between mother and child, using one of the established coding systems such as the Emotional Availability Scales (Biringen, Robinson & Emde, 2000a, 2000b), provides valuable information about the mother's emotional sensitivity to the infant's needs and communication. Better known measures such as the Strange Situation Procedure (SSP) (Ainsworth, Blehar, Waters & Wall, 1978) and the Marvin-Cassidy procedure (Cassidy & Marvin, 1992) can be used to classify attachment status. The SSP has been described previously (see Chapter 2). The Marvin-Cassidy procedure involves a video-taped series of separations and reunions between parent and infant. Biringen's Emotional Availability Scales rate video-taped interactions on the basis of parental emotional responses to the child.

Infant and child mental state assessment

It is also essential to assess mental status in the toddler and preschooler. This is important given possible experience of abuse and neglect and the effect of this on emerging representations of self, other and relationship emotional regulation and behaviour. Maltreated children may show features of generalised attachment difficulties, anxiety and features of Post-Traumatic Stress Disorder. Terr (1991) has described features of post-traumatic play in abused children and use of defences such as dissociation.

Children will communicate through play and drawing the main emotional themes concerning them, such as any traumatic experiences or issues of neglect and abandonment. Older children can be asked to describe their 'three wishes' and to draw a picture of their family that gives important insights into the child's perception of relationships.

Intervention principles

How can we intervene in this process of transgenerational transmission of personality dysfunction? Early intervention is possible if we are able to identify and target those infants and children at high risk on the basis of parental vulnerability—specifically, the parent with a background of maltreatment and abuse and personality difficulties should be a high priority for early intervention services. Programs should focus on improving the quality of infant–parent interaction and promoting the parent's capacity for empathic understanding of the infant. There are limited reports of infant–parent techniques for this high-risk population and unanswered questions as to their efficacy. The relative roles of parent psychotherapy and infant–parent work are unclear. Both approaches may be useful for particular individuals. To date, two infant–parent intervention approaches have been reported in the literature: Watch, Wait and Wonder (Muir, Lojkasek & Cohen, 1999) and Video Interaction Guidance (McDonough, 1993). These approaches are used as they focus on the attachment relationship and the improvement of parental sensitivity and capacity to respond in an empathic way to the infant's needs and communication. In high-risk situations, such as the parent with severe personality disorder, it is essential to work with the parent and infant together, as the problems are inherent in the relationship and the quality of parenting.

Infant–parent psychotherapy

Psychodynamic approaches are based on the fundamental premise that the parent must come to understand the ways in which her own past influences the current interaction with the infant. For the traumatised parent, a core clinical question is one of how to resolve traumatic experiences and associated feelings. Some parents will respond to techniques aimed at anger and affect control, encouraging more adaptive ways of managing negative affect states and dealing with impulses to self-harm. Others may require more explanatory approaches aimed at resolving past trauma and changing inner working models or representations of the self and relationships. It is currently unclear which approaches are more effective in improving parenting and empathy.

Watch, Wait and Wonder program

Watch, Wait and Wonder is a therapeutic program that involves parents observing their infant in self-initiated play activities and being instructed only to participate at the infant's initiative. Parents are encouraged to reflect on the meaning of the infant's play. Following the play activity the parent and therapist discuss the session with the aim of the parent developing an understanding of themes and relational issues in the infant's play. Preliminary research with this intervention indicates that it assists the infant in developing a more organised or secure attachment, as well as improving maternal mental health, infant mental health and increasing parenting sense of competence (Cohen et al., 1999).

Video interaction guidance

A similar technique for improving the parent's ability to respond to the infant involves the use of video playback of parent–infant interaction. This is a useful behavioural approach for parents who have difficulty understanding and processing their infant's communication. McDonough (1993, 2004) has found this approach to be as effective as psychological approaches.

EXAMPLE: ANNE AND TESSA

Anne (24 years) and her daughter Tessa (three years) were referred for psychiatric assessment by the local child-protection services following a physical assault on Tessa by Anne's boyfriend, Mark. Following the assault, Tessa was placed in temporary foster care with a court recommendation that mother and daughter be reunited if intervention went well. Anne presented as an anxious, rather depressed young woman. She had many self-inflicted scars and recited a history of severe early trauma in a detached, mechanical fashion.

Anne was the youngest of three girls, and described herself as unwanted, rejected and 'scapegoated' in her family. Constantly devalued by both parents, she described herself as a frightened, depressed child who felt that she 'must have been bad and disgusting' to attract this treatment. Punishment was harsh, unpredictable and confusing. Over recent years, Anne had 'memories' of severe beatings and other cruelties, and recalled being sexually abused by her alcoholic father from about the age of three. She frequently witnessed domestic violence between her parents.

Anne began self-mutilating in a compulsive fashion at seven, performed poorly academically and failed to make friends at school. She felt 'different' and 'alone' and began running away from home. At ten years of age, her family felt that she was 'uncontrollable' and had placed her in alternative care. This began a period of six years of multiple foster placements and disruptions for Anne, who kept returning home, only to be sent away by her family. On one such return she was raped by her father, became pregnant and decided upon a termination.

Anne's adolescence saw many failed attempts at friendships, compulsive sexually masochistic behaviour and minor substance abuse. She described herself as not being able to trust, fearful of being alone and with a profound sense of 'badness'. She became angry in an unpredictable fashion, continued to self-mutilate and at times considered suicide. She has had no full-time employment, left school at 15 years and had no stable accommodation. She has had a series of relationships with men, frequently involving violence and abuse. She had been with Mark for four years.

ASSESSMENT AND INTERVENTION

Initial assessment revealed a chronically conflictive and abusive relationship between Anne and Tessa that had culminated in a series of episodes of physical abuse by both Anne and her boyfriend Mark. Anne saw Tessa as a demanding, whiney and clingy child whom she was unable to please. She described intense feelings of hopelessness and frustration when all her efforts to please Tessa appeared to fail. The episodes of physical abuse appeared to have occurred when Anne felt she was 'just not a good mother' and was rejected by Tessa. Anne ascribed these feelings of rejection to her own rejection by her mother and wondered if Tessa 'hated' her in the same way. At other times, Anne saw Tessa as a 'chance to make things right' and establish a close relationship for the first time in her life. In this way, Anne switched between feeling overwhelmed by Tessa's demands and investing her with all her own longings for intimacy. Being close to Tessa involved Anne's fears of rejection, and she was unable to distance herself from her own abusive background, resulting in a re-enactment. Tessa herself appeared to be angry and controlling in her interactions with her mother and could be provocative and attention seeking.

Play sessions showed Tessa to be a traumatised, withdrawn child, who compulsively played out scenes of a little girl being hurt and abandoned. She rarely spoke, or left her mother's side, but told a story of a 'bad little girl called Tess' who deserved to be punished and made people angry. She spoke of 'Tess' as an imaginary friend who accompanied her, and needed to learn how to be 'good Tessa'. In play she enacted angry and aggressive outbursts of 'Bad Tess'. In the context of her frightening and confusing relationship with her mother and experiences of abuse, Tessa has a self-representation split between a good and bad child. She is traumatised and angry and disorganised in her attachment behaviours.

Tessa was assessed as being in need of protection and was maintained in foster care. During this time Tessa and Anna were seen together for intervention and Anna was supported in her decision to separate from Mark. During a course of play-based therapy Anna was able to acknowledge her own sadness about her childhood and came to see Tessa as a needy child and not merely as demanding. While Anna made some important gains in therapy, she was seen as needing ongoing support and was accepting of Tessa having regular respite care.

SUMMARY

This chapter has focused on the parenting issues for mothers with a diagnosis of borderline personality disorder. Clearly, these women are very fragile and experience high levels of inner turmoil. This distress, often a product of their own experiences of early abuse and attachment disruption in abusive relationships, can be re-enacted with their own infants. The consequences of this are infants and older children at risk of developing similar personality disturbances. Further clinical and research attention needs to be focused on this group, especially in the area of effective intervention. This may prevent the transgenerational transmission of abuse and neglect and borderline personality disorder.

ADDITIONAL READING

Akiskal, H. S. (1981). Subaffective disorders: Dysthymic, cyclothymic and bipolar II disorders in the 'borderline' realm. *Psychiatric Clinics of North America*, *4*(1), 25–46.

Batman, A., & Fonagy, P. (1999). Effectiveness of partial hospitalisation in the treatment of borderline personality disorder: A randomised controlled trial. *American Journal of Psychiatry*, *156*(10), 1563–1569.

Holmes, J. (1993). Attachment theory and personality development: The research evidence. In J. Holmes (Ed.), *John Bowlby and attachment theory* (pp. 103–124). London: Routledge.

Linehan, M. M., Schmidt, H., Craft, J. C., Kanter, J., & Comtois, K. A. (1999). Dialectical behaviour therapy for patients with borderline personality disorder and drug dependence. *American Journal of Addiction*, *8*, 279–292.

Main, M., & Hesse, E. (1990). Parents' unresolved traumatic experiences are related to infant disorganised attachment status: Is frightened and/or frightening parental behaviour the linking mechanism? In M. T. Greenberg, D. Cicchetti & E. M. Cummings (Eds.), *Attachment in the preschooler years: Theory, research, and intervention* (pp. 161–182). Chicago: University of Chicago Press.

Norton, K., & Adar, P. (1996). Personality disorder and parenting. In M. Göpfert, J. Webster & M. V. Seeman (Eds.), *Parental psychiatric disorder: Distressed parents and their families* (pp. 219–223). New York: Cambridge University Press.

van der Kolk, B. A. (1989). The compulsion to repeat the trauma: Attachment, reenactment and masochism. *Psychiatric Clinics of North America*, *12*, 389–411.

CHAPTER 15

Parenting and substance abuse

KEY CONCEPTS

- Common characteristics of women who misuse substances
- Effect of drug use on foetus and newborn
- Attachment relationships and parental substance abuse
- Infant outcome and parental substance abuse

FACTORS IN ASSESSMENT AND FORMULATION

- Ability of parent to prioritise infant needs
- Risk factors in the caregiving environment
- Effect of substance abuse on parenting capacity
- Capacity to receive support

Substance misuse in parents has both direct and indirect effects on infant mental health. Infants may be born with addiction and withdrawal symptoms, affecting sleep behaviour, responsiveness and the amount of crying. This creates additional challenges for the new parent attempting to comfort and respond to infant needs. A mother who misuses substances, despite being highly motivated to care for her baby like all new parents, may find the competing demands of her infant and her dependence needs overwhelming. The caregiving environment may be disorganised, with a risk of exposure to violence depending on the nature of the mother's social network and relationships. In this context, meeting infant physical and emotional needs is extremely challenging and infants may experience neglect, abuse and repeated separations, and develop impaired attachment relationships. Parenting capacity is directly affected by substance abuse and risk for infants is significantly increased.

Parents who misuse substances benefit from information about normal development and parenting techniques, as do all new parents. However, these parents also require ongoing support in order to manage infant needs and substance-dependency issues. There is little research available on the needs of parents who misuse substances and their infants, however, clinical experience has shown that the availability of coordinated, ongoing home-based support, as well as the characteristics of the parent and the caregiving environment, often determine the ability of the parent to provide 'good enough' parenting to the infant. There is also an opportunity around the arrival of a new baby for the parent to address some of the issues that have contributed to her substance-use patterns. With skilled and sensitive support, it may be possible for real changes to occur that benefit both the parent and her infant. Provision of early intervention in the home and a trusting, honest relationship with the parents are important aspects of providing effective support. Infant risk is a critical first stage of assessment and it is important to recognise physical effects of in-utero drug exposure.

In this chapter, we will look at the characteristics of women who misuse substances and how these traits influence parenting. We will also look at the effects of specific drugs on parental responses and the subsequent effect on the infant–parent relationship. The challenges of assessing and making decisions about the appropriateness of the caregiving environment will also be discussed.

WOMEN AND SUBSTANCE MISUSE

Misuse of drugs and alcohol is an increasing social problem. Alcohol dependence affects around 8 per cent of adults and 13 per cent use illicit drugs. These figures are likely to be underestimates. Substance misuse is common among young people. Opiate addiction represents a significant social issue and there are around 250 000 heroin users in Australia. The NSW Child Death Review Team (2000) noted that infants less than 12 months old of drug- and alcohol-dependent parents are over-represented in child death statistics. It is difficult to estimate the number of women who give birth each year with a substance-use problem, as most women do not disclose substance abuse. Women who misuse substances are less likely to have regular ante-natal care and their problems may often go undetected.

Many factors including the type of drug and the nature of its use influence the effect on the developing foetus and whether the newborn experiences withdrawal. A range of physical and developmental problems may also occur in infants.

Characteristics of women who misuse substances

Women who misuse substances often share similar characteristics as a result of their own childhood experiences, as well as the effects of their lifestyle being oriented around obtaining drugs. Many have experienced abuse in their own families and have difficulties managing difficult emotions and anxiety. Diagnoses of personality disorder, depression and anxiety disorders are common. When these women become pregnant they may have difficulty accepting the reality of the unborn child as their focus remains on their dependency needs. Conflict between the mother's dependency needs and the baby's needs can contribute to a range of emotions including shame and guilt. Parenting is a challenge for women who themselves have experienced negative care and who find the demands of nurturing the infant anxiety provoking.

Childhood traumas

Childhood traumas are common in the history of substance-abusing women who may also have role models of neglect and substance misuse. A dysfunctional family of origin, poor parenting role modelling and availability, and physical abuse are frequent, and may contribute to ongoing difficulties in forming trusting relationships and in parenting.

Psychological characteristics

Low self-esteem, depression and anxiety are common in substance-abusing women. Many have difficulty taking personal responsibility for life decisions and have a fatalistic or 'helpless' approach. Intimate relationships may be abusive and associated with domestic violence and reflect a rigid sex-role stereotype.

Socioeconomic issues

Parental drug and alcohol use affects most aspects of family functioning. Families are frequently isolated with significant financial problems as money is spent on drugs. Unemployment is common. Early onset of drug use affects school performance and is linked to limited education and opportunities for work and development. Drug users may form strong personal relationships united around a drug-using culture and become mistrustful of 'mainstream' culture. Children may be socially isolated and become involved in their parents' drug-related activities.

Pregnancy issues

Pregnancy is more likely to be unplanned and unacknowledged for women affected by substances. Women may continue to use drugs in pregnancy and deny any risk to the infant. They may have romantic and idealised ideas about motherhood and deny any potential problems. They may experience guilt and shame about the drug-exposed newborn but also ambivalence and resentment as the demands of parenting become apparent.

Use of drug and alcohol in pregnancy is associated with a range of adverse effects on the developing infant. Negative infant outcome results from the effects of the substance on foetal development, but also from lifestyle factors such as poor nutrition and low rates of ante-natal care. It is often difficult to establish the effects of a particular drug as poly-substance and alcohol abuse are common. Overall, infants exposed to illicit drugs are more likely to have intra-uterine growth retardation, preterm delivery, small head circumference and various infections. These factors are linked with poorer developmental scores at two years of age (Velleman, 2004).

Infants exposed to drugs in utero show poor regulation in the first year of life with delay in establishing sleep patterns, uncoordinated feeding and swallowing difficulties. This can contribute to failure to thrive, as can neglect and inconsistent care. Longitudinal studies suggest that as a group these infants have developmental difficulties and by the prenatal period score within the low normal range with particular difficulties in organisation and sustained attention (Velleman, 2004).

Various substances are abused singly or multiply during pregnancy. Some types of drugs have well-established effects on foetal development while others are less directly harmful.

ALCOHOL

Alcohol is a common substance of abuse and may be used with other drugs. Alcohol is a known teratogen (agent with effects on foetal development) and a Foetal Alcohol Syndrome was first described in 1973 (Jones & Smith, 1973). This pattern of abnormalities and neurological effects results from high levels of alcohol use, particularly binge-pattern drinkers. Infants affected are growth retarded with minor facial abnormalities. Heart and limb abnormalities may also occur. A less severe syndrome is more common and is associated with growth retardation and developmental delay.

OTHER DRUGS

The range of illicit drugs influences emotions, perceptions and behaviour. Parenting is also influenced by the effect of the particular drug on emotional interaction with the child. A sedative drug, for example, will make it difficult for a parent to be appropriately responsive, while a stimulant drug may make the parent irritable, erratic and overstimulating. Drugs of abuse can be divided into several groups with differing effects.

Depressant drugs

Depressants include alcohol, benzodiazepines, barbiturates and other tranquillisers. They all depress the activity of the nervous system and can produce drowsiness and sleep. Tolerance is common and withdrawal effects can be severe.

Opiates

Opiate drugs include heroin, methadone and codeine. These produce euphoria and sedation and can be fatal in overdose. Regular use produces tolerance and physical dependence. Intravenous use is associated with infection risk, particularly of hepatitis and HIV. Opiate use in pregnancy is associated with premature labour, low birthweight and infant withdrawal (Neonatal Abstinence Syndrome), which includes diarrhoea, fever, sneezing, yawning, tremors and seizures.

Stimulant drugs

Stimulant drugs include amphetamines, cocaine, ecstasy and other newer amphetamine-like substances. These drugs increase the activity of the sympathetic nervous system, producing an increase in arousal, concentration and energy. High-dose users, especially those who inject, are at risk of developing dependence. Many users 'binge' for several days and then experience fatigue and low mood. Use of alcohol and benzodiazepines is common. Many users report mental health problems such as anxiety, depression, paranoia and panic attacks. Psychosis may be induced by high doses of amphetamines.

Cocaine exposure in utero has been associated with congenital abnormalities, cerebrovascular infarction and neonatal irritability.

Hallucinogenic drugs

Hallucinogens are drugs that affect perceptual functioning and include LSD and cannabis (in high doses). Cannabis produces relaxation and euphoria, and some individuals experience paranoia and dysphoria. Cannabis dependence may develop.

Obstetric and medical complications

Obstetric complications are common with opiate use and include premature delivery, intrauterine growth retardation, malpresentation, hypertensive disease, third-trimester bleeding, nutritional deficiencies and poor ante-natal care. Medical complications of injecting drug use include endocarditis, thrombophlebitis, Hepatitis B and C, and HIV/AIDS.

Withdrawal symptoms in a newborn

Withdrawal symptoms in a newborn are common with opiates, including methadone use, and include high-pitched cry, irritability, hypertonicity and hyperflexia. Cocaine use has been associated with neonatal irritability, nasal snuffiness, jitteriness, tremor, fever, diarrhoea, vomiting, fist sucking, yawning and tachycardia.

Substance-abusing mothers are more likely to have an infant with perinatal problems and to experience birth complications. Early separations are common in cases of neonatal withdrawal and influence the parents' developing relationship with the infant. Infants affected by in-utero substances may be irritable, 'jittery' and deregulated, presenting a challenge to the drug-using parents. A parent in this situation may be intolerant of distress in his infant, anxious or even avoidant. The capacity of the drug-using parent to respond sensitively to the infant will be important in determining the quality of the attachment relationship. The degree to which the parent remains involved in drug use is also important in the developing relationship.

EFFECTS OF SUBSTANCE MISUSE ON INFANT MENTAL HEALTH

Direct effects of substance misuse refers to the specific effects of a type of drug on behaviour and emotional responsiveness. Depressants, opiates, and stimulants and hallucinogens have different biological effects on the user and the infant–parent relationship is affected by these changes. Indirect effects of substance misuse refer to the disruption to the infant–parent relationship that occurs in conjunction with the hazards of difficulty prioritising infant needs, potential exposure to violence and infant–parent separations.

Direct effects

As we have seen in the previous discussion, there are specific direct effects on the foetus as a result of the action of different drugs. Similarly, the effect of a particular type of drug on the parent using it creates a specific emotional profile or pattern of responding that over time will have effects on the infant–parent relationship.

Depressant drugs

Depressant drugs, such as benzodiazepines and barbiturates, lead to parental unavailability and insensitivity, withdrawal and irritability. The infant's experience of the parent affected by depressant drugs is one of being poorly responded to and sometimes neglected.

Opiates

Opiates, such as heroin, cause emotional blunting and sedation, withdrawal, depression or agitation in the parent. The infant experiences this as periods of neglect.

Stimulants and hallucinogens

Stimulants and hallucinogens, such as cocaine and amphetamines, lead to agitation, withdrawal, depression and dysphoria in the parent, following initial euphoria. The infant's experience of his parent affected by these drugs is of inconsistent care, depending on the parent's level of intoxication or withdrawal 'crash'.

Indirect effects

Drug use affects the structure and functioning of family relationships, with disruptions to daily routines and social isolation. Drug-related activity focuses on obtaining drugs and children may be involved in, or exposed to, drug-seeking behaviour. Exposure to aggression and violence are common, and children may experience abuse and maltreatment. Accidents and illnesses may result from poor nutrition, inadequate care and lack of supervision. Attachment disruption and separations occur when children are placed with alternative carers or when parents enter hospital or prison.

Parenting issues

Parents affected by drug use are often inconsistently available, depending on their pattern of drug use. Infants show signs of attachment insecurity and behavioural disorganisation. Relationships are often disrupted by loss of routine, parental intoxication and the parent's limited ability to focus on the child's needs. Infant outcome is worse when drug taking occurs in the home and there is conflict and domestic violence (Orford & Velleman, 1991).

Protective factors for children of drug-using parents include the presence of a non-substance-abusing adult, and activities and social supports outside the family.

ASSESSMENT, FORMULATION AND INTERVENTION

Principles of risk assessment and parenting capacity described in Chapters 3 and 4 are important in situations where a parent misuses substances. As we have seen, the substance-using parent has difficulty prioritising the infant's needs over his own, clearly leading to risks to the infant's well-being and development. The effect of drug taking and the culture surrounding it are important elements of the assessment process, as these factors will influence the nature of the risks the infant is exposed to. There is little evidence around intervention programs for this group, however, it is clear that early intervention is a priority.

Assessment principles

When considering infant–parent relationships where a parent has a substance-abuse problem, the following questions should be considered:
- How is money obtained for drug use? Are bills paid?
- Is the home sufficiently hygienic? Is there adequate food?
- Do other substance users live in the home?
- Is the house used for dealing or prostitution?
- To what extent does the provision of basic needs depend on whether or not the parent is using?
- What is the pattern, type, frequency and method of drug use?
- Are children protected from drug ingestion?
- Is use stable or chaotic?
- Does the parent experience withdrawal?
- What attempts have been made to detox?
- What has been the effect on the child of absences, criminal activity and imprisonment?
- Is drug use accompanied by psychiatric disorder and what effect does this have on the parent's cognitive state and judgements?
- Are children involved in substance misuse?
- What is the quality of the infant–parent attachment relationship?
- What is the effect on the infant's development and socialisation?
- What is the parent's capacity for education and acceptance of intervention and supervision?

Intervention principles

There is a limited evidence base about the types of support that could benefit families where parents misuse substances. Most research notes that many substance-using parents have experienced abuse in their own childhood and the substance misuse may be a way to mask the effects of this. Work with families therefore needs to afford the opportunity to deal with recollections of childhood abuse and feelings associated with this. Engagement with drug-using parents is often challenging and many are mistrustful of clinicians.

Comprehensive intervention aims to stabilise drug use and improve parenting capacity. The focus is on minimising harm to the infant resulting from insensitive care, and supporting the parent in developing an understanding of the infant's needs as well as skills in parenting.

Ideally, women with substance-use problems should be monitored throughout pregnancy by a drug service and receive appropriate counselling intervention. Comprehensive programs that also address welfare needs and any concurrent mental health issues along with drug use are more likely to be effective than multiple treatment settings. There is some evidence that home visitation parenting support may he helpful (Black et al., 1994).

EXAMPLE: EMMA

Emma is a two year old in a temporary foster placement. She was removed from the care of her parents, Jane, 27, and Andrew, 29, following police intervention as a result of domestic violence. Emma was assessed at this time as being at risk of neglect and exposure to violence and drug use. Both Jane and Andrew have substance-abuse problems and a history of multiple drug use, including heroin, methadone, cannabis, benzodiazepines and alcohol. They have had a tumultuous relationship with multiple separations and chronic conflict. Despite this, they have remained together for four years. They have been known to police and child-protection authorities for this period.

On assessment of Jane, she tends to minimise the degree of drug use and expresses anger at child-protection officers who had informed her that her drug use was putting Emma at risk of harm. Jane admits that her and Andrew's lifestyle is organised around drug-seeking and that Emma accompanies them. They have been discharged from the local methadone program for heroin use. They have major financial problems and at times are short of food. Emma has been repeatedly placed with drug-using friends when the couple 'need a break'. Emma has not been in formal child care and has no contact with her grandparents, who have now applied for care of Emma.

Jane describes a difficult childhood and states that she was rejected by her parents and did not accept their values. Despite excelling academically, she left school at 16 and drifted into a drug-using peer group. She began using opiates intermittently intravenously at 20 and despite attempts at detoxification, became a regular user at 24. She has contracted hepatitis B and C. She describes her pregnancy as unplanned and said she felt very little connection with her child-to-be. She participated in a methadone program late in pregnancy but had irregular ante-natal care. She separated from Andrew during the pregnancy but they reunited when Emma was born.

Jane describes Emma's birth as 'bad' and she found it difficult to tolerate Emma's obvious distress due to opiate withdrawal. While Emma was in ICU, Jane visited irregularly and had conflict with the staff who felt she was intoxicated on occasion. She describes Emma as 'cranky' and 'demanding' and said she was easily frustrated by her crying. Jane was assessed by the unit social worker and referred to an early parenting program and to the methadone service.

Assessment of Emma finds her to be small for her age, reserved and watchful. She avoids eye contact and is noted to be avoidant of Jane. Jane interacts with

Emma in a controlling and boisterous fashion, and does not seem to notice that Emma seems uncomfortable. In relation to Andrew, Emma appears fearful and confused. Emma agrees that she has been frightened by her parents' fighting and worried about her mother.

Factors in formulation for this case include the fact that Emma has experienced inconsistent care and neglect and has witnessed significant violence and been exposed to her parents' intoxication. It is likely that she has had disruption to routine and to stability of care. She now shows signs of acute stress and avoidance. She was made vulnerable from birth by in-utero substance exposure, neonatal withdrawal and need for treatment in intensive care. She showed early dysregulation and her mother found her difficult to parent.

Jane is challenged in her parenting by her own early experiences of rejection, poor capacity to deal with emotions and educational underachievement. She has ongoing stress related to her drug-using lifestyle and conflictive relationship. She has not been able to comply with methadone maintenance in the past, but is aware that child-protection authorities may require this.

In this case Jane is motivated to make the changes needed to care adequately for Emma, however, Emma's immediate need is for safety and protection. As in all cases such as this, the clinician is faced with challenging decisions regarding separation of infant and parent, and needs to weigh up the risk to the infant with the ability of the parent to make sufficient changes to ensure short-term safety. Longer term progress in the issues that contribute to both drug use and parenting difficulties will also affect the outcome.

SUMMARY

Parenting capacity and quality of care are directly and indirectly affected by substance use. Infants may be exposed to a variety of substances in utero with varying effects and frequently show signs of dysregulation in the first year of life. Infant outcome is also influenced by the secondary complications of drug use, such as inconsistent care, separations, neglect and poor family functioning. Infants with substance-using parents should receive a comprehensive risk assessment.

ADDITIONAL READING

Hans, S. L. (2004). When mothers use drugs. In M. Göpfert, J. Webster & M. V. Seeman (Eds.), *Parental psychiatric disorder: Distressed parents and their families* (2nd ed., pp. 203–216). Cambridge: Cambridge University Press.

Velleman, R. (2004). Alcohol and drug problems in parents: An overview of the impact on children and implications for practice. In M. Göpfert, J. Webster & M. V. Seeman (Eds.), *Parental psychiatric disorder: Distressed parents and their families* (2nd ed., pp. 185–202). Cambridge: Cambridge University Press.

CHAPTER 16

Adolescent parents

KEY CONCEPTS

- Developmental tasks of adolescence
- Increased obstetric and perinatal risks for mother and baby
- Teenage pregnancy is a risk factor for, and also occurs more often with, socioeconomic disadvantage
- Characteristics of adolescent parents

FACTORS IN ASSESSMENT AND FORMULATION

- Psychological maturity of parent(s)
- Degree of social and personal support
- Ability to access and use support

Around the world more than 13 million adolescent girls give birth each year, mostly in developing countries, and complications from pregnancy and childbirth are the leading cause of death in 15 to 19 year olds in many poorer nations. This is associated with high rates of perinatal infant mortality and maternal morbidity (Save the Children, 2004).

In developed countries approximately 5 per cent of infants are born to women and girls aged 19 and under, and rates in Australia are slightly lower than in the UK and North America, but higher than in western Europe and parts of Asia. In Australia, the adolescent birth rate is steady in recent years after a gradual decline. Abortions now exceed live births after teenage pregnancy (van der Klis, Westenberg, Chan, Dekker & Keane, 2002). Adolescent parents and their children are a group consistently identified as at high risk of psychosocial and developmental disadvantage. As parents, these young women are more likely to be single, poor and reliant on welfare support, and less likely to complete secondary or further education. There is discussion in the literature about the extent to which pregnancy and parenting contribute to these difficulties or should be seen as following from lives often already characterised by neglect, poverty and marginalisation. Teenage pregnancy is probably best understood as both a cause and effect of socioeconomic and psychosocial disadvantage (SmithBattle, 2000). Within this group of parents there is great variation in coping skills, resources and levels of functioning.

Assessment of adolescent parents and their infant's needs to include consideration of the developmental tasks or issues arising during adolescence. How pregnancy and parenting affect the teenager's emotional and social development is influenced by factors preceding the pregnancy and by the degree of support the parent(s) receive. The teenage parents' capacity to meet their infant's needs adequately depends on their level of physical health and development, their social and emotional maturity and the effectiveness of their support networks.

PSYCHOSOCIAL FACTORS INVOLVED IN TEENAGE PREGNANCY

In Australia, teenagers who give birth are more likely to be Australian born, Aboriginal and poor. American studies suggest that as many as 60 per cent of teenage mothers live below the poverty line. Pregnant teenagers seek or attend ante-natal care less often than older women. They often smoke and have poor nutrition during pregnancy. They have higher rates of perinatal complications, including long and difficult labours, premature and 'small for dates' infants, and increased perinatal mortality. This has halved in teenagers under 17 years in the past 10 years (van der Klis et al., 2002), and these complications are significantly reduced in the 20–23 year age group, indicating that maternal youth is consistently associated with perinatal complications for parents and infants.

Over 75 per cent of teenage mothers are single and about 25 per cent of fathers are never told about the pregnancy (McElroy & Moore, 1997). Teenage mothers are more likely to live in refuges or shelters than with the child's father. Teenage parents are very likely to be disadvantaged by sole parenthood, poverty and reduced socioeconomic options. They are also at high risk of domestic violence and their children are more often the subjects of child-protection notifications.

As discussed in previous chapters, socioeconomic disadvantage, including poverty, social isolation or instability, and exposure to violence are all clearly identified risk factors when considering optimal child development.

Influences on decisions about termination

Decisions about whether to keep or abort the foetus and how to manage the pregnancy are complex. They are influenced by the structure of relationships within the extended family and sociocultural background of the adolescent, but also by the young woman's psychological state of mental health. Anecdotal reports suggest that vulnerable and disadvantaged young women may be unable to realistically anticipate the long-term practicalities that being a parent involves. They may imagine the infant as a companion, someone who will always love them, significantly underestimating the extent of an infant's needs and the long-term impact on their circumstances. Adolescents with access to better education and support are more likely to make the decision to continue a pregnancy with a more realistic understanding of the implications of parenthood.

EXAMPLE: CATE AND BEN

>Cate and Ben were 15 when they started going out together. They were in Year 10 at different public high schools, bright kids but getting bored with school. Both had parents with professional training. Ben's parents had separated two years earlier and were both dating a series of new partners.
>
>Soon after they met, they began having intercourse and Cate went on the pill. In Year 11 Cate got bored with school, withdrew and began management training with a fast-food company. She did very well at this and was rapidly given increased responsibilities. She enjoyed the practical aspects of the work rather than 'sitting around talking about things'. Ben continued at school but was not very engaged. He was partying hard at the weekends and seemed in his mother's words 'in a hurry to grow up'.
>
>After a chest infection for which she was prescribed antibiotics, Cate had a period of fatigue and nausea. A pregnancy test was positive. At 17, she was 10 weeks pregnant. Ben and Cate had been together about 18 months at this time.
>
>Ben decided it was Cate's decision whether to continue the pregnancy, but he said he would support whatever she decided. They spent long hours talking about it with both sets of parents, who strongly recommended termination. The age at which a girl's mother became a parent is strongly linked to the age at which she will parent—Cate's mother had had her first child at 19, and had only later trained as a teacher. She was anxious about her daughter's education and training and wanted to protect her from the struggle she had experienced. Despite this, both sets of parents said they would support the couple emotionally and practically if they decide to keep the baby. This was a difficult time for both families, who had not known each other well before the pregnancy. Cate's mother was just entering a period of life when she was free of childrearing and able to pursue her career.

Both sets of potential grandparents were concerned about the effect of a baby on their own lives as well as on their children.

Access to ante-natal care

Even when good ante-natal care is available, adolescents are less likely than older pregnant women to use it, especially in the first half of the pregnancy. Obstacles include:
- the teenager's inability to prioritise her health care
- the sense of omnipotence that is an integral part of adolescence: the young person feels that, for her, there are no risks
- lack of age-appropriate information about pregnancy and the need for ante-natal care
- denial or late diagnosis of pregnancy
- lack of a peer group.

EXAMPLE: CATE AND BEN, CONTINUED

Cate decided to keep the baby and as they lived near the centre of a city access to ante-natal care was easy. They joined a group of four other teenage women preparing for parenthood and began to try to work out where they would live and how they would support themselves once the baby was born. Attendance at the ante-natal classes fluctuated but they made friends with another couple expecting around the same time.

Jake was born at term. The labour was long and he required a forceps delivery. Ben was present along with Cate's mother. Cate suffered a third-degree perineal tear and was anaemic after the delivery, but otherwise mother and baby were well. She established breastfeeding and continued this for six weeks. She found it difficult and painful and Jake required 'top ups' with formula. The couple moved into a small unit near to her parents. Ben left school and worked as a kitchen hand. Both families helped them furnish the house and they moved in together a few weeks before the baby was born.

Cate had access to almost optimal ante-natal care. She had a supportive, involved partner and family and easy access to high-quality care at a teaching hospital plus involvement in a teen parenting program. The labour and delivery were difficult, as was breastfeeding.

Family and social support

For all pregnant women, the quality and availability of family and social support have a major influence on the transition to parenthood and subsequent maternal and infant well-being. Single parenthood and social isolation are major risk factors for perinatal mood disorder. Pregnant young women often find themselves isolated from their peer group especially in the later stages of pregnancy. Social stigma still exists about teenage pregnancy. Most young women also have to leave school. Teenage pregnancy rates are higher in vulnerable young women with family backgrounds characterised by abuse and neglect, therefore, family support may be unavailable.

EXAMPLE: CATE AND BEN, CONTINUED

> *From the start, Jake was cared for regularly by Cate's parents and Ben's mother and sisters. When he was six months old Cate enrolled in Year 11 part-time and gradually recommenced her studies. Ben began a TAFE course in hospitality.*
>
> *They were poor and moved several times in an attempt to save money. When Jake was two and a half, they separated as Cate decided she wanted to live on her own with Jake, and Ben returned to live with his mother and sisters. He stayed several nights a week with Cate and cared for Jake at his family home on two evenings and part of the weekend. The family arranged for Jake to attend the crèche at the secondary college where Cate was going three days a week, so she could do another subject at school. Jake was reported by the day-care staff to be a toddler with lots of energy and good language skills. His parents seemed at times to overestimate his capacity to understand and reason, but overall managed him appropriately.*

This family is doing extremely well considering both parents were only 17 when Jake was born. They have had extensive family support emotionally and practically. They have been able to continue their own growing up to a degree by returning to study and having the opportunity to go out together and 'play' with their friends, knowing that Jake is well cared for by his grandparents. They have not conceived another child and diligently use contraception, while having conversations about whether it would be better as a family to have another child sooner or to leave it for a while. They live apart at present but consider themselves to be 'together'; and this is an antidote to the sudden cohabitation and responsibilities that early parenthood brought with it.

On the other hand, they are poor, have moved house several times and have not yet reached the educational levels they are capable of. Ben and Cate have had to grow up fast, but with family support, appear to have managed this huge transition relatively well.

They are atypical of adolescent parents as a group. Ben remains involved despite their separation. They have extensive family support. They are continuing their education. They have only one child.

This example provides an introduction to the issues and demonstrates that some teenage parents manage well. Despite this, it also shows the challenges teenagers may face in becoming parents at a time when this inevitably interrupts their own social and emotional development. Clinical assessment of adolescent parents requires focus on the developmental needs of both infant and parents as well as understanding of the psychological characteristics of adolescents.

IMPLICATIONS FOR INFANT MENTAL HEALTH

Young women who become pregnant and elect to keep their babies often have family backgrounds that include neglect, abuse and/or socioeconomic disadvantage. They are less likely to access adequate ante-natal care than older women, and the younger they are, the higher their risk of obstetric and perinatal complications. Psychological immaturity and a past or current history of trauma are among the factors that may make it hard for a young woman to look forward to the arrival of her baby and to anticipate the practical and emotional realities of parenthood. This means that adjustment to the realities of parenting and the capacity to put the infant's needs first may be limited.

The quality of adolescent parenting

Studies suggest that adolescent parents tend to:
- initiate less verbal interaction with their children, and as a consequence their children are at risk of delayed language and cognitive development
- have less knowledge than older parents about normal development and have unrealistic behavioural expectations of their children
- perceive their children as more difficult and less rewarding
- be less sensitive in their interactions and their children have an increased likelihood of developing an insecure (particularly, avoidant) pattern of attachment to their parents.

This is well summarised in Luster and Brophy-Herb (2000) and Zeanah, Boris and Larrieu (1997).

Attachment patterns and longitudinal risk

In families with high levels of socioeconomic risk and disadvantage, particularly where the mothers have histories of abuse and/or neglect in their own backgrounds, there is increased risk of a disorganised attachment relationship developing. This predisposes the child to long-term emotional and behavioural problems.

The parenting style of young women with multiple risk and disadvantage is observed to be more punitive and authoritarian and their children are at high risk of notification to child-protection agencies.

ASSESSMENT, FORMULATION AND INTERVENTION

Teenage parents and their infants present with the same range of difficulties as other families. This said, they tend to be a socially disadvantaged, isolated group with particular needs because of their developmental status. Assessment needs to take into account the range of biopsychosocial issues that can affect parenting and infant development. As well as this, the clinician must keep in mind the psychological tasks and characteristics of adolescents, and the need for information services and supports to be accessible and appropriately targeted to teenage parents and their infant.

Strengths and protective factors

It is always important to look for protective factors in any vulnerable family or individual presenting for assessment and help. Building on strengths provides the basis for any effective intervention and is an essential part of assessing risk, particularly in the long term.

Generally, the factors in Cate and Ben's story that were identified as protective are important for all teenage parents and their children. For all parents, these include factors in the parent, child and context that help or hinder parenting, and the physical health and development of their infant.

For the adolescent parent, protective factors are likely to support the adequate development of parent and infant (Osofsky, 1997). They include:
- goals or ambitions in relation to education and employment
- the ability to resolve personal difficulties
- the ability to use support
- the ability to limit fertility (Powell & Steelman, 1993).

Factors in the child include general resilience factors such as physical health, temperament and the 'fit' with parental expectations and abilities. Most studies suggest that involvement of a father has a positive impact on the outcome for the child.

Risk factors

Early motherhood is associated with a range of adverse outcomes for the child and the parent, as described above. Particularly vulnerable are those young women and their babies who lack enough of the protective factors listed above. These young women are already at high risk of social and psychological difficulties. They suffer social isolation or marginalisation and emotional or psychiatric illness. Maternal depression and low self-esteem are risk factors for poor infant outcomes (Osofsky, Eberhart-Wright, Ware & Hann, 1992). Having more children in rapid succession compounds the problems for parents and children.

The following example describes a high-risk teenage mother and her child.

EXAMPLE: ANGIE AND CHLOE

You are asked to assess Angie, aged 18 years, in the emergency department where she has presented with suicidal ideation. She is well known to the hospital and has had numerous crisis admissions to the adolescent ward since her mid-teens. After the birth of her daughter (who is now three years old) she had a brief psychiatric admission to a mother–baby unit and community supports were established for her with her daughter. She has otherwise remained out of hospital since Chloe's birth. She and Chloe live in supported accommodation for young mothers in an outer suburb. Community services have been involved in a monitoring capacity since Chloe was born and have organised several brief periods in foster care.

Angie has no support from her extended family. Chloe was conceived during a one-night stand and her father is unknown. Angie left home at 14 after being sexually assaulted by her older brother. Her family claimed she had lied about the assault and her brother continued living at home. She was homeless and itinerant before conceiving Chloe. Since then she has lived in supported accommodation.

Family life for Angie prior to the sexual assault was characterised by violence and neglect, with a family history of drug and alcohol abuse. She considered her maternal grandmother who lived nearby to be her 'real mother' and spent a lot of time at her place. In the past, she has been diagnosed with dysthymia and at other times major depression on a background of borderline personality traits. She has also experimented with most illicit drugs and has used marijuana regularly.

The risk factors for this mother and child are clear, and potentially overwhelming, but Angie is reported by others to have strengths, including being bright although having left school early, likeable and committed to her daughter. She has formed a useful relationship with the workers at the supported accommodation where she lives and intermittently calls the staff at the mother–baby service for advice about Chloe. She takes prescribed medications, although she also continues to use illicit drugs.

During an initial assessment of Angie in the emergency department, safety issues have to take priority. Angie's mental state, current level of functioning and current risk to herself as well as safety issues for Chloe must be considered. Where is Chloe now, who is caring for her and how has Angie's state over recent weeks affected her?

When you see Angie she is a thin young woman in track pants and a beanie, looking slightly unkempt and grubby. She appears agitated, makes little eye contact and looks unwell. She says she is having intrusive thoughts about throwing herself under a truck. She has been unable to sleep and has been smoking a few 'cones' a day 'to try to calm myself'. She feels Chloe would be better off without her. She tells you that bad things have happened to her because she is a bad person.

Chloe is with her, and, although rather grubby, is appropriately dressed and looks remarkably composed. She offers her mother a tissue at times but otherwise explores the room, looking in the desk drawers and asking if you have any jellybeans.

Angie tells you eventually that in the last month her grandmother has died and that she was physically and sexually assaulted by a man she was seeing. Chloe had been present during previous verbal arguments and physical threats but didn't witness the assault.

You say to Chloe that she seems to be trying to comfort Mummy and Chloe says, 'Yes, mummy cries all the time and she smacks me'. You ask more about this and Angie says that she has been hitting Chloe lately because Chloe has become 'too cheeky and won't do as she is told'. Angie says, 'I can't cope with Chloe anymore; I can't even cope with myself. I just think I would be better off dead'.

Angie is currently a risk to herself, with major depression and suicidal ideation in response to significant stressors including bereavement and assault. You agree with Angie that she needs time to concentrate on her own issues. This means Chloe will have to be placed in foster care while Angie has a voluntary psychiatric admission.

In the example described above there are two very vulnerable young people, one aged three and one aged 18, with apparently little social support and many risk factors. Recently, Angie has not been able to provide Chloe with the care and protection she needs. The demands on Angie to mother Chloe are currently in conflict with what she needs to do for herself. Also, Angie's history of neglect and abuse makes it more likely that she will continue to suffer mental health and drug and alcohol problems and have difficulty establishing appropriate and safe relationships for herself and her daughter. Her family history and current personal use of drugs and alcohol are a major concern.

On the other hand, Angie has remained out of hospital for most of the three years since her daughter was born, and community services have decided that, overall, she is doing an adequate job of parenting. Chloe attends a good child-care centre four days a week and is reported by the staff there to be bossy and demanding but overall doing well. Until the last few weeks Angie has been consistent in bringing Chloe to the centre and she always appears appropriately physically cared for, although the family are obviously poor.

Also, Angie has established supportive relationships with two services and her current presentation is in response to considerable stress.

To complete the assessment, information from the supported accommodation and community workers involved with Angie and Chloe is necessary to understand the current and past risk for Chloe and the length and severity of

Angie's decompensation. It is also important to find out whether community services have been involved recently and to make a decision about where Chloe should be placed while her mother is admitted to hospital, if a mother–baby unit is not an option, or inappropriate. A stable relationship with a foster carer will protect Chloe from further disruption and decrease some of the secondary or indirect risks associated with her mother's current illness and ongoing vulnerability.

Intervention principles

Principles include:
1 Addressing safety issues for parents and infants. This includes treatment of parental mental health or substance abuse problems.
2 Information, resources and support need to be developmentally appropriate and accessible, practically and financially.

Social support

Social support is crucial if adolescent parents are to function adequately. This involves a sense of being cared for and cared about as well as practical support such as child care and adequate housing.

Support and intervention services need to consider and address the needs of the young parent and her infant. Involvement of the previous generation in the form of parental support and input where appropriate may also be a valuable intervention for these families. Ideally, services need to be multidisciplinary with the ability to think and act developmentally and systemically and to provide continuity of care for a group of young people whose vulnerability often preceded their becoming parents. The flexibility to visit young parents at home or at locations of their choice enhances service involvement and the chance of successful engagement and intervention (American Academy of Paediatrics [AAP], 2001).

Population-based programs

Programs have been developed to try to reduce the number of teenage pregnancies. Overall, these programs have had little success. A recent review stated: 'Primary prevention strategies evaluated to date do not delay the initiation of sexual intercourse, improve use of birth control among young men and women, or reduce the number of pregnancies in young women' (DiCenso, Guyatt, Willan & Griffith, 2002, p. 1426).

EXAMPLE: ANGIE AND CHLOE, CONTINUED

It is necessary to re-notify Chloe as 'at risk' because of the history suggesting that Chloe has been exposed to physical abuse from her mother and violence between Angie and her boyfriend. She is presenting in a way that suggests that despite the support Angie and Chloe have received, her developmental needs, particularly for emotional support, are not being met. Also Angie reports using marijuana regularly lately and this is likely to have had a negative effect on her parenting capacity.

The case study of Angie and Chloe provides an opportunity to think about a high-risk dyad where there are serious concerns about the safety and well-being of infant and parent despite past support and intervention. Angie remains vulnerable and isolated because of her background, including past abuse. Despite this, she has strengths and presents asking for help. Chloe's emotional needs are not always her mother's priority. She presents as articulate, controlling and precocious. This dyad will need ongoing support from accessible services as well as crisis intervention. The prognosis for both of them is better if Angie avoids further pregnancies, develops stability in her social circumstances and is able to resume her own training and education as Chloe gets older.

SUMMARY

Socioeconomic isolation and disadvantage is both a risk factor for and a consequence of teenage pregnancy. The responsibilities of parenthood are difficult to meet consistently for young people for whom sole parenthood and poverty are common. There are higher rates of perinatal and obstetric complications the younger the teen parent. Support and intervention services ante- and post-natally need to be accessible and targeted to the needs of young parents and their infants, and to integrate the health, educational and social needs of this vulnerable population.

CHAPTER 17

Families with multiple adversity

KEY CONCEPTS

- High- and low-risk environments
- Cumulative effect of multiple risk factors
- The process of engagement
- Range of services and interventions offered
- Liaison with other agencies

FACTORS IN ASSESSMENT AND FORMULATION

- Assessing risk
- Assessing parenting capacity and parental empathy
- Respecting family and cultural diversity
- Changing overt behaviours and representations
- Family's capacity to work with agencies and to change
- Family and community resources available

The concept of risk in infancy was discussed in Chapter 4. In the following clinical chapters the authors explored factors in the infant, in the parent and in their relationship that contribute to vulnerability and influence infant development and mental health. Some families carry a great burden of adversity in multiple areas. This chapter attempts to provide an approach to assessment and intervention with families where risk and multiple adversity may seem overwhelming. As discussed in earlier chapters, there is no linear relationship between one particular risk factor (such as, maternal depression) and any particular infant outcome (for example, externalising behaviour problems or cognitive delay). Rather, developmental risk accumulates with the number of adverse factors or events that an infant and family experience (Ferguson & Horwood, 2003; Zeanah, Boris & Larrieu, 1997).

A number of different descriptive labels have been used to describe families

FAMILIES WITH MULTIPLE ADVERSITY

with multiple adversities and risk factors, including 'overburdened', 'multiproblem' and 'high risk'. In this chapter, we predominantly use 'overburdened' or 'high risk' to indicate both the experience of the parents and, conversely, the situation for the infant. It is the clinician's responsibility to clarify, define and prioritise the list of problems these families may present with.

As detailed in earlier chapters, the human infant is extremely vulnerable when born, utterly dependent on the immediate social environment for safety and nurturance. He is dependent on someone to care for him, usually the mother and father, who will, through nurturing and availability, facilitate self-regulation and the development of the attachment relationship (see Chapter 2). For survival, the infant is equipped with behaviours that are most likely to 'hook in the parent', to elicit those responses from the parent that will guarantee his survival.

The baby's dependence places responsibility on the environment to be safe and the parents to be available to the baby. Thus, any discussion of infant mental health has to take into account the social and physical context of the family. Where the immediate environment is not safe and/or if the mother and father are not available, physically or emotionally (that is, where the parents are not able to put the needs of their child above their own, nor realise the impact of their behaviour or lifestyle on the infant), the infant is at risk. It is relatively recently that the impact of abuse and neglect on brain development and thus all aspects of development have been detailed (Schuder & Lyons-Ruth, 2004).

This chapter will explore ways to assess and work with overburdened families to support their strengths, and where necessary make decisions about notification of children at risk, to enable increased support and child protection.

HIGH-RISK ENVIRONMENTS

For many practitioners there is the difficulty of knowing when a situation is less than 'good enough'. Perhaps the child is hurting at some level, but is the hurting enough for serious intervention or removal?

Kempe and Kempe (1978) are credited with alerting the world to the extent of child abuse and neglect by stating, 'We should stress that, when we say a *family* is untreatable, we do not mean that the parents do not deserve treatment. What we mean is that the child should not be used as the instrument of treatment...There must be a more civilized way of dealing with incurable failures than providing a martyred child' (p. 105).

A similar notion is expressed in the phrase 'babies can't wait' (Bemporad, 1995). Infancy is such a critical time for development (which occurs in interaction with a consistent, lovingly responsive parent or caregiver) that infants cannot be left in environments that do not provide such care and support while parents try to learn to be parents or amend their ways. Research on the brain has given clinicians a better understanding of the crucial role of early positive, consistent, reliable infant–parent interaction on early brain development and subsequent development and, therefore, the importance of early intervention (Siegel, 1999).

Practitioners often have difficulty quantifying or measuring an emotionally harmful interaction. The problem of defining emotional maltreatment, including active emotional abuse and passive neglect, has often been a question of whether to focus on parental behaviour considered to be damaging or to focus on child outcomes (Iwaniec, 1995). Emotional abuse is considered to be at the core of physical and sexual abuse and has more serious consequences than either physical or sexual abuse (Iwaniec, 1995).

What makes an environment high risk for an infant?

High-risk environments for infants are usually multifaceted, with, for example, psychological risks compounding or contributing to social risk or disadvantage. Extreme risk in one area is possible. Such environments include interacting risks in the biological, psychological and social domains, for example, an absence of parental empathy for the infant. Some authors (Donald & Jureidini, 2004) would argue this is the core issue in assessing risk and, while primarily related to psychological aspects of the parents, also includes their capacity to empathise with and meet the needs of this particular infant. It is also about the quality of the relationship between infant and caregivers.

The biological domain includes:
- infants with medical or developmental complications (for example, prematurity, chronic illness and frequent hospitalisations)
- parents with physical illness or disability. Some would include chronic psychiatric illness such as schizophrenia here as well as parents with intellectual disabilities.

In the psychological domain:
- parents with unrealistic expectations of their child and misperceptions of their needs, usually due to lack of knowledge of child development
- parents with a psychiatric illness, substance misuse or abuse
- parents who themselves have a history of abuse and neglect with unresolved issues of loss and trust.

The social domain includes:
- poverty and low socioeconomic status, little or no education
- parents with overwhelming external stress or trauma.

Often maltreatment is not because of malicious intent but because of characteristics of the parent—ongoing mental illness, substance abuse or poor intellectual capacity or disability. Parents are trying but the situation is not 'good enough'. It is necessary to consider whether there are mitigating circumstances that can change, but the welfare of the child has to be uppermost in any decision related to child safety.

Poverty and ethnicity

Neither poverty nor ethnicity are risk factors of themselves. However, poverty can affect the family functioning. Poverty relative to the local community affects access to services. Poverty usually involves social and geographic isolation, which in turn means deprivation of health and welfare resources. Poverty leads to stress on parents, which affects their psychological availability to their child. Poverty, lower parental education and socioeconomic status can also be consequences of inadequate or abusive experiences as a child. Disadvantage is multifactorial and, as discussed in Chapter 13, often transgenerational.

Likewise, ethnicity or minority cultural or linguistic status of itself is not a risk factor but can increase the developmental risk for infants and children by adding to social and personal isolation. Ethnicity has to be considered relative to the wider community and the wider community's tolerance of diversity (Coll & Magnuson, 2000). Ethnicity may mean belonging to a minority group. Issues of acceptance into the wider community and availability of resources in the language of the minority group may cause families to be isolated and stressed. Also, issues of loss and non-availability of appropriate parental role models and family support can mean new parents are floundering with the responsibility of their new role. There can be intergenerational conflict where new parents want to adopt parenting practices of their new culture in conflict with an older generation. Conversely, external pressure to adopt the ways of the new culture, creating fear in the minds of new migrant parents, can lead to a reluctance to accept assistance and services.

Parental factors

The contribution of parental factors to risk and parenting difficulties has been discussed in detail in earlier chapters. Current adversity or trauma, for example, exposure to domestic or community violence, depression or intoxication, limit a parent's capacity to be sensitively available and responsive to her infant. If this occurs in the context of other adversity or isolation, it is likely that social support, other figures to provide for and protect the infant, are also unavailable.

Parenting capacity, as discussed in Chapters 3 and 4, is not only about qualities of individual adults but also about their ability to meet the needs of their particular infant and to harness, if available, other personal and social resources to assist them in doing that. That is, factors in the infant, the parent, their interaction, and the personal and social context have to be considered.

As mentioned, Donald and Jureidini (2004) argue that it is the incapacity of the parents to put the needs of the child before their own that is the essential parenting factor that ultimately determines whether or not the situation is 'high risk' to the child's well-being and safety. Fonagy (1998) argues that the essential factor for secure attachment is the parent's capacity to mentalise, to ponder on the mind of the infant and to create an environment where it is safe for the child to begin to explore the mind of the parent. In some families, survival, physical and emotional, takes priority with children's emotional needs coming second to the physical imperatives of providing food, shelter, safety, and, for some, drugs or alcohol.

EFFECT OF HIGH-RISK ENVIRONMENTS ON INFANT MENTAL HEALTH

Babies and infants in high-risk environments are at risk of forming disturbed attachments with their primary caregivers because of the unavailability of a consistently nurturing parent. Infants with insecure and disorganised attachments struggle to develop emotional self-regulation, as it is within a secure attachment that the neural pathways of the brain are formed that regulate emotions and the infant's response to stressful situations (Gunnar, 2000). Major disruptions to the bond between baby and caregiver damage the foundation of his development and interfere with the infant's developmental trajectory (Schore, 2002). As discussed in Chapter 10, trauma in infancy is unique in nature; it is woven into the moment-to-moment interactions between infant and caregiver (Schuder & Lyons-Ruth, 2004).

Repeated or chronic stress is associated with disruption to the autonomic nervous system and disrupts the capacity to regulate affect (Gunnar, 2000). Schore (2002) states that all forms of psychopathology have embedded symptoms of emotion dysregulation.

Thus, behavioural outcomes of children left too long in high-risk situations can have a range of manifestations that may include:
- attachment disruption, distortion or disorder (see Chapter 2)
- externalising behaviour problems (tantrums, aggression)
- chronic depression or anxiety
- failure to meet physical, cognitive and emotional developmental milestones.

When the family environment is considered inadequate and the risk to the infant too great, or when maltreatment in any form is found to have occurred, infants and children may be removed from parental care. The intention is clearly to ensure the infant's safety and to maximise his opportunity for optimal development. For a range of systemic and practical reasons, removal from parental care is not without consequences for the infant. The effects of alternate care on the infant are discussed later in this chapter.

ASSESSMENT, FORMULATION AND INTERVENTION

As in all competent infant mental health assessments, assessment of overburdened or multiproblem families with infants must include consideration of a range of factors including the particular needs of the infants and children, parental resources and vulnerabilities, and social sources of stress and support. These families are often known to or already involved with a range of agencies and services, and assessment also includes clarification of the role of other services as well as an attempt to understand and document the success or otherwise of previous attempts at intervention.

Therefore, the challenges include:
- establishing a working alliance with the family
- collecting and organising often large amounts of information from a range of sources, including clarifying the various roles of other services and agencies
- establishing priorities for assessment and intervention.

Principles of assessment and formulation

As discussed, high-risk families include both families at risk of neglect and abuse as well as families where neglect and abuse has already occurred and the child has already been taken into care. In both situations there is a role for infant mental health workers, with a focus on the quality of the infant–parent relationship and the capacity for change in the family system.

Clinicians at times have to assess families when abuse or neglect has been notified or is confirmed to have occurred. Because of the legal as well as clinical implications of information obtained during these assessments, clinicians are required to thoroughly document information they obtain at interview and on examination, and to follow procedures designed to ensure that due process has been followed. These assessments can be distressing and at times traumatic for workers required to interview families when infants have suffered physical trauma or shocking neglect. Adequate staff support and opportunities for supervision and consultation are necessary, some would say for all infant mental health clinicians, but certainly for those dealing with child abuse and neglect.

Assessing parenting capacity once abuse or neglect has occurred

Donald and Jureidini (2004) warn of the danger of predicting parenting capacity from too narrow a base, for example, microanalysis of video-taped interactions (Osofsky & Connors, 1979), or analyses that focus on specific aspects of parent–child relationships, for example, only on the attachment of the child to the parent. In addition, the authors maintain that although many approaches to assessing parenting involve factors that influence the quality of parenting rather than the tasks of parenting 'there is no clear indication of their relative individual importance' (Donald & Jureidini, 2004, p. 6).

Some authors argue that assessment of parenting is of most use once abuse has been confirmed, for then the statutory body is in a stronger position to act upon the recommendations of the parenting assessment, for example, by insisting that the parents accept therapeutic intervention (Donald & Jureidini, 2004; Larrieu & Zeanah, 2004). The parents are aware that by accepting the recommendations they will be in a stronger position to have access to their child and possible reconciliation. There is an argument that therapeutic work with maltreating families can only begin once the parents acknowledge the seriousness of the situation, that is, that the care of their child has been considerably compromised. If there is no acknowledgement, then the infant–parent relationship is untenable and no therapeutic work should be undertaken. Unfortunately, clinicians are sometimes in a situation where abuse or neglect has occurred but no perpetrator has been identified. It may be necessary to assess and attempt to work with the family in circumstances where a high index of suspicion exists but denial by the parent(s) is pervasive.

Some services include the use of family risk checklists, self-reporting and structured interviews attempting to define and quantify family risk environment. The usefulness of such checklists depends on the relationship between interviewer and interviewee as to whether the interviewee will be honest in completing checklists. Donald and Jureidini (2004) argue that checklists are only of value if they include factors related to quality of assessment, not just the tasks of parenting, and if the questionnaire addresses the emotional relationship between the parent and the child. See Larrieu and Zeanah (2004) for an example of assessing the infant–parent relationship with a variety of structured and unstructured procedures.

Challenges of working with families with multiple adversity

Very often, families with multiple adversity are suspicious of or uncooperative with services due to their past experiences. Some of these families have a history of contact with welfare agencies, often negative, which goes back to previous generations, and family members speak of 'the welfare' in derogatory terms.

Working with high-risk families creates anxiety for workers. Many agencies are engaged and become involved and the problem list is long and daunting. In such situations, there is a danger of overlapping services, a lack of role definition for workers and agencies, conflict between agencies and a risk that the effectiveness of one intervention is cancelled by the other.

At times the priority of any one agency may not be the priority of the family. It is essential that both the family and the workers are involved together in determining goals and priorities.

Conflict between the many workers involved may arise if there are not common goals. There is a danger of those working with the adult over-identifying with the parents who are trying but not seeing the potential harm to the infant. On the other hand, workers advocating for the welfare of the infant may over-identify with the infant and fail to come alongside the parent and identify their strengths and the supports available in the infant's environment. It is often difficult to hold both the needs of the child and the needs of the parent in mind at the same time. Supervision for workers and regular meetings are necessary to enable integration of services towards a common goal.

Engagement

There are difficulties in developing a trusting relationship with families who may be suspicious of intervention workers. Often high-risk families also experience economic hardship with the consequence of insufficient funds for food, transport and housing, including attending appointments. They may be isolated geographically or socially. Families often do not have the energy to be emotionally available to their infant until some effort has been made to address their material and physical needs in a practical and immediate way.

McDonough (2004) defines a therapeutic stance 'created specifically to meet the needs of infants and their families who previously were not successfully engaged in mental health treatment or who refused treatment referral. Many of these families could be described as "overburdened"' (p. 80). The components of this approach include:

- to ask what help is wanted rather than assume that the family believes that you will be helpful to them
- to embrace a culturally sensitive non-judgemental approach in coming to know the family
- to take a cooperative egalitarian stance when identifying problems and generating potential solutions for treatment
- to emphasise family strengths but recognise family vulnerabilities.

McDonough (2004) writes that 'the majority of families…are doing the *best job they know how to do now* in caring for their children and themselves' (p. 82).

When an effort is made to work with an at-risk family in a preventive role, that is, before more serious neglect has been identified or physical abuse occurred, a range of support services are offered. These support services can include home visiting, child development education, developmental guidance, practical support designed to enhance parenting, and infant parent psychotherapy to create a space in the parent's mind for focusing on the infant's emotional needs and their relationship with the infant. The difficulty for the worker is the balance between establishing a trusting relationship with the family while at the same time being vigilant as to whether and how the infant's needs are being met. The worker needs to engage the parents, appeal to the parents' desire for the best for their child, emphasise their strengths and limitations while conveying social norms about the care and protection of infants. Parents are assisted in a non-judgemental way to be more sensitive to the impact of their behaviour on the infant.

Liaison between agencies

Clear lines of communication between workers and agencies are essential. There needs to be clear identification of the lead agency and primary worker, and specific roles of designated workers from other agencies, to avoid confusion for the family and agencies being played off against one another. Regular case conferences with the family and workers from all agencies involved are one way in which agencies keep the family and each other informed in a transparent manner. See Larrieu and Zeanah (2004) for an example of how an infant mental health team is integrated within a public sector service system and works with legal, child welfare, educational, health care and mental health care systems to provide assessment and treatment with multiproblem families where abuse of an infant or toddler has occurred.

Interventions for high–risk infants and parents

Once a family has been identified as having high risks, very often there are many services asked to be involved, including mental health consultants. Lieberman (1998) suggests there are three goals for the infant mental health consultant:
- to identify the developmental, psychological and relationship-based factors affecting the child and family's functioning
- to make short- and long-term plans for the infant in the context of these factors
- to ensure that the plans are implemented by the services involved, in particular, the child-protection and legal services.

With overburdened or multiproblem families, Larrieu and Zeanah (2004) advocate interventions that are comprehensive and operate on several levels. It may be necessary to integrate and coordinate various systems and services—legal, child protection and health—while adopting a relationship focus characteristic of infant mental health (Zeanah & Zeanah, 2001).

Home visiting is an integral part of early intervention work and acknowledges the practical difficulties these families may have in organising themselves and their resources, as well as their motivation to attend office-based appointments.

There is often insufficient agreement between the workers as to 'the best interests of the child'. Difficult choices have to be made and often it is 'the least detrimental' alternative that is searched for: how to minimise damaging psychological distress for the child and maximise optimal development.

Regular dialogue between the agencies and the family in the form of case conferences lessen the chance that the goals will be forgotten and the workers divided by the issues of the parties involved.

Early intervention programs

Early intervention programs for high-risk families take many forms. In Australia and overseas, governments have allocated resources to early intervention, recognising the importance of the early years to later development. Powerful support for the importance of early intervention programs for families identified as 'at risk' is provided in McCain and Mustard (1999). These programs usually involve several tiers of services to families. The initial tier involves pre- and post-natal health workers giving parents regular support ante-natally and in the home from a visiting nurse after the baby's birth. More intensive support, often home based, is provided to families who continue to need support or have particularly high needs.

Volunteer home-visiting programs

There are a variety of volunteer home-visiting programs throughout Australia that are appropriate for low-risk families. Such programs are often effective in engaging families and responding to changes in risk level with additional resources as required.

They incorporate the following aspects:
- trained and supported volunteers
- a buddy system where parents are linked into supportive relationships with each other
- child development education and information, sometimes delivered in group settings
- a drop-in centre or physical place for parents and infants to meet.

Therapeutic interventions

Relationship-based therapeutic work with high-risk families can take a number of forms and may be longer term. It takes time to establish a relationship, in particular when, as mentioned previously, these families have suffered disappointment, at least, from various agencies and systems.

For the infant mental health worker, the infant–parent relationship provides the primary context for therapeutic intervention to occur. The Bruschweiler-Stern and Stern model (1989) for intervention provides a framework for assessment and working with the family, taking note of the parent's representations as well as the interaction between infant and parent, and working flexibly with both.

Changing one element of the system influences the whole system. Therapy (changing internal representations) may be a longer term goal in high-risk environments. Changing overt behaviours, for example, teaching a parent how to wrap and settle her baby, may lead to changed internal representations of both infant and parent. This enables the development of the infant's self-representation of being effective in getting help when needed and the parent's representations of being able to meet her infant's needs. She becomes more able to see her infant needing her help rather than just being demanding.

McDonough (2004) suggests that the therapeutic stance taken by the Interaction Guidance approach, in conjunction with the use of brief video-taped interactions between infant and parent, provides parents with an opportunity to learn about and reflect on the infant, themselves and their interaction. McDonough (2004) emphasises that the focus on 'observable interactions between the baby and caregiver serves as the early therapeutic focus and, as such, serves as the therapeutic port of entry' (p. 79), thus, agreeing with Bruschweiler-Stern and Stern (1989) that whatever the initial focus, there is an opportunity in infant–parent therapy to change internal models as well as observable behaviour and interactions.

Another approach with high-risk families is based on attachment theory and referred to as the 'Circle of Security' (Marvin, Cooper, Hoffman & Powell, 2002). The group-based intervention of 20 weeks consists of parent education and psychotherapy designed to shift patterns of attachment and caregiver interactions to more appropriate developmental pathways in high-risk parent–infant dyads, initially with teenage parents.

See Marvin et al. (2002) for details of the conceptual background of the protocol and the protocol itself.

Alternative care

In the current social context children are not removed from parents lightly. The removal of a child into care is a difficult decision that requires thoughtful consideration of the effect of separation on the infant vis-a-vis careful assessment of the damaging physical, psychological and developmental impacts on the child of the abuse and/or neglect being experienced. A thorough assessment of the infant at the time of going into care is essential to identify specific areas of need and implement appropriate intervention.

Once a child is removed from parental care there is a break in the psychological bond between parent and infant—the foundations of the child's development have been eroded because the biological parents have not 'been good enough'. The goal is no longer the best outcome for the child, but 'the least detrimental alternative' (Bemporad, 1995, p. 3). There is a growing awareness that babies and toddlers have specific needs upon entering the alternative care system (Berrick, Needell, Barth & Jonson-Reid, 1998).

Existing bonds to parents are important to infants, notwithstanding the inadequacy of nurturance and the distortion in attachment with the parent. In the event of separation or removal of the infant, it is acknowledged that recognition and time need to be given to mourning the loss of parents and family even though they may have been inadequate.

A review (Dozier, Dozier & Manni, 2002) of the research of the last decade on how children in foster-care cope with disruptions in care noted the difficulties foster children have in forming secure attachments. The authors noted several factors that increased the infant's vulnerability. In addition to pre-fostering factors of compromised pre-natal environment, abuse and/or neglect, and disruption in their primary relationships, there was a tendency for these infants to fail to elicit nurturing from their carers, often behaving in ways that pushed foster parents away. This increased the risk of placement breakdown, adding to disruption and loss, with a greater risk of developing disorganised attachment with its likely sequela of continual difficulty in later establishing positive supportive relationships.

Alternative care is usually referred to as foster care or adoption. Foster-care arrangements include temporary, emergency or respite care as well as longer term placements, sometimes to age 18 years. Jurisdictions differ in the rules and processes governing adoption, which can include intercountry as well as local and open adoption arrangements. There is increasing recognition of children's need for security and permanence, as well as emphasis on the need for contact with birth family and culture. At times there appears in practice to be tension between these two priorities in decision making about the best interests of the child. Some children experience repeated breakdown of foster placements and are cared for in group homes or institutions, although in most western countries the number of large welfare or residential institutions for children is diminishing.

Once the decision is made to remove a child from parental care, the emphasis needs to be placed on providing the best alternative care situation, preferably where it will be possible for the infant to form a more secure attachment relationship with the carer. This has been shown to be a protective factor in the longer term (Shonkoff & Phillips, 2000; Werner, 2000).

Issues for infants and children in foster-care

There are many issues for babies and toddlers who enter the care of the welfare system, which are often unrecognised by the system, the carers or the community at large. They often experience three to four placements in their experience of care, which is the antithesis of what is considered necessary for the healthy development of babies and toddlers, that is, consistent, reliable care. Babies, in particular, are more vulnerable to abuse and neglect, which will influence their presentation into care (Wulczyn & Hislop, 2002).

At the more extreme end of the continuum of early childhood abuse and neglect, the effect on brain development is wide ranging and may permanently modify an individual's vulnerability to disorganised attachment and psychiatric disorder (Perry, 1997, 2001) and affect his long-term capacity for intimate, satisfying relationships.

A cautionary note is given to carefully assess the infant described as a 'good baby' (Perry, 2001). It may indicate what he describes as 'dissociative continuum' for children exposed to protracted neglect and/or abuse. Perry states that babies have 'early alarm stages' in which they attempt to attract the attention of their caregivers through facial expressions, body movements and, when necessary, vocalising and crying. When the caregiver comes to soothe, warm, feed or protect by flight or fight, the early alarm stages are successful. When the caregiver does not respond to the early cries, the system is not effective and the baby abandons the early alarm response, appearing 'good' or compliant. In the face of persistent threat to the infant, other neurophysiological and functional responses will be elicited, which Perry refers to as dissociative adaptations, and which include distraction, avoidance, numbing, daydreaming, fantasy and, in the extreme, fainting and catatonia.

These children are often reported to be numb or non-reactive, daydreaming or staring off with a glazed look (Perry, 2001, p. 228). The child has developed an adaptive strategy that reduces the possibility of abuse (Cousins, 2004). Common presentations when taken into care include passivity of movement, limited range of affect, trance-like states and developmental delay in terms of milestones. Such behaviour on presentation can be interpreted as that of a 'good' baby and can be a desirable attribute in terms of management, as the baby does not make demands, but is not adaptive for the infant in forming a secure attachment relationship with the new carer, and maximising developmental experiences.

Given the difficulty of interpreting the behaviour of infants there is a need for careful selection of foster parents, as well as education, training and ongoing support for foster parents to help them understand the behaviour of babies and infants entering their care.

The attachment state of mind of the caregiver plays a part in the possibility of the infant developing a more secure attachment (Dozier, Stovall, Albus & Bates, 2001). In their sample of 50 foster-family dyads, the authors used the AAI (described in Chapter 2) to assess caregivers and found that children placed with caregivers with autonomous states of mind formed secure attachments, and most children placed with caregivers with non-autonomous (insecure) states of mind formed insecure attachments. This was found regardless of what age the infants were when placed in care (they had all been in care for at least three months). The more disturbing result of this research is that the children placed with carers who had non-autonomous states of mind, either dismissing or unresolved, were likely to form disorganised attachments (72 per cent), and it is disorganised attachment that is more likely to correlate with concurrent behavioural difficulties and later psychopathology.

Thus, careful selection of foster caregivers is one factor in securing good foster care, along with training, education, emotional support and infant–parent psychotherapy for carers where appropriate. The reality, however, is that most child-welfare agencies are under-resourced, have high staff turnover and manage only intermittently to provide adequate practical and emotional support to their alternative care providers.

If reunification is a possibility, quality access of parent with child is essential to maintain the possibility of an ongoing relationship. Currently, in some situations, when reunification is a goal, access of the baby or toddler to his mother is usually only once or twice a week in a room in the office of the child-protection services in the presence of a worker, where there are a variety of people observing what is happening. Obviously, this is not the ideal place for a mother and baby to relax and be together. Meanwhile, the baby is beginning to form a relationship with and attach to the foster carer, which has to be taken into account as the baby moves between carer and biological mother.

There has to be a constant recognition of grief and loss for all the parties involved, in particular, for the baby or toddler being separated from mother and family context, no matter how inadequate that has been. If the infant experiences several placements, each placement will involve a fresh attempt at relationship with subsequent grieving and loss on separation. Foster carers need training to understand the effect of these emotional experiences on the infant and the infant's subsequent behaviour, and on themselves. They also need recognition and support as they work through their own emotional experiences of loss and transition.

The importance of establishing stability for the infant as quickly as possible is obvious, but many care and welfare systems seem unable to put this into practice. As mentioned above, there may be a conflict or tension between the infant's developmental needs and the ideal that he be restored to parental or family care. The time the legal and welfare systems need to establish more stable arrangements for the child is at odds with the infant's developmental imperatives. As a consequence, already vulnerable and traumatised infants are further disrupted during critical and vulnerable periods of their development. In this way risks become cumulative.

SUMMARY

In this chapter there has been an emphasis on identifying and working with families where infants' needs for a safe and nurturing environment are not being met. Often it is not a matter of intentional abuse or neglect but, for a range of reasons, the inability of the parent or carer to provide an environment where the infant's needs are prioritised above the needs of the parent. Issues of poverty, ethnicity, intelligence and education affect family functioning and parents' psychological well-being, increasing the risk of maltreatment. The infant's experience of neglect and abuse with its damaging psychological impact is the crucial element in identifying risk, rather than the intent or otherwise of parents, or parents' efforts at parenting.

Models of intervention and treatment are varied. Of particular importance is the fact that high-risk families engage with many agencies and systems. Coordination and clear communication between workers and agencies is essential, and the infant mental health worker's role, in particular, will involve long-term commitment. Providing appropriate alternative care, together with appropriate training and intervention with foster families, is of tremendous importance to infants already at risk, as an appropriate placement may enable the infant to develop a secure attachment relationship, with clear positive effects on development.

Finally, on a more positive note, early intervention programs aimed at reaching infants, families and communities identified as at risk, but prior to neglect or abuse occurring, have the potential to substantially improve the outcome for infants at risk.

ADDITIONAL READING

Osofsky, J. D. (Ed.). (2004). *Young children and trauma: Intervention and treatment.* New York: Guilford Press.

Glossary

Attachment behaviours Infant behaviours that promote proximity to the primary caregiver or attachment figure (such as, crying, approaching and following) with the aim of achieving feelings of safety and security.

Attachment relationship An attachment relationship is an enduring affective relationship with a particular preferred individual who provides most of the primary caregiving, usually the mother, and from whom the infant seeks security and comfort. The attachment relationship develops in the first year of life. Attachment patterns or classifications can be assessed and can be predictive of later mental health. Classifications of attachment include secure, insecure and disorganised patterns.

Biopsychosocial model Biological, psychological and sociocultural factors and the manner in which these interact and contribute to the overall developmental outcome for an infant. This model holds that developmental problems are multifactorial—that is, several factors usually interact to result in a particular problem and a variety of factors may interact to result in the same clinical presentation.

Continuity debate Debate about the significance of the infant experience, with some theorists seeing infant experience as crucial and setting lifelong, relatively unchanging patterns and others arguing that later life events can change early patterns, which infancy does not necessarily determine later outcome. The basis of the argument is the extent of 'hard-wiring' that occurs as a result of infant experience, and the extent of adaptation and flexibility that are possible in later development.

Critical periods Time periods in infant development when particular experiences are necessary for specific aspects of neuropsychological development to occur and when the brain is particularly sensitive but also vulnerable to environmental influences.

Facilitating environment The environmental circumstances, including in particular, the infant–parent relationship that supports and enables optimal development of the infant's emerging capabilities.

Formulation A formulation is an integrative statement that provides an aetiological understanding of factors contributing to the presentation. It can take different forms, but ideally includes consideration of biopsychosocial factors. This multilevel summary informs the development of a comprehensive intervention plan. Formulation differs from diagnosis in that it enables

GLOSSARY

identification and integration of a broad range of factors across several domains that interact and contribute to the presenting problems.

Goodness of fit   This term was initially coined by Thomas and Chess (1977) to refer to the interaction as they saw it, between infant temperament (genetics) and the environment (in this case the parents). It is now used more broadly to refer to the match between parental abilities, resources and expectations, and infant characteristics and needs, and includes multiple aspects of the infant–parent interaction. The parent cannot be expected to 'fit' or match the infant perfectly, and for the infant a 'tolerable' degree of dissonance is developmentally stimulating (Stern, 1985). Ideally, the family system adapts to and accommodates the varying needs and characteristics of different children. Without sufficient 'fit' the infant experiences a less than attuned or adequate environment, and this may have developmental implications.

Implicit or procedural memory   The earliest form of memory (also called non-declarative memory) that cannot be spoken about and is usually not available for conscious recall. Procedural memory is stored in brain structures and pathways that are present from birth and remain throughout life. The knowledge about how to ride a bike is an example. It differs from what is called declarative, semantic, explicit or narrative memory—experiences that can be spoken about.

Infant competencies   The innate skills and abilities infants are born with that enable them to attract and maintain the interest, attention and care of their primary caregivers.

Internal representations or internal working models   Models of the world, of ourselves and of significant others based on our experiences. These models guide and focus our subsequent experience and behaviour in relationships. It is presumed that these 'models' or representations are incorporated at a neurobiological level into neural networks and pathways linked to regulation of affect and arousal.

Internal state language   A range of words infants use, usually beginning in the third year, to describe their own emotions.

Maltreatment   Treatment of children that includes physical, sexual and emotional (psychological) abuse and parenting practices detrimental to child welfare and development. Psychological abuse includes parental behaviours that undermine the child's development and self-esteem, as well as neglect and stimulus deprivation. Child maltreatment is associated with behavioural and emotional problems and is a risk factor for adult mental health problems.

Parenting capacity   Parents' capacity to recognise and meet the child's changing physical, social and emotional needs for care and protection in a developmentally appropriate way, and to accept their responsibility for this.

Post-natal depression   A commonly used term that describes a range of mental health problems occurring in the post-partum period. The term can be misleading because it is used to cover a range of mood and anxiety disorders of varying severity, and does not represent a clear diagnosis of the maternal mental health problem.

Risk and protective factors The complex interaction of factors in the infant, factors in the carer, factors in the infant–carer interaction and factors in the broader social environment that contribute to development in infancy. Risk and protective factors may be biological and/or psychosocial. They may also be acute or longstanding.

Secure base An adult who is appropriately responsive and available to an infant for comfort and shared enjoyment.

Secure base behaviour This term was first used by Mary Ainsworth in her observations of Ugandan infants and their mothers: 'The mother seems to provide a secure base from which these excursions [infant explorations] may be made without anxiety' (Ainsworth, 1967, p. 345). Ideally, the parent is a person whom the infant knows he or she can explore from and return to for care and protection but also shared enjoyment. This exploratory coming and going behaviour is readily seen as infants gain increasing mobility.

Self-regulation Self-regulation is the process of the infant gaining regulation of his or her behaviour—physiological, social, sensory motor and emotional—to achieve functional goals such as settling to sleep, effective interaction, holding the body still so attention can be focused on a toy, task or person, and satisfactory and satisfying food intake (Siegel, 1999, and Sroufe, 1996). This occurs through the integration of social interaction experiences (infant–parent relationships) with the infant's maturing systems. Emerging self-regulation is affected by sensory motor experiences and infant maturation.

Self-representation, sense of self, self-concept Internal working models incorporate a sense of one's self and one's self in relation to others through experience with caregivers and in the environment. As with internal working models it is presumed that these 'models' or representations are incorporated at a neurobiological level into neural networks and pathways linked to regulation of affect and arousal.

State system or state organisational system The capacity of the infant–caregiver system to manage the infant's transitions through varying states of arousal (such as, deep sleep, light sleep, drowsiness, alertness, quietness, active alertness and crying).

Temperament Individual differences in neurophysiological reactivity and adaptation. Temperament has been defined as 'a behavioural and physiological profile that is under some genetic control...a changing, but coherent, profile of behaviour and emotion linked to an inherited physiology' (Kagan, 1997, p. 269). Temperament is a controversial construct because of the lack of correlation between parental and observer ratings.

GLOSSARY

Transactional model of development The transactional model of development (Sameroff & Fiese, 2000) emphasises the interaction between genetic and environmental factors over time and 'the development of the child is seen as a product of the continuous dynamic interactions of the child and the experiences provided by his or her family and social context' (p. 10).

Transgenerational transmission The transfer or repetition of relationship patterns or difficulties from one generation to the next. This includes the link between adult or parental attachment status and attachment patterns in children. Parents may reproduce patterns of behaviour from their own childhood and experiences of being parented with their own children. In situations where a parent has experienced early trauma or adverse attachment experiences, he or she may reproduce dysfunctional patterns with his or her own children or have difficulties in parenting in a way that promotes attachment security.

References

Chapter 1 Introduction to infant mental health

Als, H. (1992). Individualized, family focussed developmental care for the very low birth weight preterm infant in the NICU. In S. L. Friedman and M. D. Sigman (Eds.), *The psychological development of low birth weight children* (pp. 341–388). Norwood, NJ: Ablex.

Anders, T., Goodlin-Jones, B., & Sadeh, A. (2000). Sleep disorders. In C. H. Zeanah (Ed.), *Handbook of infant mental health* (2nd ed., pp. 326–338). New York: Guilford Press.

Barton, M. L., & Robins, D. (2000). Regulatory disorders. In C. H. Zeanah (Ed.), *Handbook of infant mental health* (2nd ed., pp. 311–325). New York: Guilford Press.

Bowlby, J. (1969). *Attachment and loss: Vol. 1. Attachment*. New York: Basic Books.

Bowlby, J. (1973). *Attachment and loss: Vol. 2. Separation: Anxiety and anger*. New York: Basic Books.

Cicchetti, D., & Cohen, C. (Eds.). (1995). *Developmental psychopathology: Vol 1. Theory and method*. New York: John Wiley.

Fairbairn, D. W. (1952). *Psychoanalytic studies of the personality*. London: Tavistock Publications.

Field, T. M., Schanberg, S. M., Scafirdi, F., Bauer, C. R., Vega-Lahr, N., Garcia, R., Nystrom, J., & Kuhn, C. M. (1986). Tactile/Kinesthetic stimulation effects on preterm neonates. *Paediatrics*, 77, 654–658.

Ferguson, D. W., & Horwood, L. J. (2003). Resilience to childhood adversity: Results of a 21-year study. In S. S. Luthar (Ed.), *Resilience and vulnerability: Adaptation in the context of childhood adversities* (pp. 130–155). Cambridge: Cambridge University Press.

Fonagy, P., Steele, M., Steele, H., Moran, G., & Higgitt, A. C. (1991). The capacity for understanding mental states: The reflective self in parent and child and its significance for security of attachment. *Infant Mental Health Journal*, 12(3), 201–218.

Fonagy, P., & Target, M. (1996). Playing with reality: I. Theory of mind and the normal development of psychic reality. *International Journal of Psychoanalysis*, 77(Pt 2), 217–233.

Fox, N. A., Henderson, H. A., Rubin, K. H., Calkins, S. D., & Schmidt, L. A. (2001). Continuity and discontinuity of behavioral inhibition and exuberance: Psychophysiological and behavioral influences across the first four years of life. *Child Development*, 72(1), 1–21.

Freud, S. (1922). *Beyond the pleasure principle* (C. J. Hubback, Trans., 2nd ed.). London: International Psycho-analytical Press.

Goldberg, S. (2000). *Attachment and development*. New York: Oxford University Press.

Greenspan, S., & Wieder, S. (1993). Regulatory disorders. In C. H. Zeanah (Ed.), *Handbook of infant mental health* (pp. 280–290). New York: Guilford Press.

Kagan, J. (1997). Temperament. In J. D. Noshpitz, S. Greenspan, S. Wieder & J. Osofsky (Eds.), *Handbook of child and adolescent psychiatry: Vol. 1. Infancy and preschoolers: Development and syndromes* (pp. 268–275). New York: Wiley.

Kagan, J., Snidman, N., & Arcus, D. (1998). Childhood derivatives of high and low reactivity in infancy. *Child Development*, 69, 1483–1493.

Klein, M. & Riviero, J. (1937). *Love, guilt and reparation*. London: Hogarth Press.

Kohnstamm, G. A., Bates, J. E., & Rothbart, M. K. (Eds.). (1989). *Temperament in childhood*. New York: Wiley.

REFERENCES

Lieberman, A., & Slade, A. (1997a). The first year of life. In J. D. Noshpitz, S. Greenspan, S. Wieder & J. Osofsky (Eds.), *Handbook of child and adolescent psychiatry: Vol. 1. Infancy and preschoolers: Development and syndromes* (pp. 3–10). New York: Wiley.

Lieberman, A., & Slade, A. (1997b). The second year of life. In J. D. Noshpitz, S. Greenspan, S. Wieder & J. Osofsky (Eds.), *Handbook of child and adolescent psychiatry: Vol. 1. Infancy and preschoolers: Development and syndromes* (pp. 56–62). New York: Wiley.

Mahler, M. S., Pine, F., & Bergman, A. (1975). *The psychological birth of the human infant: Symbiosis and individuation.* New York: Basic Books.

Maldonado-Duran, M., & Sauceda-Garcia, J. M. (1996). Excessive crying in infants with regulatory disorders. *Bulletin of the Menninger Clinic, 60*(1), 62–78.

Miller, P. H. (2002). *Theories of developmental psychology* (4th ed.). New York: Worth.

Murray, L., & Andrews, L. (2001). *Your Social Baby: Understanding babies' communication from birth.* Melbourne: ACER Press.

Sameroff, A. J., & Fiese, B. H. (2000). Models of development and developmental risk. In C. H. Zeanah (Ed.), *Handbook of infant mental health* (2nd ed., pp. 3–19). New York: Guilford Press.

Sameroff, A. J., McDonough, S. C., & Rosenblum, K. L. (Eds.). (2004). *Treating parent infant relationship problems: Strategies for intervention.* New York: Guilford Press.

Schore, A. N. (1994). *Affect regulation and the origin of the self: The neurobiology of emotional development.* Hillsdale, NJ: Erlbaum.

Shore, R. (1997). *Rethinking the brain: New insights into early development.* New York: Families and Work Institute.

Siegel, D. J. (1999). *The developing mind: Towards a neurobiology of interpersonal experience.* New York: Guilford Press.

Sroufe, L. A. (1996). *Emotional development: The organization of emotional life in the early years.* Cambridge: Cambridge University Press.

Stern, D. (1985). *The interpersonal world of the infant: A view from psychoanalysis and developmental psychology.* New York: Basic Books.

Thomas, A., & Chess, S. (1977). *Temperament and development.* New York: Brunner/Mazel.

Trevarthen, C. (2001). Intrinsic motives for companionship in understanding: Their origin, development, and significance for infant mental health. *Infant Mental Health Journal, 22*(1), 95–131.

Winnicott, D. W. (1978). *The child, the family and the outside world.* Harmondsworth, Middlesex: Penguin Books. (Original work published 1964.)

Zeanah, C. H., Boris, N. W., & Larrieu, J. A. (1997). Infant development and developmental risk: A review of the past 10 years. *Journal of the American Academy of Child and Adolescent Psychiatry, 36*(2), 165–178.

Chapter 2 Attachment: theory, disruptions and disorders

Ainsworth, M. D., Blehar, M. C., Waters, E., & Wall, S. (1978). *Patterns of attachment: A psychological study of the strange situation.* Hillsdale, NJ: Lawrence Erlbaum Associates.

American Psychiatric Association. (1980). *Diagnostic and statistical manual of mental disorders* (3rd ed.). Washington, DC: Author.

American Psychiatric Association. (1987). *Diagnostic and statistical manual of mental disorders* (3rd rev. ed.). Washington, DC: Author.

American Psychiatric Association. (1994). *Diagnostic and statistical manual of mental disorders* (4th ed.). Washington, DC: Author.

Bowlby, J. (1944). Forty-four juvenile thieves: Their characteristics and home life. *International Journal of Psycho-Analysis, 25,* 19–25.

Bowlby, J. (1951). *Maternal care and mental health: A report prepared on behalf of the World Health Organisation as a contribution to the United Nations Programme for the welfare of homeless children.* Geneva: World Health Organization.

REFERENCES

Burlington, D., & Freud, A. (1944). *Infants without families.* New York: International Universities Press.

Crittenden, P. A. (1992). Quality of attachment in the preschool years. *Development and psychopathology, 4*, 209–241.

Fonagy, P. (2001). *Attachment theory and psychoanalysis.* New York: Other Press.

Fonagy, P., & Target, M. (1997). Attachment and reflective function: Their role in self organisation. *Development and Psychopathology, 9*(4), 679–700.

Fonagy, P., & Target, M. (2000). The place of psychodynamic theory in developmental psychopathology. *Development and Psychopathology, 12*(3), 407–425.

Fraiberg, S. (Ed.). (1980). *Clinical studies in infant mental health: The first year of life.* New York: Basic Books.

Fraiberg, S., Adelson, E., & Shapiro, V. (1975). Ghosts in the nursery: A psychoanalytic approach to impaired infant–mother relationships. *Journal of the American Academy of Child Psychiatry, 14*(3), 387–422.

George, C., Kaplan, N., & Main, M. (1996). *The Adult Attachment Interview* (3rd ed.). Unpublished manuscript, University of California, Berkeley.

Hesse, E. (1999). The Adult Attachment Interview: Historical and current perspectives. In J. Cassidy & P. Shaver (Eds.), *Handbook of attachment: Theory, resources, and clinical applications* (pp. 395–433). New York: Guilford Press.

Hodges, J., & Tizard, B. (1989). Social and family relationships of ex-institutional adolescents. *Journal of Child Psychology and Psychiatry and Allied Disciplines, 30*(1), 77–97.

Holmes, J. (2001). *The search for the secure base: Attachment theory and psychotherapy.* London: Brunner-Routledge.

Lieberman, A. F., & Zeanah, C. H. (1995). Disorders of attachment in infancy. *Child and Adolescent Psychiatric Clinics of North America, 4*(3), 571–587.

Lieberman, A. F., & Zeanah, C. H. (1999). Contributions of attachment theory to infant–parent psychotherapy and other interventions with infants and young children. In J. Cassidy & P. Shaver (Eds.), *Handbook of attachment: Theory, research, and clinical applications* (pp. 555–574). New York: Guilford Press.

Lyons-Ruth, K., & Jacobovitz, D. (1999). Attachment disorganisation: Unresolved loss, relational violence and lapses in behavioural and attentional strategies. In J. Cassidy & P. Shaver (Eds.), *Handbook of attachment theory and research* (pp. 520–554). New York: Guilford.

Main, M., & Goldwyn, R. (1994). *Adult attachment scoring and classification systems* (2nd ed.). Unpublished manuscript, University of California, Berkeley.

Muir, E., Lojkasek, M., & Cohen, N. J. (1999). *Watch, wait, and wonder: A manual describing a dynamic infant-led approach to problems in infancy and early childhood.* Toronto: Hincks-Dellcrest Institute.

Sameroff, A. J., McDonough, S. C., & Rosenblum, K. L. (Eds.) (2004). *Treating parent–infant relationship problems: Strategies for intervention.* New York: Guilford Press.

Stern, D. (1985). *The interpersonal world of the infant: A view from psychoanalysis and developmental psychology.* New York: Basic Books.

Stern, D. (1995). *The motherhood constellation: A unified view of parent–infant psychotherapy.* New York: Basic Books.

van IJzendoorn, M. H. (1995). Adult attachment representations, parental responsiveness, and infant attachment: A meta-analysis on the predictive validity of the Adult Attachment Interview. *Psychological Bulletin, 117*(3), 387–403.

Zeanah, C. H. (1996). Beyond insecurity: A reconceptualisation of attachment disorders of infancy. *Journal of Consulting and Clinical Psychology, 64*(1), 42–52.

Zeanah C. H., & Boris, N. W. (2000). Disturbances and disorders of attachment in early childhood. In C. H. Zeanah (Ed.), *Handbook of infant mental health* (pp. 353–368). New York: Guilford Press.

REFERENCES

Zeanah, C. H., Boris, N. W., Bakshi, S., & Lieberman, A. (2000). Attachment disorders of infancy. In J. D. Osofosky & H. E. Fitzgerald (Eds.), *World Association for Infant Mental Health (WAIMH) Handbook of infant mental health: Vol. 4. Infant mental health in groups at high risk* (pp. 93–122). New York: Wiley.

Chapter 3 Principles of assessment in infant mental health

Brazelton, T. B., & Nugent, J. K. (1995). *Neonatal Behavioural Assessment Scale* (3rd ed.). London: Mac Keith Press.

Fraiberg, S. (1980). *Clinical studies in infant mental health.* New York: Basic Books.

Sameroff, A. J., & Fiese, B. H. (1990). Transactional regulation and early intervention. In S. J. Meisels & J. P. Shonkoff (Eds.), *Handbook of early childhood intervention* (pp. 119–149). New York: Cambridge University Press.

Sameroff, A. J., & Fiese, B. H. (2000). Models of development and developmental risk. In C. H. Zeanah (Ed.), *Handbook of infant mental health* (2nd ed., pp. 3–19). New York: Guilford Press.

Winnicott, D. W. (1987). The ordinary devoted mother. In C. Winnicott, R. Shepherd & M. Davis (Eds.), *Babies and their mothers* (pp. 3–14). Reading, MA: Addison-Wesley.

Zeanah, C. H., Boris, N. W., & Larrieu, J. A. (1997). Infant development and developmental risk: A review of the past 10 years. *Journal of the American Academy of Child and Adolescent Psychiatry, 36*(2), 165–178.

Chapter 4 Assessing risk in infancy

Donald, T., & Jureidini, J. (2004). Parenting capacity. *Child Abuse Review, 13,* 5–17.

Egeland, B., Bosquet, M., & Chung, A. L. (2002). Continuities and discontinuities in the intergenerational transmission of child maltreatment: Implications for breaking the cycle of abuse. In K. Brown, H. Hanks, P. Stratton & C. Hamilton (Eds.), *Early prediction and prevention of child abuse: A handbook* (pp. 217–232). New York: Wiley and Sons.

Ferguson, D. W., & Horwood, L. J. (2003). Resilience to childhood adversity: Results of a 21-year study. In S. S. Luthar (Ed.), *Resilience and vulnerability: Adaptation in the context of childhood adversities* (pp. 130–155). Cambridge: Cambridge University Press.

Hoghughi, M. (1997). Parenting at the margins: Some consequences of inequality. In K. N. Dwivedi (Ed.), *Enhancing parenting skills: A guide book for professionals working with parents* (pp. 21–41). Chichester: Wiley.

Jones, D. (2001). The assessment of parental capacity. In J. Horwath (Ed.), *The child's world: Assessing children in need* (pp. 225–272). London: Jessica Kingsley.

Kaufman, J., & Zigler, E. (1987). Do abused children become abusive parents? *American Journal of Orthopsychiatry, 57*(2), 186–192.

Luthar, S. S., & Zelazo, L. B. (2003). Research on resilience: An integrative review. In S. S. Luthar (Ed.), *Resilience and vulnerability: Adaptation in the context of childhood adversities* (pp. 510–549). Cambridge: Cambridge University Press.

Luthar, S. S. (Ed.). (2003). *Resilience and vulnerability: Adaptation in the context of childhood adversities.* Cambridge: Cambridge University Press.

Reder, P. (2003). Does the past predict the future? In P. Reder, S. Duncan & C. Lucey (Eds.), *Studies in the assessment of parenting* (pp. 229–246). New York: Brunner-Routledge.

Reder, P., Duncan, S., & Lucey, C. (Eds.). (2003a). *Studies in the assessment of parenting.* New York: Brunner-Routledge.

Reder, P., Duncan, S., & Lucey, C. (2003b). What principles guide parenting assessments? In P. Reder, S. Duncan & C. Lucey (Eds.), *Studies in the assessment of parenting* (pp. 3–26). New York: Brunner-Routledge.

Sameroff, A., Gutman, L. M., & Peck, S. C. (2003). Adaptation among youth facing multiple risks: Prospective research findings. In S. S. Luthar (Ed.), *Resilience and vulnerability: Adaptation in the context of childhood adversities* (pp. 364–391). Cambridge: Cambridge University Press.

Sturge, C., & Glasser, D. (2000). Contact and domestic violence: The expert's court report. *Family Law, 30,* 615–626.

Thompson, R. A. (1999). Early attachment and later development. In J. Cassidy & P. R. Shaver (Eds.), *Handbook of attachment: Theory, research and clinical applications* (pp. 265–286). New York: Guilford Press.

Zeanah, C. H., Boris, N. W., & Larrieu, J. A. (1997). Infant development and developmental risk: A review of the past 10 years. *Journal of the American Academy of Child and Adolescent Psychiatry, 36*(2), 165–178.

Chapter 5 Pregnancy, labour and birth

Boyce, P., & Condon, J. (2000). Traumatic childbirth and the role of debriefing. In B. Raphael & J. P. Wilson (Eds.), *Psychological debriefing: theory, practice and evidence* (pp. 272–280). Cambridge: Cambridge University Press.

Brockington, I. F. (1996). *Motherhood and mental health.* Oxford: Oxford University Press.

Condon, J. T., & Corkingdale, C. (1997). The correlates of antenatal attachment in pregnant women. *British Journal of Medical Psychology, 70*(4), 359–372.

Glover, V. (1997). Maternal stress or anxiety in pregnancy and emotional development of the child. *British Journal of Psychiatry, 171,* 105–106.

Glover, V., & O'Conner, T. G. (2002). Effects of antenatal stress and anxiety: Implications for development and psychiatry. *British Journal of Psychiatry, 180,* 389–391.

Hepper, P. G. (1989). Foetal learning: Implications for psychiatry? *British Journal of Psychiatry, 155,* 289–293.

Hrasky, M., & Morice, R. (1986). The identification of psychiatric disturbance in an obstetric and gynaecological population. *Australian and New Zealand Journal of Psychiatry, 20*(1), 63–69.

Newport, D. J., Wilcox, M. M., & Stowe, Z. N. (2001). Antidepressants during pregnancy and lactation: Defining exposure and treatment issues. *Seminars in Perinatology, 25*(3), 177–190.

O'Hara, M. (1997). The nature of postpartum depressive disorders. In L. Murray & P. J. Cooper (Eds.), *Postpartum depression and child development* (pp. 3–31). New York: Guilford Press.

Orr, S. T., & Miller, C. A. (1995). Maternal depressive symptoms and the risk of poor pregnancy outcome: Review of the literature and preliminary findings. *Epidemiological Review, 17*(1), 165–171.

Sacker, A., Done, D. J., & Crowe, T. J. (1996). Obstetric complications in children born to parents with schizophrenia: A meta-analysis of case control studies. *Psychological Medicine, 26*(2), 279–287.

Stern, D. N. (1995). *The motherhood constellation: A unified view of parent–infant psychotherapy.* New York: Basic Books.

Van Egeren, L. (1998). The development of the parenting alliance over the transition to parenthood. *The Signal, 6*(2), 1–10.

van IJzendoorn, M. H. (1992). Intergenerational transmission of parenting: A review of studies in nonclinical populations. *Developmental Review, 12*(1), 76–99.

Winnicott, D. W. (1964). *The child, the family and the outside world.* Harmondsworth, Middlesex: Penguin Books.

Winnicott, D. W. (1987). The ordinary devoted mother. In C. Winnicott, R. Shepherd & M. Davis (Eds.), *Babies and their mothers* (pp. 3–14). Reading, MA: Addison-Wesley.

REFERENCES

Chapter 6 Biomedical problems in infancy

Als, H. (1982). Toward a synactive theory of development: Promise for the assessment and support of infant individuality. *Infant Mental Health Journal, 3*(4), 229–243.

Als, H. (1986). A synactive model of neonatal behavioral organization: Framework for the assessment of neurobehavioral development in the premature infant and for support of infants and parents in the neonatal intensive care environments. In J. K. Sweeney (Ed.), *The high-risk neonate: Developmental therapy perspectives* (pp. 3–53). New York: The Haworth Press.

Als, H. (1991). Neonatal organization of the newborn: Opportunity for assessment and intervention. *National Institute on Drug Abuse Research Monograph, 114*, 106–116.

Als, H. (1998). Developmental care in the newborn intensive care unit. *Current Opinion in Pediatrics, 10*(2), 138–142.

Als, H., & Gilkerson, L. (1997). The role of relationship-based developmentally supportive newborn intensive care in strengthening outcome of preterm infants. *Seminars in Perinatology, 21*(3), 178–189.

American College of Obstetricians and Gynecologists. (1999). ACOG educational bulletin: Special problems of multiple gestation. International Journal of Gynaecology and Obstetrics, 64(3), 323–333.

Bennett, F. C. (1988). Neurodevelopmental outcome in low-birthweight infants: The role of developmental interventions. *Clinics in Critical Care Medicine, 13*, 221–249.

Benton, A. L. (1940). Mental development of prematurely born children. *American Journal of Orthopsychiatry, 10*, 719–746.

Brazelton, T. B. (1993). Touchpoints: The essential reference guide to your child's emotional and behavioural development. Sydney: Doubleday.

Brazelton, T. B., Als, H., Tronick, E., & Lester, B. M. (1979). Specific neonatal measures: The Brazelton Neonatal Behavioural Assessment Scale. In J. D. Osofsky (Ed.), *The handbook of infant development* (pp. 185–215). New York: Wiley.

Brazelton, T. B., & Nugent, J. K. (1995). *Neonatal Behavioural Assessment Scale* (3rd ed.). London: Mac Keith Press.

Brazy, J. E., Eckerman, C. O., Oehler, J. M., Goldstein, R. F., & O'Rand, A. M. (1991). Nursery Neurobiologic Risk Score: Important factors in predicting outcome in very low birth weight infants. *Journal of Paediatrics, 118*(5), 783–792.

Brisch, K. H. (2003). *Attachment disorders in preterm infants: Neurological implications.* Paper presented at the International Conference of Infant Development in Neonatal Intensive Care. London.

Brisch, K. H., Bechringer, D., Betzler, S., & Heinemann, H. (2003). Early preventive attachment oriented psychotherapeutic intervention program with parents of a very low birthweight premature infant: Results of attachment and neurological development. *Attachment and Human Development, 5*(2), 120–135.

Browne, J. V. (2003). New perspectives on premature infants and their parents. *Zero to Three, 24*(2), 4–12.

Dolby, R., Warren, B., Meade, V., & Heath, J. S. (1987, May). *Preventive Care for Low Birthweight Infants.* Paper presented at the International Physiotherapy Conference, Sydney.

Douglas, J. W. (1975). Early hospital admissions and later disturbances of behaviour and learning. *Developmental Medicine and Child Neurology, 17*(4), 456–480.

Drillien, C. M. (1964). *The growth and development of the prematurely born infant.* Edinburgh: Livingstone.

Feldman, R., & Eidelman, A. I. (2003). Skin-to-skin contact (Kangaroo Care) accelerates autonomic and neurobehavioural maturation in preterm infants. *Developmental Medicine and Child Neurology, 45*(4), 274–281.

REFERENCES

Feldman, R., Weller, A., Sirota, L., & Eidelman, A. I. (2003). Testing a family intervention hypothesis: The contribution of mother–infant skin-to-skin contact (Kangaroo Care) to family interaction, proximity, and touch. *Journal of Family Psychology, 17*(1), 94–107.

Gillberg, C., & Coleman, M. (1992). *The biology of the autistic syndromes* (2nd ed.). London: Mac Keith Press.

Kanner, L. (1943). Autistic disturbances of affective contact. *Nervous Child, 2*, 217–250.

Keren, M., Feldman, R., Eidelman, A. I., Sirota, L., & Lester, B. (2003). Clinical interview for high-risk parents of premature infants (CLIP) as a predictor of early disruptions in the mother–infant relationship at the nursery. *Infant Mental Health Journal, 24*(2), 93–110.

Kopp, C. B. (1987). Developmental risk: Historical reflections. In J. D. Osofsky (Ed.), *The handbook of infant development* (2nd ed., pp. 881–912). New York: Wiley.

Lambrenos, K., Weindling, A. M., Calam, R., & Cox, A. D. (1996). The effect of a child's disability on mother's mental health. *Archives of Disease in Childhood, 74*(2), 115–120.

Lampe, J., Trause, M. A., & Kennell, J. (1977). Parental visiting of sick infants: The effect of living at home prior to hospitalisation. *Pediatrics, 59*(2), 294–296.

Lorenz, J. M., Wooliever, D. E., Jetton, J. R., & Paneth, N. (1998). A quantitative review of mortality and developmental disability in extremely premature newborns. *Archives of Pediatrics and Adolescent Medicine, 152*(5), 425–435.

Mangelsdorf, S. C., Plunkett, J., Dedrick, C., Berlin, M., Meisels, S. J., McHale, J. L., et al. (1996). Attachment security in very low birth weight infants. *Developmental Psychology, 32*(5), 914–920.

Marvin, R. S., & Pianta, R. C. (1996). Mothers' reactions to their child's diagnosis: Relations with security of attachment. *Journal of Clinical Child Psychology, 25*(4), 436–445.

Mayes, L. C., Gabriel, H. P., & Oberfield, R. (2002). Prematurity, birth defects, and early death: Impact on the family. In M. Lewis (Ed.), *Child and adolescent psychiatry: A comprehensive textbook* (3rd ed., pp. 1123–1135). Philadelphia: Lippincott Williams & Wilkins.

McCormick, M. C., Shapiro, S., & Starfield, B. H. (1980). Rehospitalisation in the first year of life for high-risk survivors. *Pediatrics, 66*(6), 991–999.

Minde, K. (1993). Prematurity and serious medical illness in infancy: Implications for development and intervention. In C. H. Zeanah (Ed.), *Handbook of infant mental health* (pp. 87–105). New York: Guilford Press.

Minde, K. (2000). Prematurity and serious medical conditions in infancy: Implications for development, behaviour and intervention. In C. H. Zeanah (Ed.), *Handbook of infant mental health* (2nd ed., pp. 176–194). New York: Guilford Press.

Minde, K., Perrotta, M., & Hellmann, J. (1988). The impact of delayed development in premature infants on mother–infant interaction: A prospective investigation. *Journal of Pediatrics, 112*(1), 136–142.

Montrasio, V. (1997). A developmental approach for premature children. *The Signal, 5*, 7–13.

Quinton, D., & Rutter, M. (1976). Early hospital admissions and later disturbances of behaviours: An attempted replication of Douglas' findings. *Developmental Medicine and Child Neurology, 18*, 447–459.

Sizun, J., Ratynski, N., & Boussard, C. (1999). Humane neonatal care initiative, NIDCAP and family-centred neonatal intensive care. Neonatal Individualized Developmental Care and Assessment Program. *Acta Paediatrica, 88*(10), 1172.

Stratton, P. (Ed.). (1982). *Psychobiology of the human newborn*. Chichester: Wiley.

Symington, A., & Pinelli, J. (2003). *Developmental care for promoting development and preventing morbidity in preterm infants. The Cochrane Database of Systematic Reviews, Issue 4*. Retrieved 27 January 2005 from http://www.cochrane.org/cochrane/revabstr/ab001814.htm.

Tjossem, T. D. (Ed.). (1976). *Intervention strategies for high risk infants and young children*. Baltimore: University Park Press.

REFERENCES

Tracey, N. (Ed.). (2000). *Parents of premature infants: Their emotional world.* London: Whurr.

Veddovi, M., Gibson, F., Kenny, D. T., Bowen, J., & Starte, D. (2004). Preterm behaviour, maternal adjustment and competencies in the newborn period: What influence do they have 12 months postnatal? *Infant Mental Health Journal, 25*(6), 580–599.

Volpe, J. J. (1998). Neurological outcome of prematurity. *Archives of Neurology, 55*(3), 297–300.

Wolke, D. (1998). Psychological developmental of prematurely born children. *Archives of Disease in Childhood, 78*(6), 567–570.

Chapter 7 Sleeping

Ainsworth, M. D., Blehar, M. C., Waters, E., & Wall, S. (1978). *Patterns of attachment: A psychological study of the strange situation.* Hillsdale, NJ: Lawrence Erlbaum Associates.

Anders, T., Goodlin-Jones, B., & Sadeh, A. (2000). Sleep disorders. In C. H. Zeanah (Ed.), *Handbook of infant mental health* (2nd ed., pp. 326–338). New York: Guilford Press.

Barton, M., & Robins, D. (2000). Regulatory disorders. In C. H. Zeanah (Ed.), *Handbook of infant mental health* (2nd ed., pp. 311–325). New York: Guilford Press.

Bayley, N. (1993). *Bayley Scales of Infant Development* (2nd ed.). San Antonio: Psychological Corporation.

Greenspan, S. (1989). *The development of the ego: Implications for personality theory, psychopathology, and the psychotherapeutic process.* Madison, CT: International Universities Press.

Greenspan, S., & Wieder, S. (1993). Regulatory disorders. In C. H. Zeanah (Ed.), *Handbook of infant mental health* (pp. 280–290). New York: Guilford Press.

Griffiths, R. (1984). *The abilities of young children.* High Wycombe, UK: Test Agency.

Mahler, M. S., Pine, F., & Bergman, A. (1975). *The psychological birth of the human infant: Symbiosis and individuation.* New York: Basic Books.

Minde, K. (1997). Sleep disorders in infants and young children. In J. D. Noshpitz, S. Greenspan, S. Wieder & J. Osofsky (Eds.), *Handbook of child and adolescent psychiatry: Vol. 1. Infancy and Preschoolers: Development and Syndromes* (pp. 492–507). New York: Wiley.

Mosko, S., McKenna, J., Dickel, M., & Hunt, L. (1993). Parent–infant co-sleeping: The appropriate context for the study of infant sleep and implications for Sudden Infant Death Syndrome (SIDS) research. *Journal of Behavioural Medicine, 16*(6), 589–610.

Stein, M. T., Colaruso, C. A., McKenna, J. J., & Powers, N. G. (2001). Cosleeping (bedsharing) among infants and toddlers. *Pediatrics, 107*(4), 873–877.

Stern, D. N. (1995). *The motherhood constellation: A unified view of parent–infant psychotherapy.* New York: Basic Books.

Chapter 8 Feeding

Barr, R. G., & Young, S. N. (1999). A two-phase model of the soothing taste response: Implications for a taste probe of temperament and emotion regulation. In M. Lewis & D. Ramsay (Eds.), *Soothing and Stress* (pp. 109–137). Mahwah, NJ: Lawrence Erlbaum Associates.

Benoit, D., Wang, E. E., & Zlotkin, S. H. (2000). Discontinuation of enterostomy tube feeding by behavioural treatment in early childhood: A randomized controlled trial. *Journal of Pediatrics, 137*(4), 498–503.

Bernbaum, J. C., Pereira, G. R., Watkins, J. B., & Peckham, G. J. (1983). Nonnutritive sucking during gavage feeding enhances growth and maturation in premature infants. *Pediatrics, 71*(1), 41–45.

Blass, E. M. (1997). Milk-induced hypoalgesia in human newborns. *Pediatrics, 99*(6), 825–829.

Brazelton, T. B. (1984). *Neonatal Behavioural Assessment Scale* (2nd ed.). London: Spastics International Medical Publications.

REFERENCES

Brisch, K. H. (2002). *Treating attachment disorders: From theory to therapy* (K. Kronenberg, Trans.). New York: Guilford Press.

Casey, P. H. (1999). Failure to thrive. In M. D. Levine, W. B. Carey & A. C. Crocker (Eds.), *Developmental–behavioural pediatrics* (3rd ed., pp. 397–405). Philadelphia: Saunders.

Chatoor, I. (1986). *Mother–Infant/Toddler Feeding Scale: Birth to three years*. Washington, DC: Children's Hospital National Medical Center.

Chatoor, I., Ganiban, J., Colin, V., Plummer, N., & Harmon, R. J. (1998). Attachment and feeding problems: A reexamination of nonorganic failure to thrive and attachment insecurity. *Journal of the American Academy of Child and Adolescent Psychiatry, 37*(11), 1217–1224.

Chatoor, I., Ganiban, J., Harrison, J., & Hirsch, R. (2001). Observation of feeding in the diagnosis of posttraumatic feeding disorder in infancy. *Journal of the American Academy of Child and Adolescent Psychiatry, 40*(5), 595–602.

Chatoor, I., Ganiban J., Hirsch, R., Borman-Spurrell, E., & Mrazek, D. A. (2000). Maternal characteristics and toddler temperament in infantile anorexia. *Journal of the American Academy of Child and Adolescent Psychiatry, 39*(6), 743–751.

Chatoor, I., Getson, P., Menvielle, E., Brasseaux, C., O'Donnell, R., Rivera, Y., et al. (1997). A feeding scale for research and clinical practice to assess mother–infant interactions in the first three years of life. *Infant Mental Health Journal, 18*(1), 76–91.

Chatoor, I., Loeffler, C., McGee, M., & Menvielle, E. (1998). *Observational Scale for Mother–Infant Interaction during Feeding: Manual* (2nd ed.). Washington, DC: Children's National Medical Center.

Corbett, S. S., Drewett, R. F., & Wright, C. M. (1996). Does a fall down a centile chart matter? The growth and development sequelae of mild failure to thrive. *Acta Paediatrica, 85*(11), 1278–1283.

Derivan, A. T. (1982). Disorders of bonding. In P. J. Accardo (Ed.), *Failure to thrive in infancy and early childhood: A multidisciplinary team approach* (pp. 91–103). Baltimore: University Park Press.

de Vries, J. I., Visser, J. H., & Prechtl, H. F. (1984). Fetal motility in the first half of pregnancy. In H. F. R. Prechtl (Ed.), *Continuity of neural functions from prenatal to postnatal life: Vol. 4. Clinics in Developmental Medicine No. 94* (pp. 46–64). Oxford: Blackwell Scientific.

Dowling, S. (1977). Seven infants with esophageal atresia: A developmental study. *The Psychoanalytic Study of the Child, 32*, 215–256.

Dowling, S. (1980). Going forth to meet the environment: A developmental study of seven infants with esophageal atresia. *Psychosomatic Medicine, 42*(Suppl. 1), 153–161.

Drotar, D., Eckerle, D., Satola, J., Pallotta, J., & Wyatt, B. (1990). Maternal interactional behavior with nonorganic failure-to-thrive infants: A case comparison study. *Child Abuse and Neglect, 14*(1), 41–51.

Duniz, M., Scheer, P. J., Trojovsky, A., Kaschnitz, W., Kvas, E., & Macari, S. (1996). Changes in psychopathology of parents of NOFT (non-organic failure to thrive) infants during treatment. *European Child and Adolescent Psychiatry, 5*(2), 93–100.

Dunitz-Scheer, M. (2002, March). *Feeding the difficult neonate: Impact and practical guidelines*. Paper presented at the Perinatal Society of Australia and New Zealand 16th Annual Congress, Christchurch, New Zealand.

Dunitz-Scheer, M., Wilken, M., Walch, G., Schein, A., & Scheer, P. (2000). Wie kommen wir von der Sonde los?! Diagnostische Überlegungen und therapeutische Ansätze zur interdisziplinären Sondenentwöhnung im Säuglings-und Kleinkindalter [How can we get rid of the tube? Diagnostic considerations and therapeutic beginnings to interdisciplinary probe curing in babies and infants]. *Die Kinderkrankenschwester, 19*(11), 448–456.

REFERENCES

Dunn, W. (2002). *Infant/Toddler Sensory Profile: User's Manual*. San Antonio, TX: The Psychological Corporation.

Field, T. (1999). Sucking and massage therapy reduce stress during infancy. In M. Lewis & D. Ramsay (Eds.), *Soothing and Stress* (pp. 157–169). Mahwah, NJ: Lawrence Erlbaum Associates.

Field, T., Ignatoff, E., Stringer, S., Brennan, J., Greenberg, R., Widmayer, S., et al. (1982). Nonnutritive sucking during tube feedings: Effects on preterm neonates in an intensive care unit. *Pediatrics, 70*(3), 381–384.

Hepper, P. G. (1996). Fetal memory: Does it exist? What does it do? *Acta Paediatrica, 416*(Suppl.), 16–20.

Hooker, D. (1969). *The prenatal origin of behaviour*. New York: Hafner Publishing Company. (Original work published 1952.)

Humphrey, T. (1968). The development of mouth opening and related reflexes involving the oral area of the human fetuses. *Alabama Journal of Medical Sciences, 5*(2), 126–157.

Kennedy, C., & Lipsitt, L. P. (1993). Temporal characteristics of non-oral feedings and chronic feeding problems in premature infants. *Journal of Perinatal and Neonatal Nursing, 7*(3), 77–89.

Lehtonen, J., Kononen, M., Purhonen, M., Partanen, J., Saarikoski, S., & Launiala, K. (1998). The effect of nursing on the brain activity of the newborn. *The Journal of Pediatrics, 132*(4), 646–651.

Lubbe, T. (1996). Who lets go first? Some observations on the struggles around weaning. *Journal of Child Psychotherapy, 22*(2), 195–203.

Lucarelli, L., Ambruzzi, A. M., Cimino, S., D'Olimpio, F., & Finistrella, V. (2003). Feeding disorders in infancy: An empirical study on mother–infant interactions. *Minerva Pediatrica, 55*(3), 253–259.

Macfarlane, A. (1975). Olfaction in the development of social preferences in the human neonate. *Ciba Foundation Symposium, 33*, 103–117.

Main, M., & Goldwyn, R. (1991). *Adult attachment scoring and classification systems*. Unpublished manuscript, University College, London.

Marchi, M., & Cohen, P. (1990). Early childhood eating behaviours and adolescent eating disorders. *Journal of the American Academy of Child and Adolescent Psychiatry, 29*(1), 112–117.

Marlier, L., Schaal, B., & Soussignan, R. (1998). Neonatal responsiveness to the odor of amniotic and lacteal fluids: A test of perinatal chemosensory continuity. *Child Development, 69*(3), 611–623.

Menahem, S. (1994). Conservation-withdrawal reaction in infancy? An underdescribed entity. *Child Care, Health and Development, 20*(1), 15–26.

Meyer, E. C., Coll, C. T., Lester, B. M., Boukydis, C. F., McDonough, S. M., & Oh, W. (1994). Family-based intervention improves maternal psychological well-being and feeding interaction of preterm infants. *Pediatrics, 93*(2), 241–246.

Mizuno, K., & Ueda, A. (2001). Development of sucking behavior in infants who have not been fed for 2 months after birth. *Pediatrics International, 43*(3), 251–255.

Mizuno, K., & Ueda, A. (2005). Neonatal feeding performance as a predictor of neurodevelopmental outcome at 18 months. *Developmental Medicine and Child Neurology, 47*, 299–304.

Morris, S. E., & Klein, M. D. (2000). *Pre-feeding skills: A comprehensive resource for mealtime development* (2nd ed.). Tucson, AZ: Therapy Skill Builders/Harcourt.

Oates, R. K. (1996). *The spectrum of child abuse: Assessment, treatment and prevention*. New York: Bruner/Mazel.

Polan, H., & Ward, M. J. (1998). Role of the mother's touch in failure to thrive: A preliminary investigation. *Journal of the American Academy of Child and Adolescent Psychiatry, 33*(8), 1098–1105.

REFERENCES

Ramsey, M., Gisel, E. G., McCusker, J., Bellavance, F., & Platt, R. (2002). Infant sucking ability, non-organic failure to thrive, maternal characteristics, and feeding practices: A prospective cohort study. *Developmental Medicine and Child Neurology, 44*(6), 405–414.

Raphael-Leff, J. (1993). *Pregnancy: The inside story*. London: Sheldon.

Reilly, S. M., Skuse, D. H., Wolke, D., & Stevenson, J. (1999). Oral-motor dysfunction in children who fail to thrive: Organic or non-organic? *Developmental Medicine and Child Neurology, 41*(2), 115–122.

Salzberger-Wittenberger, I., Henry, G., & Osborne, E. (1983). *The emotional experience of learning and teaching*. London: Routledge & Kegan Paul.

Sayre, J. M., Pianta, R. C., Marvin, R. S., & Saft, E. W. (2001). Mothers' representations of relationships with their children: Relations with mother characteristics and feeding sensitivity. *Journal of Pediatric Psychology, 26*(6), 375–384.

Senez, C., Guys, J. M., Mancinic, J., Paz Paredes, A., Lena, G., & Choux, M. (1996). Weaning children from tube to oral feeding. *Child's Nervous System, 12*(10), 590–594.

Sewell, J., Tsitsikas, H., & Bax, M. (1982). Comparison of the Brazelton NBAS with health visitors' assessments of the nursing couple. *Developmental Medicine and Child Neurology, 24*(5), 615–625.

Spitz, R. A. (1945). Hospitalism: An inquiry into the genesis of psychiatric conditions in early infanthood. *The Psychoanalytic Study of the Child, 1*, 53–74.

Stein, A., Murray, L., Cooper, P., & Fairburn, C. G. (1996). Infant growth in the context of maternal eating disorders and maternal depression: A comparative study. *Psychological Medicine, 26*(3), 569–574.

Stein, A., Woolley, H., Cooper, S. D., & Fairburn, C. G. (1994). An observational study of mothers with eating disorders and their infants. *The Journal of Child Psychology and Psychiatry, 35*(4), 733–748.

Stern, D. N. (1985). *The interpersonal world of the infant: A view from psychoanalysis and developmental psychology*. New York: Basic Books.

Stevenson, M. B., Roach, M. A., ver Hoeve, J. N., & Leavitt, L. A. (1990). Rhythms in the dialogue of infant feeding: Preterm and term infants. *Infant Behavior and Development, 13*(1), 51–70.

Ward, M. J., Lee, S. S., & Lipper, E. G. (2000). Failure-to-thrive is associated with disorganized infant–mother attachment and unresolved maternal attachment. *Infant Mental Health Journal, 21*(6), 428–442.

Welch, K., Pianta, R. C., Marvin, R. S., & Saft, E. W. (2000). Feeding interactions for children with cerebral palsy: Contributions of mothers' psychological state and children's skills and abilities. *Journal of Developmental and Behavioural Pediatrics, 21*(2), 123–129.

Winnicott, D. W. (1964). *The child, the family and the outside world*. Harmondsworth, Middlesex: Penguin Books.

Winnicott, D. W. (1982). The depressive position in normal emotional development. In D. W. Winnicott (Ed.), *Through paediatrics to psycho-analysis* (pp. 262–277). London: The Hogarth Press and the Institute of Psycho-Analysis. (Original work published 1975.)

Winnicott, D. W. (1996). The bearing of emotional development on feeding problems. In R. Shepherd, J. Johns & H. R. Taylor (Eds.), *D. W. Winnicott: Thinking about children* (pp. 39–41). Reading, MS: Addison-Wesley. (Original work published 1967.)

Wolf, L. S., & Glass, R. P. (1992). *Feeding and swallowing disorders in infancy: Assessment and management*. Tucson, AZ: Therapy Skill Builders.

Wolke, D. (1996). Failure to thrive: The myth of maternal deprivation syndrome. *The Signal, 4*(3&4), 1–6.

REFERENCES

Chapter 9 Behavioural and emotional difficulties in toddlers

Ainsworth, M. D., Blehar, M. C., Waters, E., & Wall, S. (1978). *Patterns of attachment: A psychological study of the strange situation.* Hillsdale, NJ: Lawrence Erlbaum Associates.

American Psychiatric Association. (1994). *Diagnostic and statistical manual of mental disorders* (4th ed.). Washington, DC: Author.

Baker, L., & Cantwell, D. P. (1987). A prospective psychiatric follow-up of children with speech and language disorders. *Journal of the American Academy of Child and Adolescent Psychiatry, 26,* 546–553.

Beitchman, J. H., Nair, R., Clegg, M., & Patel, P. G. (1986). Prevalence of speech and language disorders in 5-year-old kindergarten children in the Ottawa Carlton region. *Journal of Speech and Hearing Disorders, 51,* 98–110.

Cynader, M., & Frost, B. (1999). Mechanisms of brain development: Neuronal sculpting by the physical and social environment. In D. Keating & C. Hertzman (Eds.), *Developmental health and the wealth of nations: Social, biological, and educational dynamics* (pp. 153–184). New York: Guilford Press.

Dionne, G., Tremblay, R., Boivin, M., Laplante, D., & Perusse, D. (2003). Physical aggression and expressive vocabulary in 19-month-old twins. *Developmental Psychology, 39*(2), 261–273.

Erikson, E. (1950). *Childhood and society.* New York: Norton.

Fonagy, P., Steele, M., Steele, H., Moran, G. S., & Higgitt, A. (1991). The capacity for understanding mental states: The reflective self in parent and child and its significance for security of attachment. *Infant Mental Health Journal, 12*(3), 201–218.

Forehand, R., King, H. E., Peed, S., & Yoder, P. (1975). Mother–child interactions: Comparison of a non-compliant clinic group and a non-clinic group. *Behaviour Research and Therapy, 13*(2–3), 79–84.

Lieberman, A. F. (1993). *The emotional life of the toddler.* New York: Free Press.

Lieberman, A. F. (1994). The emotional life of the toddler. *The Signal, 2*(4), 1–4.

Minton, C., Kagan, J., & Levine, J. A. (1971). Maternal control and obedience in the two-year-old. *Child Development, 42,* 1873–1894.

Patterson, G. R. (1980). Mother: The unacknowledged victims. *Monographs of the Society for Research in Child Development, 45*(5, Serial No. 186).

Sameroff, A. J., & Fiese, B. H. (2000). Models of development and developmental risk. In C. H. Zeanah (Ed.), *Handbook of infant mental health* (2nd ed., pp. 3–19). New York: Guilford Press.

Stern, D. (1985). *The interpersonal world of the infant: A view from psychoanalysis and developmental psychology.* New York: Basic Books.

Stern, D. (1995). *The motherhood constellation: A unified view of parent–infant psychotherapy.* New York: Basic Books.

Tremblay, R. E. (2004). Decade of behavior distinguished lecture: Development of physical aggression during infancy. *Infant Mental Health Journal, 25*(5), 399–407.

Tremblay, R. E., Nagin, D. S., Séguin, J. R., Zoccolillo, M., Zelazo, P., Boivin, M., et al. (2004). Physical aggression during early childhood: Trajectories and predictors. *Pediatrics, 114*(1), 43–50.

Zero to Three. (1995). *Diagnostic Classification: 0–3. Diagnostic classification of mental health and developmental disorders of infancy and early childhood.* Arlington, VA: Author.

Chapter 10 Consequences of trauma

De Bellis, M., Baum, A., Birmaher, B., Matcheri S., Keshavan, C. H., Eccard, A. M., et al. (1999). Developmental traumatology part 1: Biological stress systems. *Biological Psychiatry, 45*(10), 1259–1270.

REFERENCES

Gunderson, J. G., & Sabo, A. (1993). The phenomenological and conceptual interface between borderline personality disorder and PTSD. *American Journal of Psychiatry, 150*(1), 19–27.

Perry, B. D., Pollard, R. A., Blakely, T. L., Baker, W., & Vigilante, D. (1995). Childhood trauma, the neurobiology of adaptation and 'use-dependent' development of the brain: How 'states' become 'traits'. *Infant Mental Health Journal, 16*(4), 271–291.

Chapter 11 Gender development and identity

American Psychiatric Association (1994). *Diagnostic and statistical manual of mental disorders* (4th ed.). Washington, DC: Author.

Butler, J. P. (1990). *Gender trouble: Feminism and the subversion of identity.* New York: Routledge.

Colapinto, J. (2000). *As nature made him: The boy who was raised as a girl.* Sydney: Harper Collins.

Fast, I. (1984). *Gender identity: A differentiation model.* Hillsdale, NJ: The Analytic Press.

Herdt, G. (Ed.). (1994). *Third sex, third gender: Beyond sexual dimorphism in culture and history.* New York: Zone Books.

Laqueur, T. W. (1990). *Making sex: Body and gender from the Greeks to Freud.* Cambridge, MA: Harvard University Press.

Mead, M. (1949). *Male and female: a study of the sexes in a changing world.* New York: William Morrow.

Money, J., & Ehrhardt, A. A. (1972). *Man and woman, boy and girl: The differentiation and dimorphism of gender identity from conception to maturity.* Baltimore: John Hopkins University Press.

Newman, L. (2002). Sex, gender and culture: Issues in the definition, assessment and treatment of gender identity disorder. *Clinical Child Psychology and Psychiatry, 7*(3), 352–359.

Stoller, R. J. (1968). *Sex and gender: On the development of masculinity and femininity.* London: Hogarth Press.

Swaab, D. F., & Fliers, E. (1985). A sexually dimorphic nucleus in the human brain. *Science, 228*(4703), 1112–1115.

Zucker, K. J., & Bradley, S. J. (1995). *Gender identity disorder and psychosexual problems in children and adolescents.* New York: Guilford Press.

Chapter 12 Perinatal mental illness

American Psychiatric Association. (1994). *Diagnostic and statistical manual of mental disorders* (4th ed.). Washington, DC: Author.

Appleby, L., Warner, R., Whitton, A., & Faragher, B. (1997). A controlled study of fluoxetine and cognitive-behavioural counselling in the treatment of postnatal depression. *British Medical Journal, 314*(7085), 932–936.

Austin, M. P., & Mitchell, P. B. (1998). Psychotropic medications in pregnant women: Treatment dilemmas. *Medical Journal of Australia, 169*(8), 428–431.

Brockington, I. (1996). *Motherhood and mental illness.* Oxford: Oxford University Press.

Castle, D. J., McGrath, J., & Kulkarni, J. (Eds.). (2000). *Women and schizophrenia.* Cambridge: Cambridge University Press.

Cooper, P., Campbell, E. A., Day, A., Kennerley, H., & Bond, A. (1988). Non-psychotic psychiatric disorder after childbirth: A prospective study of prevalence, incidence, course and nature. *British Journal of Psychiatry, 152,* 799–806.

Cooper, P. J., & Murray, L. (1995). Course and recurrence of postnatal depression: Evidence for the specificity of the diagnostic concept. *British Journal of Psychiatry, 166*(6), 191–195.

Cooper, P. J., & Murray, L. (1997). The impact of psychological treatments of postnatal depression on maternal mood and infant development. In L. Murray & P. J. Cooper (Eds.), *Postpartum depression and child development* (pp. 201–220). London: Guilford Press.

REFERENCES

Cox, J. L., Holden, J. M., & Sagovsky, R. (1987). Detection of postnatal depression: Development of the 10-item Edinburgh Postnatal Depression Scale. *British Journal of Psychiatry, 150*, 782–786.

Cox, J. L., Murray, D., Chapman, G. (1993). A controlled study of the onset, duration and prevalence of postnatal depression. *British Journal of Psychiatry, 163*, 27–31.

Cross-National Collaborative Group. (1992). The changing rate of major depression: Cross-national comparisons. *Journal of the American Medical Association, 268*(21), 3098–3105.

Field, T. (1998). Maternal depression effects on infants and early interventions. *Preventive Medicine, 27*(2), 200–203.

Hay, D. (1997). Postpartum depression and cognitive development. In L. Murray & P. J. Cooper (Eds.), *Postpartum depression and child development* (pp. 85–110). London: Guilford Press.

Holden, J. M., Sagovsky, R., & Cox, J. L. (1989). Counselling in a general practice setting: Controlled study of health visitor intervention in treatment of postnatal depression. *British Medical Journal, 298*(6668), 223–226

Jones, I., & Craddock, N. (2001). Familiality of the puerperal trigger in bipolar disorder: Results of a family study. *American Journal of Psychiatry, 158*(6), 913–917.

Kendell, R. E., Chalmers, J. C., & Platz, C. (1987). Epidemiology of puerperal psychosis. *British Journal of Psychiatry, 150*, 662–673.

Kowalenko, N., Barnett, B., Fowler, C., & Matthey, S. (2000). The perinatal period: Early interventions for mental health. In R. Kosky, A. O'Hanlon, G. Martin & C. Davis (Eds.), *Clinical approaches to early intervention in child and adolescent mental health* (Vol. 4). Adelaide: Australian Early Intervention Network for Mental Health in Young People.

Kurstjens, S., & Wolke, D. (2001). Effects of maternal depression on cognitive development of children over the first 7 years of life. *Journal of Child Psychology and Psychiatry, 42*(5), 623–636.

Lovestone, S., & Kumar, K. (1993). Postnatal psychiatric illness: The impact on partners. *The British Journal of Psychiatry, 163*, 210–216.

McMahon, C., Barnett, B., Kowalenko, N., Tennant, C., & Don, N. (2001). Postnatal depression, anxiety and unsettled infant behaviour. *Australian and New Zealand Journal of Psychiatry, 35*(5), 581–588.

Milgrom, J., Burrows, G. D., Snellen, M., Stamboulakis, W., & Burrows, K. (1998). Psychiatric illness in women: A review of the function of a specialist mother–baby unit. *Australian and New Zealand Journal of Psychiatry, 32*(5), 680–686.

Morgan, M., Matthey, S., Barnett, R., & Richardson, C. (1997). A group programme for postnatally distressed women and their partners. *Journal of Advanced Nursing, 26*(5), 913–920.

Murray, L., & Cooper, P. J. (1997). The role of infant and maternal factors in postpartum depression, mother–infant interactions, and infant outcomes. In L. Murray & P. J. Cooper (Eds.), *Postpartum depression and child development* (pp. 111–135). New York: Guilford Press.

O'Hara, M. (1997). The nature of postpartum depressive disorder. In L. Murray & P. J. Cooper (Eds.), *Postpartum depression and child development* (pp. 3–31). New York: Guilford Press.

Orr, S. T., & Miller, C. A. (1995). Maternal depressive symptoms and the risk of poor pregnancy outcome: Review of the literature and preliminary findings. *Epidemiological Reviews, 17*(1), 165–171.

Royal Women's Hospital, Pharmacy Department. (2001). *Drugs and pregnancy*. Melbourne: Author.

Sacker, A., Done, D. J., & Crow, T. J. (1996). Obstetric complications in children born to parents with schizophrenia: A meta-analysis of case-control studies. *Psychological Medicine, 26*(2), 279–287.

Scottish Intercollegiate Guidelines Network. (2002). *Postnatal depression and puerperal psychosis: SIGN publication 60*. Retrieved 12 January 2005, from http://www.sign.ac.uk/guidelines/fulltext/60/index.html.

Seifer, R., & Dickstein, S. (2000). Parental mental illness and infant development. In C. H. Zeanah (Ed.), *Handbook of infant mental health* (2nd ed., pp. 145–160). New York: Guilford Press.

Wisner, K. L., Perel, J. M., & Findling, R. L. (1996). Antidepressant treatment during breast-feeding. *American Journal of Psychiatry, 153*(9), 1132–1137.

Wisner, K. L., Zarin, D. A., Holmboe, E. S., Applebaum, P. S., Gelenberg, A. J., Leonard, H. L., et al. (2000). Risk-benefit decision making for treatment of depression during pregnancy. *American Journal of Psychiatry, 157*(12), 1933–1940.

Yoshida, K., Smith, B., & Kumar, R. (1999). Psychotropic drugs in mothers' milk: A comprehensive review of assay methods, pharmacokinetics and of safety of breast-feeding. *Journal of Psychopharmacology, 13*(1), 64–80.

Chapter 13 Parents abused as children

Belsky, J. (1993). Etiology of child maltreatment: A developmental-ecological analysis. *Psychological Bulletin, 114*(3), 413–434.

Belsky, J., & Vondra, J. (1989). Lessons from child abuse: The determinants of parenting. In D. Cicchetti & V. Carlson (Eds.), *Child maltreatment: Theory and research on the causes and consequences of child abuse and neglect* (pp. 153–202). Cambridge: Cambridge University Press.

Briere, J. (1989). *Therapy for adults molested as children: Beyond survival*. New York: Springer.

Egeland, B., Bosquet, M., & Chung, A. L. (2002). Continuities and discontinuities in the intergenerational transmission of child maltreatment: Implications for breaking the cycle of abuse. In K. Brown, H. Hanks, P. Stratton & C. Hamilton (Eds.), *Early prediction and prevention of child abuse: A handbook* (pp. 217–232). New York: Wiley and Sons.

Egeland, B., Jacobovitz, D., & Sroufe, L. A. (1988). Breaking the cycle of abuse. *Child Development, 59*(4), 1080–1088.

Fonagy, P., Steele, M., Steele, H., Moran, G., & Higgitt, A. C. (1991). The capacity for understanding mental states: The reflective self in parent and child and its significance for security of attachment. *Infant Mental Health Journal, 12*(3), 201–218.

Fonagy, P., Steele, M., Steele, H., Higgitt, A., & Target, M. (1994). The Emanuel Miller Memorial Lecture 1992: The theory and practice of resilience. *Journal of Child Psychology and Psychiatry, 35*(2), 231–257.

Fraiberg, S., Adelson, E., & Shapiro, V. (1975). Ghosts in the nursery: A psychoanalytic approach to the problems of impaired infant–mother relationships. *Journal of the American Academy of Child Psychiatry, 14*(3), 387–421.

Glasser, D. (2000). Child abuse and neglect and the brain: A review. *Journal of Child Psychology and Psychiatry, 41*(1), 97–116.

Herrenkohl, E. C., Herrenkohl, R. C., & Toedter, L. J. (1983). Perspectives on the intergenerational transmission of abuse. In D. Finkelhor, R. J. Gelles, G. T. Hotaling & M. A. Straus (Eds.), *The dark side of families: Current family violence research* (pp. 305–317). Beverly Hills, CA: Sage.

Herzog, E. P., Gara, M. A., & Rosenberg, S. (1992). The abused child as parent: Perception of self and other. *Infant Mental Health Journal, 13*(1), 83–98.

Gara, M. A., Rosenberg, S., & Herzog, E. P. (1996). The abused child as parent. *Child Abuse and Neglect, 20*(9), 797–807.

Lyons-Ruth, K., Bronfman, E., & Atwood, G. (1999). A relational diathesis model of hostile-helpless states of mind: Expressions in mother–infant interaction. In J. Solomon & C. George (Eds.), *Attachment Disorganisation* (pp. 33–69). New York: Guilford Press.

REFERENCES

Kaufman, J., & Zigler, E. (1987). Do abused children become abusive parents? *American Journal of Orthopsychiatry, 57*(2), 186–192.

Main, M., & Hesse, E. (1990). Parents' unresolved traumatic experiences are related to infant disorganised attachment status: Is frightened and/or frightening parental behaviour the linking mechanism? In M. T. Greenberg, D. Cicchetti & E. M. Cummings (Eds.), *Attachment in the preschooler years: Theory, research, and intervention* (pp. 161–182). Chicago: University of Chicago Press.

McGloin, J. M., & Widom, C. S. (2001). Resilience among abused and neglected children grown up. *Development and Psychopathology, 13*(4), 1021–1038.

Perry, B. D., Pollard, R. A., Blakely, T. L., Baker, W. L., & Vigilante, D. (1995). Childhood trauma, the neurobiology of adaptation, and 'use-dependent' development of the brain: How 'states' become 'traits'. *Infant Mental Health Journal, 16*(4), 271–291.

Putallaz, M., Costanzo, P. R., Grimes, C. L., & Sherman, D. M. (1998). Intergenerational continuities and their influences on children's social development. *Social Development, 7*(3), 389–427.

Reder, P. (2003). Does the past predict the future? In P. Reder, S. Duncan & C. Lucey (Eds.), *Studies in the assessment of parenting* (pp. 229–246). New York: Brunner-Routledge.

Rogosch, F. A., Cicchetti, D., & Aber, J. L. (1995). The role of child maltreatment in early deviations in cognitive and affective processing abilities and later peer relationship problems. *Development and Psychopathology, 7*, 591–609.

Stern, D. N. (1995). *The motherhood constellation: A unified view of parent–infant psychotherapy*. New York: Basic Books.

van IJzendoorn, M. H. (1995). Adult attachment representations, parental responsiveness, and infant attachment: A meta-analysis on the predictive validity of the Adult Attachment Interview. *Psychological Bulletin, 117*(3), 387–403.

van IJzendoorn, M. H., & Bakermans-Kranenburg, M. J. (1997). Intergenerational transmission of attachment: A move to the contextual level. In L. Atkinson & K. J. Zucker (Eds.), *Attachment and psychopathology* (pp. 135–170). New York: Guilford Press.

Chapter 14 Parents with personality disorder

Ainsworth, M. D., Blehar, M. C., Waters, E., & Wall, S. (1978). *Patterns of attachment: A psychological study of the strange situation*. Hillsdale, NJ: Lawrence Erlbaum Associates.

American Psychiatric Association. (1994). *Diagnostic and statistical manual of mental disorders* (4th ed.). Washington, DC: Author.

American Psychiatric Association. (2001). *Practice guidelines for the treatment of patients with borderline personality disorder*. Washington, DC: Author.

Beebe, B., & Lachmann, F. (2002). *Infant research and adult treatment: Co-constructing interactions*. Hillsdale, NJ: The Analytic Press.

Biringen, Z., Robinson, J. L., & Emde, R. N. (2000a). Appendix A: The Emotional Availability Scales (2nd ed.; an abridged Infancy/Early Childhood Version). *Attachment and Human Development, 2*(2), 251–255.

Biringen, Z., Robinson, J. L., & Emde, R. N. (2000b). Appendix B: The Emotional Availability Scales (3rd ed.; an abridged Infancy/Early Childhood Version). *Attachment and Human Development, 2*(2), 256–270.

Bowlby, J. (1988). *A secure base: Parent–child attachment and healthy human development*. New York: Basic Books.

Cassidy, J., & Marvin, R. S. (1992). *A system for classifying individual differences in the attachment-behaviour of 2 1/2 to 4 1/2 year old children*. Unpublished coding manual, University of Virginia, Charlottesville.

REFERENCES

Cohen, N. J., Muir, E., Parker, C., Lojkasek, M., Muir, R., Barwick, M., et al. (1999). Watch, wait, and wonder: Testing the effectiveness of a new approach to mother–infant psychotherapy. *Infant Mental Health Journal*, 20(4), 429–451.

Fonagy, P., Steele, M., Steele, H., Leigh, T., Kennedy, R., Mattoon, G., et al. (1995). Attachment, the reflective self, and borderline states: The predictive specificity of the Adult Attachment Interview and pathological emotional development. In S. Goldberg, R. Muir & J. Kerr (Eds.), *Attachment theory* (pp. 233–278). Hillsdale, NJ: The Analytic Press.

George, C., Kaplan, N., & Main, M. (1996). *The Adult Attachment Interview* (3rd ed.). Unpublished manuscript, Department of Psychology, University of California, Berkeley.

Hoffman-Judd, P., & McGlashan, T. H. (2003). *A developmental model of borderline personality disorder: Understanding variations in course and outcome.* Arlington, VA: American Psychiatric Publishing, Inc.

Kaufman, J., & Zigler, E. (1987). Do abused children become abusive parents? *American Journal of Orthopsychiatry*, 57(2), 186–192.

Ludolph, P. S., Westen, D., Misle, B., Jackson, A., Wixom, J., & Wiss, F. C. (1990). The borderline diagnosis in adolescents: Symptoms and developmental history. *American Journal of Psychiatry*, 147(8), 470–476.

Main, M., & Goldwyn, R. (1991). *Adult attachment scoring and classification systems.* Unpublished manuscript, University College, London.

McDonough, S. (1993). Interaction guidance: Understanding and treating early infant–caregiver relationship disturbances. In C. Zeanah (Ed.), *Handbook of infant mental health* (pp. 414–426). New York: Guilford Press.

McDonough, S. (2004). Interaction guidance: Promoting and guiding the caregiving relationship. In A. Sameroff, S. McDonough & K. Rosenblum (Eds.), *Treating parent–infant relationship problems: Strategies for intervention* (pp. 79–96). New York: Guilford Press.

Muir, E., Lojkasek, M., & Cohen, N. (1999). *Watch, wait, and wonder: A manual describing a dyadic infant-led approach to problems in infancy and early childhood.* Toronto: Hincks-Dellcrest Institute.

Newman, L., & Stevenson, C. (in press). Parenting and borderline personality disorder: Ghosts in the nursery. *Clinical Child Psychology and Psychiatry*.

Ogata, S. N., Silk, K. R., Goodrich, S., Lohr, N. E., Westen, D., & Hill, E. M. (1990). Childhood sexual and physical abuse in adult patients with borderline personality disorder. *American Journal of Psychiatry*, 147(8), 1008–1013.

Perry, B. D., & Pollard, R. (1998). Homeostasis, stress, trauma, and adaptation: A neurodevelopmental view of childhood trauma. *Child and Adolescent Psychiatric Clinics of North America*, 7(1), 33–51.

Schore, A. N. (2001). The effects of early relational trauma on right brain development, affect regulation, and infant mental health. *Infant Mental Health Journal*, 22(1), 201–269.

Solomon, J., & George, C. (1999). The place of disorganization in attachment theory: Linking classic observations with contemporary findings. In J. Solomon & C. George (Eds.), *Attachment disorganization* (pp. 3–32). New York: Guilford Press.

Terr, L. C. (1991). Childhood traumas: An outline and overview. *American Journal of Psychiatry*, 148(1), 10–20.

Trull, T., Stepp, S., & Durrett, C. (2003). Research on borderline personality disorder: An update. *Current Opinion in Psychiatry*, 16(10), 77–82.

Winnicott, D. (1960). The theory of the parent–child relationship. *International Journal of Psychoanalysis*, 41, 585–595.

Zanarini, M. C., Gunderson, J. G., Marino, M. F., Schwartz, E. O., & Frankenburg, F. R. (1989). Childhood experiences of borderline patients. *Comprehensive Psychiatry*, 30(1), 18–25.

REFERENCES

Zeanah, C. H., Benoit, D., Hirshberg, L., & Barton, M. L. (1993). *Working model of the child interview: Rating scales and classifications.* Unpublished manuscript, Louisiana State University School of Medicine, New Orleans.

Chapter 15 Parenting and substance abuse

Black, M. M., Nair, P., Kight, C., Wachtel, R., Roby, P., & Schuler M. (1994). Parenting and early development among children of drug-abusing women: Effects of home intervention. *Pediatrics, 94*(4), 440–448.

Jones, K. L., & Smith, D. W. (1973). Recognition of the Fetal Alcohol Syndrome in early infancy. *Lancet, 2,* 999–1001.

Orford, J., & Velleman, R. (1991). The environmental intergenerational transmission of alcohol problems: A comparison of two hypotheses. *British Journal of Medical Psychology, 64*(Pt. 2), 189–200.

NSW Child Death Review Team. (2000). *1999–2000 Report.* Sydney: NSW Commission for Children and Young People.

Velleman, R. (2004). Alcohol and drug problems in parents: An overview of the impact on children and implications for practice. In M. Gopfert, J. Webster and M. Seeman (Eds.). *Parental psychiatric disorder. Distressed parents and their families* (2nd ed.). Cambridge University Press.

Chapter 16 Adolescent parents

American Academy of Paediatrics: Committee on Adolescence and Committee on Early Childhood and Adoption, and Dependent Care. (2001). Policy Statement: Care of adolescent parents and their children. *Pediatrics, 107*(2), 429–434.

DiCenso, A., Guyatt, G., Willan, A., & Griffith, L. (2002). Interventions to reduce unintended pregnancies among adolescents: A systematic review of randomised controlled trials. *British Medical Journal, 324*(7351), 1426–1434.

Luster, T., & Brophy-Herb, H. (2000). Adolescent mothers and their children. In J. D. Osofsky & H. E. Fitzgerald (Eds.), *World Association for Infant Mental Health (WAIMH) Handbook of infant mental health, Vol. 4: Infant mental health in groups at high risk* (pp. 369–413). New York: Wiley.

McElroy, S., & Moore, K. (1997). Trends over time in teenage pregnancy and childbearing: The critical changes. In R. Maynard (Ed.), *Kids having kids: Economic costs and social consequences of teen pregnancy* (pp. 23–53). Washington, DC: Urban Institute Press.

Osofsky, J. D. (1997). Psychosocial risks for adolescent parents and infants: Clinical implications. In J. D. Noshpitz, S. Greenspan, S. Wieder & J. D. Osofsky (Eds.), *Handbook of child and adolescent psychiatry: Vol. 1: Infants and preschoolers: Development and syndromes* (pp. 191–202). New York: Wiley.

Osofsky, J. D., Eberhart-Wright, A., Ware, L. M., & Hann, D. M. (1992). Children of adolescent mothers: A group at risk for psychopathology. *Infant Mental Health Journal, 13*(2), 119–131.

Powell, B., & Steelman, L. C. (1993). The educational benefits of being spaced out: Sibship density and educational progress. *American Sociological Review, 58*(3), 367–381.

Save the Children. (2004). *State of the World's Mothers 2004. Children having children: Where young mothers are most at risk.* Retrieved 14 December 2004 from http://www.savethechildren.org.

SmithBattle, L. (2000). The vulnerabilities of teenage mothers: Challenging prevailing assumptions. *Advances in Nursing Science, 23*(1), 29–40.

van der Klis, K. A., Westenberg, L., Chan, A., Dekker, G., & Keane, R. (2002). Teenage pregnancy: Trends, characteristics and outcomes in South Australia and Australia. *Australian and New Zealand Journal of Public Health, 26*(2), 125–131.

Zeanah, C. H., Boris, N. W., & Larrieu, J. A. (1997). Infant development and developmental risk: A review of the past 10 years. *Journal of the American Academy of Child and Adolescent Psychiatry*, *36*(2), 165–178.

Chapter 17 Families and multiple adversity

Bemporad, S. (1995). Babies can't wait: Infants and toddlers in the child protection system. *The Signal*, *3*(3), 1–4.

Berrick, J., Needell, B., Barth, R., & Jonson-Reid, M. (1998). *The tender years: Toward developmentally-sensitive child welfare services for very young children*. Oxford: Oxford University Press.

Bowlby, J. (1969). *Attachment and loss: Vol. 1. Attachment*. New York: Basic Books.

Bruschweiler-Stern, N., & Stern, D. (1989). A model for conceptualizing the role of the mother's representational world in various mother–infant therapies. *Infant Mental Health Journal*, *10*(3), 142–156.

Coll, C. G., & Magnuson, K. (2000). Cultural differences as sources of developmental vulnerabilities and resources. In J. P. Shonkoff & S. J. Meisels (Eds.), *Handbook of early childhood intervention* (2nd ed., pp. 94–114). Cambridge: Cambridge University Press.

Cousins, C. (2004). When is it serious enough? The protection of children of parents with a mental health problem, tough decisions and avoiding a 'martyred' child. *Australian e-Journal for the Advancement of Mental Health*, *3*(2), 1–8.

Donald, T., & Jureidini, J. (2004) Parenting capacity. *Child Abuse Review*, *13*(1), 5–17.

Dozier, M., Dozier, D., & Manni, M. (2002). Attachment and biobehavioral catch-up: The ABC's of helping infants in foster care cope with early adversity. *Zero to Three*, *22*(5), 7–13.

Dozier, M., Stovall, K. C., Albus, K. E., & Bates, B. (2001). Attachment for infants in foster care: The role of caregiver state of mind. *Child Development*, *72*(5), 1467–1477.

Ferguson, D. W., & Horwood, L. J. (2003). Resilience to childhood adversity: Results of a 21-year study. In S. S. Luthar (Ed.), *Resilience and vulnerability: Adaptation in the context of childhood adversities* (pp. 130–155). Cambridge: Cambridge University Press.

Fonagy, P. (1998). Prevention, the appropriate target of infant psychotherapy. *Infant Mental Health Journal*, *19*(2), 124–150.

Gunnar, M. R. (2000). Early adversity and the development of stress reactivity and regulation. In C. A. Nelson (Ed.), *The effects of early adversity on neurobehavioral development. The Minnesota Symposia on Child Psychology* (Vol. 31, pp. 163–200). Mahwah, NJ: Lawrence Erlbaum.

Iwaniec, D. (1995). *The emotionally abused and neglected child: Identification, assessment and intervention*. Chichester: Wiley.

Kempe, R. S., & Kempe, C. H. (1978). *Child abuse*. Cambridge, MA: Harvard University Press.

Larrieu, J. A., & Zeanah, C. H. (2004). Treating parent–infant relationships in the context of maltreatment: An integrated systems approach. In A. Sameroff, S. McDonough & K. Rosenblum (Eds.), *Treating parent–infant relationship problems: Strategies for intervention* (pp. 243–265). New York: Guilford Press.

Lieberman, A. F. (1998). The trials and rewards of being a clinical consultant to child protective services. *Zero to Three*, *19*(3), 14–18.

Marvin, R., Cooper, G., Hoffman, K., & Powell, B. (2002). The Circle of Security project: Attachment-based intervention with caregiver-pre-school child dyads. *Attachment and Human Development*, *4*(1), 107–124.

McCain, M. N., & Mustard, J. F. (1999). *Early years study: Revising the real brain drain*. Toronto, ON: Publications Ontario.

McDonough, S. (2004). Interaction guidance: Promoting and guiding the caregiving relationship. In A. Sameroff, S. McDonough & K. Rosenblum (Eds.), *Treating parent–infant relationship problems: Strategies for intervention* (pp. 79–96). New York: Guilford Press.

REFERENCES

Osofsky, J. D., & Connors, K. (1979). Mother–infant interaction: An integrative review of a complex system. In J. D. Osofsky (Ed.), *Handbook of infant development* (pp. 519–548). New York: Wiley.

Perry, B. (1997). Incubated in terror: Neurodevelopmental factors in the 'Cycle of Violence'. In J. Osofsky (Ed.), *Children in a violent society* (pp. 124–189). New York: Guilford Press.

Perry, B. (2001). The neurodevelopmental impact of violence in childhood. In D. Schetky & E. P. Benedek (Eds.), *Textbook of child and adolescent forensic psychiatry* (pp. 221–238). Washington, DC: American Psychiatric Press.

Schore, A. N. (2002). Dysregulation of the right brain: A fundamental mechanism of traumatic attachment and the psychopathogenesis of posttraumatic stress disorder. *Australian and New Zealand Journal of Psychiatry, 36*(1), 9–30.

Shonkoff, J., & Phillips, D. (Eds.). (2000). *From neurons to neighbourhoods: The science of early child development*. Washington, DC: National Academy Press.

Schuder, M., & Lyons-Ruth, K. (2004). 'Hidden trauma' in infancy: Attachment, fearful arousal, and early dysfunction of the stress response system. In J. Osofsky (Ed.), *Young children and trauma: Intervention and treatment* (pp. 69–106). New York: Guilford Press.

Siegel, D. J. (1999). *The developing mind: Toward a neurobiology of interpersonal experience*. New York: Guilford Press.

Werner, E. (2000). Protective factors and individual resilience. In J. P. Shonkoff & S. J. Meisels (Eds.), *Handbook of early childhood intervention* (2nd ed., pp. 115–134). Cambridge: Cambridge University Press.

Wulczyn, F., & Hislop, K. (2002). Babies in foster care: The numbers call for attention. *Zero to Three, 22*(5), 14–15.

Zeanah, C. H., Boris, N. W., & Larrieu, J. A. (1997). Infant development and developmental risk: A review of the past 10 years. *Journal of the American Academy of Child and Adolescent Psychiatry, 36*(2), 165–178.

Zeanah, C. H., & Zeanah, P. D. (2001). Towards a definition of infant mental health. *Zero to Three, 22*(1), 13–20.

Glossary

Ainsworth, M. (1967). *Infancy in Uganda: Infant care and the growth of love*. Baltimore: John Hopkins University Press.

Kagan, J. (1997). Temperament. In J. D. Noshpitz, S. Greenspan, S. Wieder & J. Osofsky (Eds.), *Handbook of child and adolescent psychiatry: Vol. 1. Infancy and preschoolers: Development and syndromes* (pp. 268–275). New York: Wiley.

Sameroff, A. J., & Fiese, B. H. (2000). Models of development and developmental risk. In C. H. Zeanah (Ed.), *Handbook of infant mental health* (2nd ed., pp. 3–19). New York: Guilford Press.

Siegel, D. J. (1999). *The developing mind: Towards a neurobiology of interpersonal experience*. New York: Guilford Press.

Sroufe, L. A. (1996). *Emotional development: The organization of emotional life in the early years*. Cambridge: Cambridge University Press.

Stern, D. (1985). *The interpersonal world of the infant: A view from psychoanalysis and developmental psychology*. New York: Basic Books.

Thomas, A., & Chess, S. (1977). *Temperament and development*. New York: Brunner/Mazel.

Index

abandonment, 37, 95, 173, 240
abnormality, 79, 95, 104, 253, 254
Aborigines, 262
abortions *see* termination
abuse
    assessment and intervention, 22, 43, 47, 228–9, 245, 277–8
    attachment, 32, 36
    clinical presentations, 147, 220–7
    environmental factors, 218
    foster-care, 180, 283
    risk and protective factors, 58, 60, 63–6, 173–4
    and substance abuse, 256
    see also maltreatment; neglect
abuse, parent's, 62, 80–1, 170, 217–30
    assessment, 220, 227–8
    consequences, 218–20
    intervention, 228–30
    memory, recollection, reflection, 224–6, 230, 257
    parenting difficulties, 226–7
    personality disorders, 239, 242
    risk and protective factors, 221–3, 227
adjustment disorders, sleep, 119
adolescent parents, 62, 64, 90, 261–71
    assessment, 267–70
    attachment, 266
    intervention, 267–71, 282
    risk and protective factors, 267–70
adolescent pregnancy, 261, 262–6
adolescents, 236
adoption, 70, 79, 283
adoptive parents, 60, 71
adrenal glands, 186, 236
Adult Attachment Interview, 29–30, 141, 220, 245
affect, negative, 179
affect recognition and regulation, 7, 174, 238—9
agency liaison, 280
aggression, 164, 179, 244, 256
agoraphobia, 205
Ainsworth, M., 27
Ainsworth Strange Situation Procedure *see* Strange Situation Procedure
alcohol, 251, 252, 253, 254

alternative care, 282–3, 285
ambivalence, maternal, 212
amphetamines, 254
anal stage, development, 6
androgen, 186
anorexia, 142
anorexia, infantile, 139, 142
ante-natal care, 215, 254
    adolescent pregnancy, 262, 264
    failure to attend, 207
    high-risk families, 280–1
    substance abuse, 251
ante-natal period, 70–83
    mental health, 77–83
    screening, 78, 204
anti-depressant medications, 213–16
anti-psychotic medications, 210
anxiety, 33, 53, 76–7, 79–80, 101, 141, 173, 181, 202, 205–9, 252
arousal, infant, 8
artificial reproduction technology, 71
attachment
    anxiety, 31, 32
    behaviours, 15, 168, 287
    brain development, 175
    development, 78, 175
    high-risk environment, 97, 177, 276
    history, 37, 170–2
    parents and carers, 245, 266, 284–5
    patterns, 27–8, 29, 31–5
        disorganised/disoriented, 27–9, 31–2, 100, 173, 243
        insecure, 27–9, 32, 100, 175
        organised, 31
        secure, 5, 15, 27–9, 100, 175, 283
    personality disorders, 236, 238, 240, 242
    risk factors, 90–1, 97, 177, 266, 284–5
attachment disorders, 32–8, 179
    abuse, 218, 219, 224
    alternative criteria, 34–5
        disrupted, 35
        non-attachment, 34
        secure base, 34
    assessment, formulation, 32, 37
    defining, 31–5
    feeding, 139, 141
    intervention principles, 37–8

INDEX

multiple diversity, 276
reactive attachment disorders, 33
risk factors, 58–9, 62, 178, 256, 283
attachment, interview *see* Adult Attachment Interview
attachment relationships, 4, 12, 15, 19, 35, 87, 98, 116–17, 122, 173, 287
attachment theory, 3, 6–7, 9, 26–30, 35–9, 175
attention, 174, 244
autistic spectrum disorders, 97
autonomic nervous system, 88
Axis II, Relationship Classification, 163

baby blues, 204–9
barbiturates, 253, 255
barium swallow, 140, 148
Bayley Scales of Infant Development, 124, 131, 181
behaviour
assessing, 124
difficulties, 60, 62, 163–4, 179, 180
questionnaire, 100
risk factors, 18, 99–100
sleep, 120–1, 126–8
behavioural inhibition, 18
Behavioural Rating Scale, 124
benzodiazepines, 253, 254, 255
bereavement, 81, 207
bilingual children, 167
biological development, and GID, 191
biological risk factors, 97, 99
biological stress, 177
biomedical problems in infancy, 87–110
biopsychosocial framework, 42, 43, 50-51
biopsychosocial model, 20, 287
bipolar disorder, 82, 210
Biringen's Emotional Availability Scales, 245
birth, 73, 102, 254–5
birth abnormality *see* abnormality
birth family contact, 283
birth order, 51
birthweight, 90
blues *see* baby blues
body rhythms, 113
bonding, 98
Borderline Personality Disorder, 207, 231, 238–40, 241–4
Bowlby, J., 6–7, 16, 26–7, 30–1, 38
boys and maternal depression, 208
BPD *see* Borderline Personality Disorder
brain damage, 60
brain development, 7, 9, 11–12, 21, 23, 25–6, 97, 112, 138
attachment, 175

experience-dependent, 8, 174–5
trauma, 182, 283–4
brain research, 5, 8–9
brain structure and function, 8, 177–8
breastfeeding, 112, 136, 140, 146, 207
prescribing, 214–16
psychotropic medications, 214–16
breastmilk, expressing, 151
breathing, 134
Bruschweiler-Stern and Stern, 281, 282

caesarean delivery, 73, 82–3, 121, 148
cannabis, 254
caregiver
assessment, 38, 124
attachment relationship, 15
capacity, 8, 38
loss of, 35
personality disorders, 241–4
premature infant, 100–2
role, 12, 13, 15, 41
caregiver, alternate, 35, 36
see also adoptive parents; foster parents
case conferences, 280, 281
cerebral disorders in premature infants, 94, 101
cerebral palsy, 91, 98, 133, 140, 141
cerebrovascular infarction, 254
change, capacity for, 60, 63–6
child abuse *see* abuse; malnutrition; neglect
child deaths, 251, 261
child mental health, 245
child protection, 59, 79, 258
child-protection notifications, 262, 266
child-welfare agencies, 285
circadian rhythm *see* diurnal clock
clinging, 34
clinician, 48–9, 230, 278–80
co-sleeping, 117–18
cocaine, 254
codeine, 254
coding systems, 245
cognition, 23, 238
development, 10, 134, 138
cognitive therapy, 214
communication, 144, 245
infant–parent, 8, 52–4
parent sensitivity, 62
toddlers, 165
communication, non-verbal *see* non-verbal communication
community agencies, 214
community psychiatric services, 214
community support, 63, 103
community-based practitioners, 84
conception, 70, 79

INDEX

confidentiality, 48
congenital abnormality *see* abnormality
consent, 82, 85
conservation-withdrawal reaction, 138
continuity debate, 19, 287
coping capacities, infant, 56
cortisol, 176, 177, 236
counselling, 206, 257
counselling, non-directive, 214
critical period, 287
cultural contact, 283
cultural factors, 50, 188, 189
cultural isolation *see* isolation
cystic fibrosis, 95

defence mechanisms, 176, 235
definitions, 185
deformity *see* abnormality
delinquency, 95
delusions, 212
depressant drugs, 253, 255
depression, 77, 141, 142, 177, 181, 201, 204–5, 211
    abuse, 220, 222
    parental, 43, 45, 53, 121, 123
    substance abuse, 252, 255
depression, ante-natal, 84–5, 98
depression, post-natal, 63, 81-82, 84, 101–2, 202–9, 288–9
    group programs, 213
developmental context, 42
developmental delay or disturbance, 20, 87, 89, 97–8
    assessment, 104–6, 123–4, 131
    intervention, 106–10
    risk and protective factors, 7, 60, 99–104, 253
developmental outcomes, adverse, 4
developmental psychology, 7, 9
developmental psychopathology, 7
diabetes, 79
Diagnostic and Statistical Manual *see* DSM
diet *see* nutrition
disability, 58, 60, 79–80, 97
discontinuity, 19, 221
dissociation, 64, 176
dissociative continuum, 284
diurnal clock, 113–14
domestic violence, 59, 173, 256, 262
    see also violence
Down's Syndrome, 97
drug and alcohol exposure in utero, 60, 90, 215, 251–5
    see also substance abuse
DSM classification system, 31, 202
DSM-III, 31, 33, 139

DSM-IV, 33, 139, 190, 206, 237–40
dummy, 151
dynamic psychotherapy, 214
dysphagia, 134, 150
dysthymia, 205

early childhood clinic, 43
early childhood development, 4
    disturbances, 19, 20–1
    intervention models, -23
    psychosocial model, 20
    see also infant development
Early Childhood Nurse, 170
early discharge program, 210
early intervention programs, 280, 281
early parenting program, 258
eating disorders, 141, 142
ecstasy, 254
Edinburgh Postnatal Depression Scale, 204, 209
education programs, child development, 281, 282
educational opportunities, 51
ELBW *see* extremely low birthweight
electro-convulsive therapy, 206
emotional information, 44
Emotional Availability Scales, 245
emotional changes at pregnancy, 73–5, 76–83
emotional development, 10, 11–19
    abuse, 218–19
    attachment, 175
    risk factors, 59, 62, 235–6
emotional distress
    hospitalisation, 95–6
    premature infants, 100
emotional processing and control, 157–60
emotional withdrawal, 34, 81–2, 101, 179
empathy, 14, 15, 157, 161, 178, 225
    infant–parent, 53, 61, 64, 235, 242, 243, 274
employment, 51
endocarditis, 254
endocrinology, 235
environmental factors
    aggressive behaviour, 164
    assessment, 124
    personality, 232
    risk, 21, 62, 97
    sleep, 117–18
EPDS *see* Edinburgh Postnatal Depression Scale
ES *see* Edinburgh Postnatal Depression Scale
ethnicity, 275
extremely low birthweight, 89, 94, 99

313

INDEX

eye contact, 98

facilitating environment, 287
failure to thrive, 138–40, 142, 147, 179
failure to thrive, non-organic, 138–9
family
    environment, 146
    history of illness, 50, 79
    multiple-adversity, 272–86
family-clinician relationship, 48, 49, 279–80
family functioning
    assessment, 43
    conflicts, 59, 80
    interactions, 48
    interventions, 22, 278–85
    premature infant, 92–4, 98–100
    substance abuse, 252, 256
    support with parenting, 81
family networks, 41, 50, 62
fathers, 71, 74, 81, 127
feeding, 14, 133–52
    developing skills, 134–7
    infant–parent relationship, 136–7
    influences on, 134–7
    motor functions, 134–5
feeding difficulties, 91, 137–40, 179
    assessment, 140, 144–7
    failure to thrive, 138–40
    infant characteristics, 143
    infant–parent fit, 143–52
    intervention principles, 147–8, 149–52
    physical disorders, 137–8
    premature infants, 91
    risk and protective factors, 140–4
feeding, non-oral, 150–2
fertilisation, 186
fight or flight reaction, 236
'fit', parent and infant, 52, 78
foetal abnormality fears, 72
Foetal Alcohol Syndrome, 253
foetal complications, 215
foetal development, 70, 72, 77–9, 135, 251
food refusal, 142
formulation, 287
foster-care, 134, 180, 223, 283–5
foster-carers, 33, 60, 284–285
freeze or play dead response, 236
Freud, S., 5–6, 10, 184
FTT *see* failure to thrive

gag reflex, 135, 140, 151
gastro-oesophageal reflux, 137, 138
gastroschisis, 149
gastrostomy, 152
gender, 51
    definition, 185

gender-aberrant behaviour, 194, 195
gender constancy, 187
gender dysphoria, 183, 190–3
    multicultural context, 193–7
gender identity
    assessment, cross-cultural, 193–7
    caregiver's beliefs, 187–8
    definition, 185
    problems, 189–93
    society and culture, 187–8
Gender Identity Disorder, 190, 192–3
    biological determinist models, 190–2
    developmental approach, 197
    ethnomethodological approach, 196–8
    infant–parent relationships, 192
    intervention, 196–8
    sociocultural models, 191
gender labelling, 187
gender role, definition, 185
gender stability, 187
gender variability, 187
general practitioners, 46, 214
genetic abnormalities, 94, 95, 97, 104
    in-utero identification, 104
genetic endowment, 60
genetic factors, 50, 51, 79, 88, 232, 233
genetic sex, 186
genitalia, ambiguous, 186
gestational age, 90
GID *see* Gender Identity Disorder
glossary, 287–90
good baby, 284
good-enough mother, 111, 176
goodness of fit, 51, 60, 287
GOR *see* gastro-oesophageal reflux
grandparents, 65
grief, 98, 285
grief, unresolved, 45, 81, 85
Griffiths Mental Development Scales, 124, 181
group homes, 283
group therapy, 23, 214, 282
growth retardation, 149, 253
guilt, 129, 252

hallucinations, 212
hallucinogenic drugs, 254, 255
hand dexterity, 131
hand-to-mouth activity, 134–7
hand-to-mouth play, 150, 151
handling techniques for premature infants, 109
health visitors, 214
hepatitis, 254, 258
hereditary disorders, 79, 50–1, 88, 232–3
hermaphroditism, 186, 188

INDEX

heroin, 251, 254, 255
high-risk environments, 273–6
    assessment, formulation, 277-280
    infant mental health, 276–7
    intervention, 280–5
high-risk family *see* multiple adversity family
history, clinical, 44
history taking, 49–52
    background, 50
    current problem, 50
HIV/AIDS, 254
holding and wrapping, 17, 105, 113–14, 120, 125
home-visiting, 23, 280, 281
homophobia, 4
hormones, 175, 177, 205, 235–6
hospitalisation, 91–3, 95, 98, 103, 119
    psychological effects, 95–7
    toddlers, 168–9
hospitalism, 138
hostility, mother–child, 212–13
hostility, parent to child, 59
housing, 51, 64
HPA, 177, 235
human development, stage theories, 10–11
hyperactivity, 100
hyperalertness, 109
hypersensitivity, 134
hypertensive disease, 254
hyperthyroidism, 63
hypothalamic pituitary adrenal, 177, 235

ICD-10, 33
identity development, 6, 239, 240
imagined baby, 73, 74–5
immigrants *see* migrants
implicit or procedural memory, 288
impulse control, 164, 174, 238, 239
in-utero exposure to drugs and other toxins, 50, 60, 215, 251, 254, 255
indiscriminate sociability, 33, 34
infant
    addiction, 250
    feeding, 137
    needs, 56
    perinatal mental illness, 208
    research, 7–8, 9
    responsiveness, 52
    withdrawal symptoms, 250, 251
    see also newborns
infant competencies, 8, 288
    affective interactions, 8
    communicate emotions, 8
    proto-conversation, 8
    self-regulation, 8
    social interaction, 8
infant development, 4, 12–14, 23
    3 months, 12
    6–12 months, 12
    9–12 months, 12–13
    first year, 12–13, 156
    second year, 13–14, 156
    stages, 10–19
    third year, 14, 156–7
    fourth year, 14, 157
    see also toddler
infant development assessment, 20, 47, 54–7, 104–5
    risk factors, 58–66
    socioeconomic factors, 62
    substance abuse, 250–5
infant development and sex, 184–9
infant mental health, 4–9
    adolescent pregnancy, 266
    assessment, 41–57, 245–6
        context and principles, 41–2
        formulation, 45–6
        information sources, 44
        process, 42–6
    clinical assessment, 47–57
        history taking, 49–52
        interview, 47-51
    drug abuse, 255–6
    high-risk environments, 276–7
    intervention, 21–3
        family, 22–3, 281–2
        group therapies, 23
        infant focused, 21–2
        infant–parent, 22–3
        population-based, 23
    parental disorder, 243–4
    risk assessment, 41, 45–6
infant–carer interaction, 8, 19, 55
infant–parent interaction
    assessment, 47, 52–4, 59, 61–2, 245
    feeding difficulties, 143–7
    pregnancy, 77, 78
    psychotherapy, 246
    sleep, 115–18, 121–2
infant–parent relationship, 8, 62–6, 144, 282
    at birth, 73
    drug abuse, 255
    feeding, 136-137
    Gender Identity Disorder, 192
    'good enough', 111
    high-risk environment, 274–6
    hospitalisation, 96–7
    intervention, 22–3, 35–6
    personality disorders, 242
infant–parent therapies, 35
infantile anorexia, 139, 142

INDEX

infants, premature *see* premature infants
infertility, 71, 79, 186
informed consent, 82, 85
insecurity, 33
institutional care, 283
institutionalised children, 33, 34
intellectual impairment, 95
intelligence quotient see IQ
Interaction Guidance, 282
internal representation, 15
internal representations or internal working model, 288
internal state language, 288
interpersonal functioning, 50, 75–6, 203, 238, 240
intersex disorders, 183, 186–7
intersexuality, 182–3, 186–7
intersubjectivity, 13
intervention
    ante-natal psychological risk, 84–6
    assessment, 54–7
    attachment disorders, 37–8
    infant development, 21–3
    therapeutic, 54–7
    types, 84
    multiple adversity family, 278–80
interview, clinical assessment, 47–52
intra-psychic factors, 50
intra-uterine growth retardation, 253, 254
intravenous drug use, 254
IQ, 99
isolation, 63, 78, 81–2, 98, 162, 219, 256, 264, 271, 275

kangaroo care, 92
Klinefelter's Syndrome, 186

labour, 72–3, 78–80, 82–3, 91
    premature, 254
lactation, 205, 214–15
lactation service, 46
language, 157, 158
    infant–parent, 52–4
    parental, 52, 82
    toddlers, 160, 165
language development, 13, 14, 244
limbic system, 175, 177–8, 235
listening, 48, 79
loss, 32, 35, 38, 79–80, 81, 285
low-birthweight infants, 94, 99, 254
    see also extremely low-birthweight infants; very low-birthweight infants
LSD, 254

maladaptive behaviours, 22, 236, 240

maladaptive coping strategies, 176
maladjustment, 27
malnutrition, 138, 139–40
maltreatment, 32, 60, 174, 245, 256, 274, 288
    parent's abuse as child, 218–30
    see also abuse; neglect
mandatory reporting, 58
mania, 206, 210
marital relationship, 207
marital satisfaction and parenthood, 76, 123
marriage, 59, 128
Marvin-Cassidy procedure, 245
maternal age, 207
maternal changes at pregnancy, 71–3
maternal deprivation, 27, 138
maternal health threats, 78–9
maternal morbidity, 261
maternal psychological adjustment at pregnancy, 73–5, 77–85, 101–2
maternal rejection, 101
maternal relationship with unborn child, 70, 74–5
maternal stress, 70
maturation, 18
medico-legal reports, 47
memory, 14, 174, 288
men, 71, 74, 203, 231
    depression, 81, 208–9
Mental Development Index, 124
mental health
    intervention, 84–6
    population, 9
    pregnancy, 77–82
        risk factors, 78–83
    traumatic experiences, 178
mental health, infant see infant mental health
mental illness, 59, 65
    see also psychiatric illness
Mental and Motor Bayley Development Scales, 110
methadone, 254, 258
midwives, 214
migrants, 82, 207
miscarriage, 78, 79–80
mobility, 12–13, 157, 158
mood disorders, 63, 121, 179, 202, 205, 206, 238, 265
mood, post-natal disorder, 208, 211
mother–baby units, 212, 214
mother–child relationship, 100, 121–2, 128–9, 146, 161–2
    see also infant–child relationship
motor skills, 8, 88, 130, 134, 143, 146

INDEX

mourning, 35, 38, 81, 283
multicultural context, gender dysphoria, 193–7
multidisciplinary approach, 3
multiple adversity family, 46, 272–86
    assessment, 277–8
    intervention, 278–80
multiple births, 97, 207
multiproblem family *see* multiple adversity family
muscle tone, 109

NBAS *see* Neonatal Behavioural Assessment Scale
NBRS, 90
neglect, 140, 162
    attachment, 33, 34, 37–8, 173, 175, 177
    consequences, 218–20
    infant mental health, 43, 47
    risk factors, 58–60, 63–6, 258, 277–8, 283, 285
neglect, emotional, 21, 62
neglect, parent's, 217–30
Neonatal Abstinence Syndrome, 254
Neonatal Behavioural Assessment Scale, 55–7, 104–5, 109, 145
    Organizational Process-State Control, 146–7
Neonatal Intensive Care Unit, 90, 92, 93, 100, 101, 106
neonatal irritability, 254
neonatal toxicity, 215
neonatal treatment, 90
neurobehavioural responses, 148–50
neurobiology, 5, 8–9
    developmental, 3
neurodevelopment problems, 90, 100–1
neurological development, 18, 21
neurological functioning
    assessment, 56
    feeding, 136, 140–1
    personality, 233–4
    premature birth, 90–1, 101
neuronal pathways, 174, 235
neurophysiological development, 77
neuropsychiatric disorders, 94, 99
neuropsychological development, 11–12
neurosis, 121
neurotransmitter system, 177
Newborn Individualised Development Care and Assessment Program, 92
newborns
    communication strategies, 11
    neurobehavioural development, 88–9
    sleeping patterns, 112–14, 125

NICU *see* Neonatal Intensive Care Unit
NIDCAP, 92
night feeds, 131
NOFT *see* failure to thrive, non-organic
non-oral feeding *see* feeding, non-oral
non-psychotic depression *see* depression, post-natal
non rapid eye movement sleep, 114, 119, 125
non-verbal communication, 53
NREM sleep *see* non rapid eye movement sleep
NSW Child Death Review Team, 251
Nursery Neurobiological Risk Score, 90
nutrition, 140, 215, 256, 262
    prematurity, 90
    in utero, 60

OA *see* oesophageal atresia
object relations theory, 6, 9
Observational Scale for Mother–Infant Interaction During Feeding, 144
observations, clinician's, 44, 49
Obsessive Compulsive Disorder, 205
obstetric complications, 207, 215, 254
obstetric history, 78, 79–80, 104
obstetric loss, 72, 78, 79–80
obstetric management, 72, 85
obstetricians, 214
occupational therapist, 121
oesophageal atresia, 137, 150
opiates, 251, 254, 255
oral hypersensitivity, 150, 151
oral reflexes, 134
oral stage, development, 6
oropharyngeal trauma, 140, 142
orthopaedic abnormalities, 95
over-friendliness in children, 33
overburdened family *see* multiple adversity family

paediatric physiotherapy, 47, 109
panic disorder, 205
parent, 41, 42, 51, 61–2
    abused as child, 62, 80–1, 217–30
    adjustment difficulties, 203–5
    age, 62, 64
    attachment history, 170, 245
    education, 282
    expectations, 55, 60, 61, 226
    family background, 52
    psychological factors, 51, 62
    unresolved issues, 224–5, 242
    see also caregiver
parent psychopathology, 139–44

317

INDEX

parent–infant interaction *see* infant–parent interaction
parenthood
   adjustment and change, 71
   transition to, 70–83
parenting, 170, 175
   assessment, 104, 278
   behaviour, 30
   capacity, 60–2, 64–5, 224, 244–6, 275, 277–8, 288
   difficulties, 226–7
   emotional tasks, 38
   quality, 51
   roles and responsibilities, 81
   substance abuse, 250, 256
   toddlers, 161–3
parenting alliance, 75–6
perinatal illness, 89, 94–7
   drug abuse, 251, 253–6
   psychological effects, 95–6
   see also newborns
perinatal infant mortality, 261, 262
perinatal mental illness, 201–16
   adjustment difficulties, 203–4
   assessment, 204, 209–12, 213
   breastfeeding, 215–16
   effect on infant and family, 208–9
   intervention, 213–15
   occurrence, 202–3
   risk and protective factors, 207, 212–13
   screening tools, 209–12
perpetuating factors, 45
personality, 178, 207
personality development, 32, 82, 219, 232–6
personality disorder, 231–48
   assessment, presentation, 241–2, 244–6
   infant mental health, 243–4
   intervention, 246–8
   risk factors, 32, 59, 82, 176, 178, 203, 219, 233, 244
   substance abuse, 252
   types, 237–41
phallic/genital stage, 6
pharmacists, 214
physiological regulation of infant, 12
physiotherapy, 47, 109
play, 8, 13, 130, 245
population-based programs
   adolescent parenting, 270–1
   targeted interventions, 23
post-natal depression *see* depression, post-natal
post-partum psychosis *see* psychosis, post-partum
post-traumatic feeding disorder, 142, 150, 151

Post-Traumatic Stress Disorder, 37, 176, 180, 181, 205, 222, 240, 245
poverty, 51, 63, 262, 275
powerlessness, 38
pre-eclampsia, 79
precipitating factors, 45
predisposing factors, 45
pregnancy
   adjustment to, 70–3, 75
      psychological, 73–5, 76–83
   adverse experiences, 104
   personality disorders, 241–2
   prescribing, 214–15
   risk and protective factors, 83, 84
   stages, 71–3
      first trimester, 71–2
      second trimester, 72
      third trimester, 72–3, 215
   substance abuse, 251–5, 257, 259
   unplanned, 102
premature infants, 18, 87, 88, 89–98, 207
   assessment, 98, 104–5
   Australia, statistics, 89–90
   caregiver relationship, 92–4, 100–2
   development, 91, 98
   hospital care, 91–4, 103
   intervention, 106–10
   risk and protective factors, 58, 60, 90, 99–104
   sleep patterns, 115–16, 120
   substance abuse, 253, 254
prenatal diagnosis, 149
prescribing
   breastfeeding, 214–16
   pregnancy, 85, 214–15
prescribing guidelines, 214
protective factors, 45, 50
psychiatric illness, 59, 65, 82, 201, 274
   risk factors, 99–100, 219
psychiatrists, 214
psychoanalytic theory, 5–6, 9, 35, 187
psychological adjustment to pregnancy, 73–5, 82
   assessment, 83
   intervention, 84–6
   risk factors, 78–83
psychological distress, 202–3
psychological functioning, 90–1, 252
psychologists, 214
Psychomotor Development Index, 124
psychopathology, parent, 62
psychosexual stages of development, 6, 10
psychosis, 82, 210, 214, 254
psychosis, post-partum, 205–6
psychosocial development, 11, 15–18, 21
psychotherapies, 128–9

INDEX

psychotropic medication, 82, 214–15
PTFD *see* post-traumatic feeding disorder
puerperal psychosis *see* psychosis, post-partum

rapid eye movement sleep, 114–15, 119, 125
rapport, parent and worker, 55
Reactive Attachment Disorder (RAD), 33
'readiness for motherhood', 101
referral, 105, 167
Reflective Self Function, 29–30
reflexive function, 29
refugees, 207
regression, 179
regulatory disorders, 120–1, 163
relationships, 221
    abuse, 218–2
    assessment process, 42, 52–3
    personality, 235, 238, 242
    pregnancy, 75–6, 78
    quality, 5, 50, 62, 64, 81, 121
    therapeutic interventions, 281–2
relationships, reciprocal, 37
REM sleep *see* rapid eye movement sleep
remediation in intervention, 21
removal from parents, 64, 282
respite care, 180
risk, definitions, 59, 66
risk and protective factors, definition, 289
risk assessment, 40, 41, 42, 50, 58–66, 99–104
risk-taking, 240
rooting and sucking, 135
routines, 62, 130
Royal Women's Hospital, 214

same-sex female partnerships, 71
schizophrenia, 205
Scottish Intercollegiate Guidelines Network, 215
secure base behaviour, 289
sedatives, 253
self, 219, 234–5, 244
self-awareness, 13, 15
    self-assertion, 157, 158–9
self-blame, 38
self-endangerment, 34
self-esteem, 211, 240
self-harm, 65, 238, 246
self-medication, 215
self-reflective capacity, 14, 29–30, 62, 64, 224, 230
self-regulation, 11, 12, 16–17, 78, 88, 100, 103, 173, 289
    caregiving environment, 17
    parental, 62

    sleep, 115, 119
self-representation, 16, 289
sensitisation, 143
sensory impairment, 90, 92, 120–1
sensory motor experiences, 17
separation, 14, 26–7, 81, 223
    parent–infant, 59, 97, 99, 121, 124, 255, 282–3
separation anxiety, 159, 161, 169, 196
sex
    biological development, 184–9
    definitions, 185
    male and female differentiation, 186–7
sex development, 186
sex and gender, 184–9
'sex-determining region' gene, 186
sexual abuse, 218
sexual differentiation, 186
sexual orientation, 185
shy–extroverted continuum, 18
shyness and social withdrawal, 18
siblings and infant illness, 96
sick infants, 60
sleep
    assessment, 122–4
    behavioural approaches, 126–31
    developmental guidance, 125–6
    formulation principles, 124–5
    infant–parent interaction, 115–18
    intervention, 125–32
    patterns, 112–17, 125
    problems, 118–22
    psychotherapeutic approaches, 128–9
    regulation-based approach, 129–31
sleep disturbance, 76, 82, 103, 105, 111, 205, 207
small for dates, 89
small for gestational age, 89
smoking, 90, 262
social and cultural expectation
    gender identity, 188
social factors and family, 50, 93
social functioning, 60
    and personality disorders, 238
    traumatic experiences, 178
social instability, 59
social isolation *see* isolation
social services, 214
social support, 62, 63, 103, 207
    adolescent parenting, 270
social worker, 93, 258
socioeconomic status, 76
    infant health and development, 50, 90, 95
    maternal depression, 208
    risk factors, 63, 252, 262, 274

319

INDEX

sole parenthood, 262, 264
speech pathologist, 165, 167–8
spoiling, 120
SRY gene, 186
stability of caregiving, 65
stage theories of development, 10–11
state system or state organisational system, 289
stigmatisation, 38
stillbirth, 79
stimulants, 253, 254, 256
stimulation, 8, 56, 88
stomach size, 112
Strange Situation Procedure (SSP), 27–9, 32, 100, 116, 245
stress, 61, 63, 88, 98, 207, 259, 276
    attachment, 32, 177
    personality, 235
    trauma, 173, 177–8, 180
stress hormones, 175, 177, 235–6
substance abuse, 62, 64, 65
    abuse, 219
    assessment, 238, 240, 256–7
    intervention, 257–9
    parenting, 250–9
    pregnancy, 90, 215
sucking, 91, 134, 141, 151
suicide, 65, 215, 239
    see also self-harm
swallowing, 91, 134, 135, 140
sympathetic nervous system, 254
systems theory, 9

teenagers see adolescents
teething, 118
television, 171
temperament, 18, 51, 59–60, 143, 163, 169, 232–3, 289
teratogenesis, 214–15, 253
termination, 79, 85, 262, 263–4
'terrible twos', 14, 162
testicular feminisation, 187
'theory' of mind, 14
Therapeutic Goods administration, 214
therapeutic interventions, 228, 281–282
therapeutic relationship, 47, 49
thrombophlebitis, 254
toddlers
    assessment, 163–7
    attachment, 167, 168, 170–2
    behaviour, 13–15, 155–72
    development, 157–61, 166
    environmental factors, 166
    intervention, 167–72

language, 165, 168–9
    parenting tasks, 161–3, 169
    relationship and interaction, 167
tranquillisers, 253
transactional model of development, 42, 290
transgenerational issues, 30, 62, 220
    personality dysfunction, 236–7, 246, 290
transient disturbances, 118–19
trauma, 173–82
    assessment, 179–80
    attachment, 32, 178
    effect, 176–8, 179
    intervention, 37, 38, 181
    mental illness, 176, 178, 207
    parent, 102, 225
    personality disorders, 235, 239–40, 242–4
    risk factors, 60, 78–80, 82, 252
triplets see multiple births
Turner's Syndrome, 186
twins see multiple births

ultradian clock, 114–15
unemployment, 63, 252

very low birthweight, 89, 90, 94, 99, 101
Video Interaction Guidance, 246
video-taped interactions, 22, 27, 55, 245–8, 282
violence, 51, 59, 64, 180, 256, 258
VLBW see very low birthweight
voice recognition, 17
volunteers, 214, 281
vulnerabilities and strengths, 42

'Watch, Wait and Wonder', 35, 246–7
weaning, 136, 144
welfare agencies, 278
withdrawal see emotional withdrawal
withdrawal syndromes, 215, 253, 254–5
women
    interpersonal changes, 75–76
    physical and emotional changes, 71–3
    psychological adjustment, 73–5
    substance misuse, 251–5
    transition to parenthood, 70–83
work and parenthood, 76
workers and agencies, 278–9
Working Model of the Child Interview, 245

X chromosome, 186

Y chromosome, 186

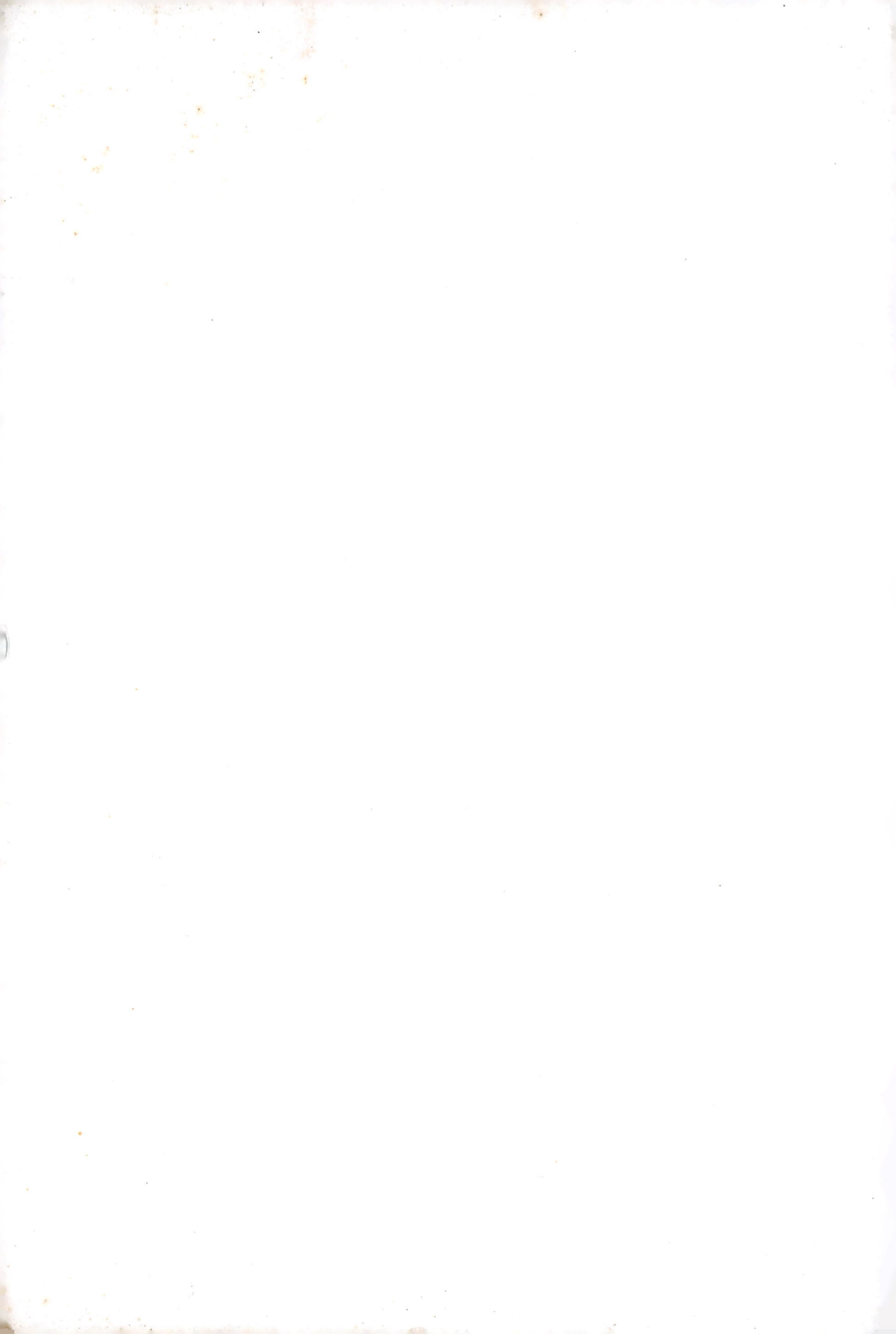